Endocrine
Physiology

The Mosby Physiology Monograph Series

Each book in this series presents normal physiology and selectively includes pathophysiology, with clinical examples highlighted in boxes/tables throughout. Chapters are summarized with key points, key words and concepts are listed, and each book contains a set of self-study problems. Two-color diagrams throughout the books illustrate basic concepts.

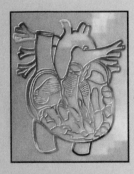

Berne and Levy:
Cardiovascular Physiology,
8th Edition

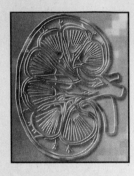

Koeppen and Stanton:
Renal Physiology,
3rd Edition

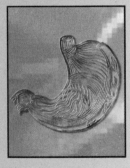

Johnson:
Gastrointestinal Physiology,
6th Edition

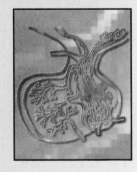

Porterfield:
Endocrine Physiology,
2nd Edition

Coming Soon:
Blaustein: *Cellular Physiology*

A book designed to help medical students "bridge the divide between basic biochemistry, molecular and cell biology . . . and organ system physiology."

Endocrine Physiology

Second Edition

Susan P. Porterfield, PhD
Professor of Physiology and Endocrinology
Associate Dean for Curriculum
Medical College of Georgia
Augusta, Georgia

M Mosby

A Harcourt Health Sciences Company

St. Louis   London   Philadelphia   Sydney   Toronto

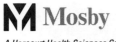

A Harcourt Health Sciences Company

Vice President and Publisher: Anne S. Patterson
Editor: William Schmitt
Project Manager: John Rogers
Senior Production Editor: Helen Hudlin
Design: Stephanie Foley
Cover Design: Rokusek Design
Design Coordinator: Mark Oberkrom

Mosby, Inc.
A Harcourt Health Sciences Company
11830 Westline Industrial Drive
St. Louis, Missouri 63146

21254168

Printed in the United States of America

ISBN 0-323-01128-4

01 02 03 04 CL/F 9 8 7 6 5 4 3 2

To
my children, James and Amy,
and my parents,
Leigh and Virginia Payne and Ralph and Audrey Porterfield,
for the love, encouragement, and support
they have provided me during my career

Preface

This book was written to introduce students to the study of the endocrine system. The endocrine system has such divergent effects that endocrine actions permeate all disciplines of the practice of clinical medicine. Therefore the study of the endocrine system can be fascinating, challenging, and clearly clinically relevant. Although this book was designed for preclinical medical students, it is also useful for graduate, allied health, and nursing students.

Endocrine Physiology is the culmination of 20 years of experience teaching first-year medical students. Because the endocrine system must typically be presented concisely in the first-year curriculum, this book is designed for a rapid, basic introduction to the endocrine system. Major pathologic conditions of the endocrine system are used as a vehicle for teaching its physiology. Expeditious review of the material is facilitated by inclusion of objectives, summary boxes, highlighted words, a list of key words and concepts, and a summary at the conclusion of each chapter. Study questions are provided in both short-answer and single-best-answer formats.

■ ACKNOWLEDGMENTS

I would like to thank Dr. Ruth-Marie Fincher for her encouragement and direction during the production of this book. Drs. Janis Work, Tom Wiedmeier, Chester Hendrich, Tom Weidman, Tom Abney, and Tom Mills provided invaluable assistance in manuscript review. Dr. Clarence Joe graciously provided multiple radiographs included in the textbook, and Dr. Dale Sickles and Mr. Gregory Oblak provided assistance with the histologic sections.

Susan P. Porterfield

Contents

Endocrine Physiology

CHAPTER 1

Introduction to the Endocrine System

Objectives

1. Identify the chemical nature of the major hormones.

2. Describe how this chemical nature influences hormone synthesis, transport, storage, mechanism and site of action, and appropriate route of exogenous hormone administration.

3. Explain the significance of hormone binding to serum proteins.

4. Describe the major theories for the mechanism of hormone action and list those hormones that are identified predominantly with each of these mechanisms.

5. Explain the impact of hormonal rhythms on endocrine function.

THE MATERIAL IN THIS CHAPTER COV-ers generalizations common to all hormones or to specific groups of hormones. The chemical nature of the hormones and their mechanisms of action are covered. This presentation provides the generalized information necessary to categorize the hormones and to make predictions about the most likely characteristics of a given hormone. Some of the exceptions to these generalizations are discussed later.

Both the endocrine and the nervous systems represent communication systems in the body. Scientists originally considered these systems fairly distinct, and the nervous system was considered a faster communication system than the endocrine system. This distinction is becoming increasingly blurred. Furthermore, components of the endocrine system such as the adrenal medulla have neurologic origins. The adrenal medulla produces the compound norepinephrine, which is also a nervous system neurotransmitter. In many ways the chromaffin cells of the adrenal medulla are homologous to postganglionic neurons of the sympathetic nervous system. Catecholamine receptors do not distinguish between norepinephrine of neural origin and norepinephrine of adrenal origin; hence, the empiric statement that endocrine responses are slower than neural responses is not always correct. The hypothalamus produces the two peptide hormones—antidiuretic hormone (ADH) and oxytocin—as well as the hypothalamic releasing or inhibiting hormones (or factors). Because the hypothalamus is neural tissue, these hormones are considered neural hormones. The hypothalamus constitutes a major control center for the endocrine system, and many factors stimulating or inhibiting the endocrine system act through altering the function of hypothalamic neurons.

A hormone was originally defined as a chemical substance produced by a ductless endocrine gland and secreted into the blood, which carried it to a specific target organ to produce an effect. This definition is now known to be an oversimplification. Some hormones act within the organ of synthesis without ever entering the blood. Hormones acting on the secretory cell itself have **autocrine actions** and hormones acting on contiguous cells have **paracrine actions.** Somatostatin produced in pancreatic delta cells is thought to influence insulin secretion (beta cells) and glucagon secretion (alpha cells) through paracrine effects within the islets of Langerhans. In fact, gap junctions allow peptide movement between these cells.

Both the nervous system and the endocrine system maintain the constancy of the **"internal milieu,"** or **homeostasis.** Endocrine organs produce their hormones according to the dictates of finely regulated feedback control systems that are tuned to set-points. These set-points may be altered by circadian rhythms (24-hour cycles or diurnal rhythms), seasonal cycles, the environment, the nervous system, and other influences. In addition, the endocrine system regulates growth, maturation, reproduction, and even behavior.

■ CHEMICAL NATURE OF HORMONES

Hormones are classified biochemically as **steroids, proteins/peptides,** or **amines.** The chemical nature of a hormone often determines how it is carried in the blood, its circulating half-life ($t_{1/2}$), and its cellular mechanism of action.

Steroids

Steroids are produced by the adrenal cortex, ovaries, testes, and placenta (Box 1-1). They include the active metabolites of vitamin D. Steroids are generally derived from cholesterol and have the **cyclopentanoperhydrophenanthrene ring,** (or a derivative thereof) as their core (Figure 1-1). They tend to be fat soluble and cross cell membranes relatively easily.

Consequently, steroids have intracellular receptors. Furthermore, because of their nonpolar nature, they are not readily soluble in blood and therefore are transported bound to proteins. Glandular storage of steroids is minimal because they easily diffuse out of cells. These compounds are absorbed fairly readily in the gastro-

---

BOX 1-1

Steroid Hormones

- Are derived from the cyclopentanoperhydrophenanthrene ring
- Have intracellular receptors
- Are nonpolar
- Usually circulate protein-bound in blood
- Are not stored in the endocrine gland
- Can often be administered orally

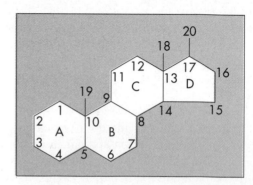

Figure 1-1 ■ Cyclopentanoperhydrophenanthrene ring.

intestinal tract and therefore often may be administered orally.

Proteins/Peptides

Because most protein/peptide hormones are destined for secretion outside the cell, they are synthesized and processed differently than proteins destined to remain within the cell (Box 1-2). The hormones are synthesized on the polyribosome as larger preprohormones or prehormones (Figure 1-2). The nascent peptides have at their N-terminal a group of 15 to 30 amino acids called the **signal peptide**. A sig-

---

BOX 1-2

Protein/Peptide Hormones

- Are synthesized as prehormones or prepro-hormones
- Are stored in membrane-bound granules
- Are relatively polar
- Often circulate in blood unbound
- Cannot be administered orally
- Usually have cell membrane receptors

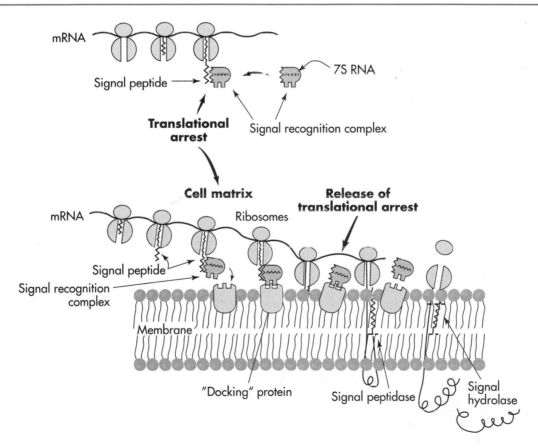

Figure 1-2 ■ Synthesis of protein and peptide hormones. (Redrawn from Wilson JD, Foster DW, Kronenberg HM, Larsen PR, editors: *Williams' textbook of endocrinology,* ed 9, Philadelphia, 1998, WB Saunders.)

nal recognition complex (a complex of six proteins and a ribonucleic acid [RNA]) binds to the N-terminal of the nascent peptide after about 70 amino acids have been polymerized. This stops further translation until the signal recognition complex binds to a **docking protein** located on the cytosolic face of the endoplasmic reticulum. This binding releases the translational block. The growing polypeptide is directed through the endoplasmic reticular membrane into the cisternae. It is released from the signal peptide by a **signal peptidase** located on the cisternal surface of the membrane. The polypeptide is then transported in the cisternae to the Golgi apparatus, where it is packaged into a membrane-bound secretory vesicle and released into the cytoplasm. The carbohydrate moiety of glycoproteins is added in the Golgi apparatus.

The original gene transcript is called either a **prehormone** or a **preprohormone** (Figure 1-3). Removing the signal peptide produces either the prohormone or the hormone. A **prohormone** is a polypeptide that requires further cleavage before the mature hormone is pro-

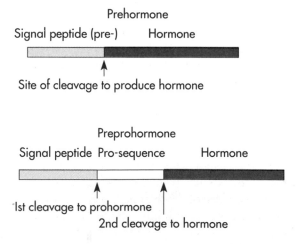

Prehormone

Signal peptide (pre-)   Hormone

↑
Site of cleavage to produce hormone

Preprohormone

Signal peptide   Pro-sequence   Hormone

↑   ↑
1st cleavage to prohormone |
2nd cleavage to hormone

Figure 1-3 ▪ Structure of prehormones and preprohormones.

duced. Often this final cleavage occurs while the prohormone is within the Golgi apparatus or the secretory granule. For example, insulin is produced as preproinsulin, cleaved to proinsulin in the endoplasmic reticulum, and packaged in secretory vesicles as proinsulin. While in the secretory vesicle, a portion of the center of the single chain (connecting [C] peptide) is cleaved to produce the insulin molecule, which contains two peptide chains. The mature secretory vesicle contains equimolar amounts of insulin and C peptide. Sometimes prohormones contain multiple hormones such as the compound pro-opiomelanocortin, which contains the amino acid sequences of adrenocorticotropic hormone (ACTH), melanocyte-stimulating hormone (MSH), lipotropin (LTH), endorphins, and enkephalins.

Protein/peptide hormones are stored in the gland as membrane-bound secretory granules and are released by **exocytosis.** Exocytosis requires energy, Ca^{2+}, and an intact cytoskeleton (microtubules, microfilaments). Protein/peptide hormones are soluble in aqueous solvents and, with the notable exceptions of the insulin-like growth factors (IGFs) and growth hormone (GH), circulate in the blood predominantly in an unbound form and therefore tend to have short t½s. Many of these protein hormones are small enough to appear in the urine in a physiologically active form. For example, follicule-stimulating hormone (FSH) and luteinizing hormone (LH) are present in urine. Urine of postmenopausal women is an excellent source of gonadotropins because postmenopausal serum gonadotropin levels are high. Pregnancy tests using human urine are based on the urinary presence of the placental hormone human chorionic gonadotropin (hCG).

Proteins/peptides are readily digested if administered orally. Hence, they must be administered by injection or, in the case of small peptides, through a mucous membrane (sublingually or intranasally). Because proteins/ peptides do not cross cell membranes readily, they tend to interact with membrane receptors. The second-messenger hypothesis was proposed to link membrane receptor binding and intracellular effects.

Amines

Amines include thyroid hormones and catecholamines, both of which are derived from tyrosine (Boxes 1-3 and 1-4). Thyroid hormones cross cell membranes by both diffusion and transport systems. They are stored extracellularly in the thyroid as an integral part of the glycoprotein molecule **thyroglobulin.** Thyroid hormones are sparingly soluble in blood and aqueous fluids and are transported in blood

bound (>99%) to serum-binding proteins. They have long $t_{1/2}$s (thyroxine [T_4] = 7 days; triiodothyronine [T_3] = 24 hours). These hormones can cross the cell membrane, and their receptors are primarily intracellular. Thyroid hormones can be administered orally, and sufficient hormone is absorbed intact to make this an effective mode of therapy. Catecholamines, on the other hand, are very different biologically. They do not cross cell membranes readily and hence produce their actions though membrane receptors. They are soluble in blood and circulate either unbound or loosely bound to albumin. They have short $t_{1/2}$s. These hormones are stored intracellularly in discrete secretory granules.

Eicosanoids

Eicosanoids are compounds that are formed from polyunsaturated fatty acids with 18, 20, and 22 carbons. Arachidonic acid is the most important precursor of this group of compounds. This group includes **prostaglandins, leukotrienes, thromboxanes,** and **prostacyclin.** These compounds are not typically considered hormones and are thus not listed Box 1-5. They are synthesized throughout the body, and their primary actions are autocrine or paracrine. Hormones often regulate the synthesis of these compounds. While most eicosanoids, like catecholamines and protein/peptide hormones, act by means of cell surface receptors, a few act through nuclear receptors.

■ TRANSPORT OF HORMONES

Many hormones are transported in the blood bound to plasma proteins. Protein and polypeptide hormones are generally transported free in the blood. Other hormones, most notably steroids and thyroid hormones, are transported bound to plasma proteins. There is an equilibrium between the concentrations of bound hormone (HP), free hormone (H), and plasma protein (P); if free hormone levels drop, hormone

---

BOX 1-3

Thyroid Hormones

- Are derived from tyrosine
- Cross cell membranes
- Are transported in blood bound to proteins
- Have intracellular receptors
- Are stored in the follicle
- Can be administered orally

BOX 1-4

Catecholamines

- Are derived from tyrosine
- Do not cross cell membranes readily
- Have cell surface receptors
- Are transported in blood free or only loosely associated with proteins
- Are stored in membrane-bound granules
- Could be administered orally but in their native form their half-life is too short to be effective

BOX 1-5

Classes of Hormones Based on Structure

Glycoproteins	Polypeptides	Steroids	Amines
Follicle-stimulating hormone (FSH)	Adrenocorticotropic hormone (ACTH)	Aldosterone	Epinephrine
	Angiotensin	Cortisol	Norepinephrine
Thyroid-stimulating hormone (TSH)	Calcitonin, parathyroid hormone (PTH)	Estradiol	Thyroxine (T_4)
	Cholecystokinin (CCK)	Progesterone	Triiodothyronine (T_3)
Luteinizing hormone (LH)	Melanocyte-stimulating hormone (MSH)	Testosterone	
Human chorionic gonadotropin (hCG)	Nerve growth factor (NGF), insulin-like growth factor (IGF), epidermal growth factor (EGF)	Vitamin D	
	Oxytocin, antidiuretic hormone (ADH)		
	Relaxin, secretin		
	Somatostatin		
	Releasing hormones		
	Prolactin, growth hormone (GH)		

will be released from the binding proteins. This relationship may be expressed as

$$[H] \times [P] = [HP] \ or \ K = \frac{[H] \times [P]}{[HP]}$$

where K = the dissociation constant.

The free hormone is the biologically active form for both target organ action and feedback control. Consequently, in evaluating hormonal status, one must sometimes determine free hormone levels rather than just total hormone levels.

Protein binding serves several purposes. It prolongs the circulating $t_{1/2}$ of the hormone. Many of these hormones cross cell membranes readily and would either enter the cells or be lost through the kidney were they not protein bound. The bound hormone represents a "reservoir" of hormone and as such can serve to "buffer" acute changes in hormone secretion. Some hormones, such as steroids, are sparingly soluble in blood and protein binding facilitates their transport.

■ RESPONSE TO HORMONES

Although hormones are frequently carried throughout the body, response specificity results from hormone receptor specificity. Serum hormone concentrations are extremely low (10^{-11} to 10^{-9} M); therefore, these receptors must have a **high affinity** for the hormone. The actual nature of the response is genetically determined. Because the hormonal response typically results from the interaction between receptor and hormone, disease states can involve the receptors as well as the synthesis and secretion of the hormone. If an individual lacks receptors for a given hormone, the hormone will not exert its normal physiologic actions. For example, in androgen insensitivity syndrome, the testes produce androgens, but the androgen receptors are deficient. Consequently, the steroidal effects are those that occur when androgens are absent. The functional androgen deficiency and the estrogens derived from testicular and adrenal androgens produce feminization even though the individual has an XY genotype.

Some hormones are converted to a more potent form at sites peripheral to the endocrine organ. For example, testosterone is converted to the potent androgen dihydrotestosterone in tissues like the prostate gland. Although the predominant hormone secreted by the thyroid is T_4, the predominant cellular response is based on the intracellular level of T_3. Most of this T_3 is produced by peripheral deiodination by the enzyme 5′-monodeiodinase. Regulation of the activity of this enzyme can alter the response to thyroid hormones.

Concept of Spare Receptors

Nuclear receptors are present in relatively small numbers, so the number of receptors generally determines the magnitude of the response. However, cell surface receptors are often present in larger numbers than are needed for a maximal response. For example, a maximal response to insulin can occur when only 15% to 20% of the receptors are bound. The additional receptors, over and above the number necessary to produce a maximal response, are referred to as **spare receptors.** The significance of hormone systems exhibiting spare receptors is that with these systems the response to a hormone is limited less by the number of receptors than by the hormone affinity of the receptors.

■ MECHANISM OF HORMONE ACTION

The mechanisms whereby hormones regulate cellular function are not unique to hormones. Cell signaling can occur by regulating intracellular calcium availability, cAMP level, and phosphatidylinositol turnover even in lower organisms such as bacteria.

Most, but not necessarily all, action of hormones are mediated by their interactions with receptors. Receptor binding initiates intracellular cell-signaling events that direct the hormone's action. Hormone receptors are large proteins or glycoproteins. For catecholamines

and peptide/protein hormones, these receptors are usually found on the cell surface. For steroid hormones, the receptors are found in the nucleus. For thyroid hormones, the major receptors are in the nucleus, but receptors have also been found in the mitochondria and even the plasmalemma. Hormones noncovalently bind with high affinity to the receptors.

Many hormones can regulate their own receptor concentrations. When hormone levels are high, tissue receptor numbers decrease. This is referred to as **down regulation** of receptor levels. There are multiple mechanisms for this phenomenon. The presence of the hormone can sometimes decrease receptor synthesis. In other instances, binding of the hormone to the receptor leads to receptor-mediated endocytosis (internalization) of the hormone-receptor (HR) complex. Internalization decreases receptor availability on the cell surface and can lead to catabolism of the receptor. The concept that rising hormone levels can decrease receptor availability in some systems is important clinically because many disease states produce receptor down regulation. Some hormones (i.e., gonadotropin-releasing hormone [GnRH]) show pulsatile secretion such that down regulation is minimized.

Hormones Acting Through Membrane Receptors

A hormone can produce its effects through binding to plasma receptors and initiating a cascade of responses that ultimately alter intracellular events. This proposed mechanism is called the *second-messenger hypothesis.* The hormone is the first messenger because it carries the "information" to the target organ. Hormone binding to the receptor initiates ultimately the intracellular production of compounds like **cyclic adenosine monophosphate (cAMP)** that are the **second messengers.** These compounds direct the events within the cell. There are at least

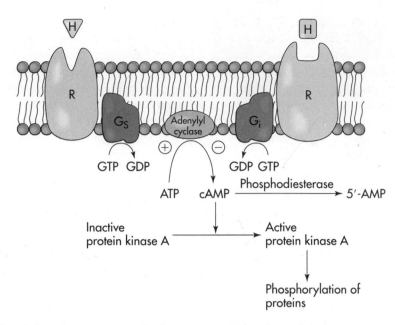

Figure 1-4 ■ **Adenylyl cyclase system. The hormone *(H)* binds to the receptor *(R)*, which interacts with either a G$_s$ or a G$_i$ protein. Association with a G$_s$ protein activates adenylyl cyclase, which increases cAMP production and thereby activates protein kinase A. Association with a G$_i$ subunit decreases cAMP production. *GTP,* Guanosine triphosphate; *GDP,* guanosine diphosphate; *ATP,* adenosine triphosphate; *cAMP,* cyclic adenosine monophosphate; *5′-AMP,* 5′-adenosine monophosphate.**

four different types of membrane spanning receptors. These include those receptors using G proteins (GTP-binding protein),[1] receptors regulating ion channels,[2] receptors containing tyrosine kinase,[3] and receptors associated with tyrosine kinase.[4]

① *Receptors Using G Proteins* This is the largest group and the receptor usually spans the membrane 7 times. This group includes the receptors regulating cyclic nucleotide production (adenylyl or guanylyl cyclase activity) as well as the receptors regulating phospholipid turnover. The **adenylyl cyclase system** is given as an example of the former type. There are three membrane components in the adenylyl cyclase system. They are the receptor, the **G protein,** and the catalytic subunit (adenylyl cyclase).

The hormone binds to the receptor, and the HR unit associates with the G protein. Such

binding stimulates the G protein to release guanosine diphosphate (GDP), which is followed by the uptake of guanosine triphosphate (GTP) from the cytosol. On binding GTP, the G protein affinity for the receptor decreases, while the affinity for the catalytic subunit (adenylyl cyclase) increases. Binding of the G protein to the catalytic subunit results in activation (or inactivation) of adenylyl cyclase and subsequent formation of cAMP. The G protein contains a GTPase that hydrolyzes GTP in approximately 15 seconds. GTP hydrolysis decreases the G protein's affinity for the catalytic subunit and hence terminates the cycle.

There are multiple types of G proteins. The G protein described previously is called **G$_s$** because it couples receptor binding with stimulation of adenylyl cyclase. When receptor systems contain **G$_i$,** receptor binding results in inhibi-

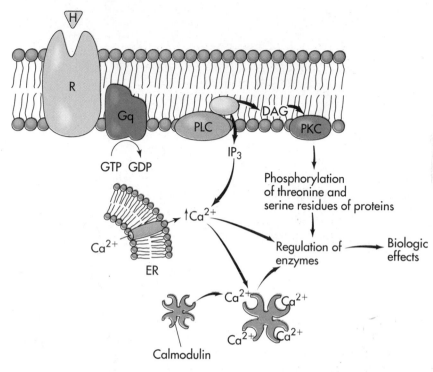

Figure 1-5 ■ Activation of phosphatidylinositol system. Hormone *(H)* binding to the receptor *(R)* activates phospholipase C *(PLC)* via G_q (or other similar G protein). This results in phosphatidylinositol bisphosphate *(PIP_2)* hydrolysis to produce inositol triphosphate *(IP_3)* and diacylglycerol *(DAG)*. IP_3 releases Ca^{2+} from endoplasmic reticulum *(ER)*. DAG activates protein kinase C *(PKC)*. GTP, Guanosine triphosphate; *GDP*, guanosine diphosphate.

tion of adenylyl cyclase. G_q couples receptors with activation of **phospholipase C (PLC)** to activate the **phosphatidylinositol system** (see discussion of phosphatidylinositol turnover following).

A rise in cytosolic cAMP level activates **protein kinase A,** and the latter mediates the biologic response by phosphorylating proteins at threonine and serine residues (Figure 1-4). Some of these proteins are enzymes, such as glycogen phosphorylase, and some are regulatory proteins, such as **transcription factors,** which can alter gene expression. The enzyme **phosphodiesterase** catalyzes the breakdown of cAMP to 5'-AMP.

Methylxanthines such as caffeine and theophylline are phosphodiesterase inhibitors and can potentiate the actions of hormones acting through cAMP.

There is also a receptor regulating phosphatidylinositol turnover. In this system, hormone binding to the receptor, acting through a G protein (often G_q), activates the enzyme PLC, which mediates the breakdown of membrane **phosphatidylinositol bisphosphate (PIP_2)** to **inositol triphosphate (IP_3)** and **diacylglycerol (DAG)** (Figure 1-5). IP_3 mobilizes calcium from intracellular stores (predominantly in the endoplasmic reticulum and the mitochondria). This calcium can act as a second messenger (see

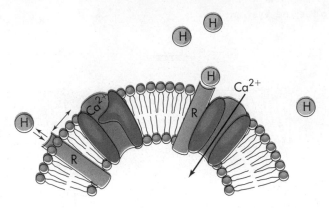

Figure 1-6 ■ Activation of calcium-calmodulin system. Hormone receptors *(R)* can bind hormone *(H)* and control opening of calcium channels in cell membrane.

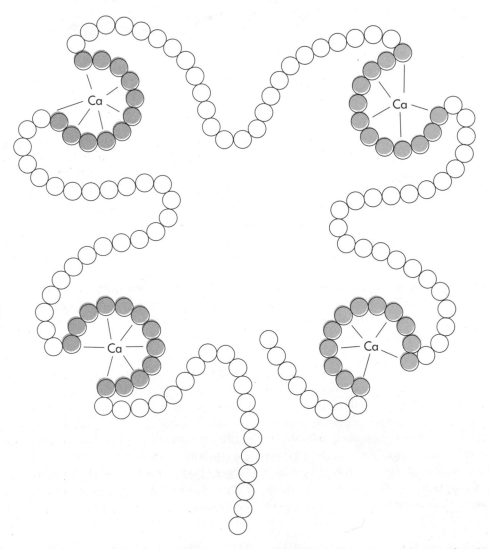

Figure 1-7 ■ Calmodulin is a protein capable of binding up to four calcium molecules.

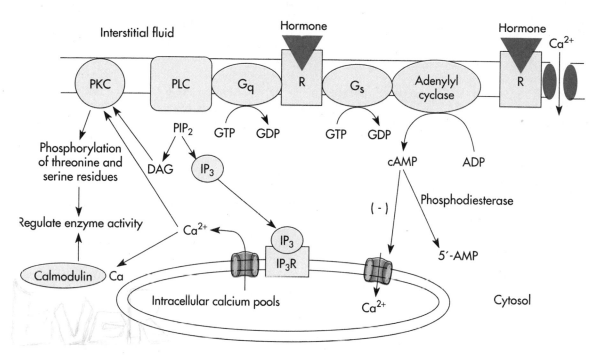

Figure 1-8 ■ Summary of mechanisms of hormone action involving cAMP, calcium, and phosphatidylinositol turnover. *PKC,* Protein kinase C; *PLC,* phospholipase C; *R,* receptor; *PIP₂,* phosphatidylinositol bisphosphate; *GTP,* guanosine triphosphate; *GDP,* guanosine diphosphate; *cAMP,* cyclic adenosine monophosphate; *ADP,* adenosine diphosphate; *DAG,* diacylglycerol; *IP₃,* inositol triphosphate; *IP₃R,* IP₃ receptor; *5'-AMP,* 5'-adenosine monophosphate.

discussion of ion channels following). Diacylglycerol activates the calcium-dependent enzyme **protein kinase C,** which catalyzes phosphorylation of threonine and serine residues in some enzymes, thereby regulating their activities. The G protein G_q serves as a transducer in this system, as G_s and G_i do in the adenylyl cyclase system.

②*Receptors Regulating Ion Channels* Hormone binding to these receptors opens ion channels, the most common of which are calcium channels (the calcium-calmodulin system). In the latter situation, hormone binding to the receptor opens the calcium channels and intracellular calcium levels rise (Figure 1-6). Intracellular calcium, particularly calcium associated

with mitochondria and endoplasmic reticulum, might be mobilized by IP_3. Many of the actions of calcium occur after binding to the protein **calmodulin.** Figure 1-7 demonstrates how hormone binding to a receptor can open calcium channels to increase calcium influx. Calmodulin is capable of binding up to four calcium molecules. Calmodulin is sometimes bound to enzymes; when calcium binds to the enzyme-bound calmodulin, enzyme activity is altered.

A summary of how hormones affect cAMP, calcium, and phosphatidylinositol turnover is provided in Figure 1-8.

③*Receptors Containing Tyrosine Kinase* This family of hormones includes insulin, insulin-like growth factor (IGF-I), epidermal

Tyrosine Kinase – Containing   Tyrosine Kinase – Associated
Receptor   Receptor

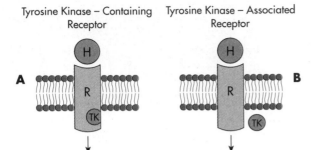

Figure 1-9 ■ Phosphorylation-mediated actions of tyrosine kinase–containing (A) and tyrosine kinase–associated (B) receptors. *H,* hormone; *R,* receptor; *TK,* tyrosine kinase

growth factor (EGF), and platelet-derived growth factor (PDGF). These receptors consist of ligand-binding domains external to the membrane, membrane-spanning domains, and cytosolic domains containing as an integral part of the receptor the enzyme **tyrosine kinase** (Figure 1-9, *A*). When the hormone binds to the receptor, the tyrosine kinase on the cytosolic domain is activated. Activation of tyrosine kinase has two effects: (1) the kinase phosphorylates tyrosine residues in the receptor itself and this **autophosphorylation** can potentiate the signal, and (2) the kinase can phosphorylate **tyrosine residues** on other intracellular proteins, including enzymes, and thereby regulate their activity. The other two classes of kinases that are cell signal regulators—protein kinases A and C—phosphorylate serine and threonine residues rather than tyrosine residues.

④ *Receptors Associated With Tyrosine Kinase* This group includes GH, PRL, cytokines, and erythropoietin. These receptors are similar to the tyrosine kinase–containing receptors in that there are external ligand-binding domains, membrane spanning domains, and cytosolic domains. The receptor does not contain tyrosine kinase activity, but rather it interacts with cyto-

solic proteins containing tyrosine kinase activity (Figure 1-9, *B*).

• • •

These systems are interrelated and frequently hormone actions involve one or more systems.

Hormones that act on the cell surface can regulate gene expression by modifying **transcription factors** (see appendix at the end of the chapter and Figure 1-10). These modifications can involve calcium-induced changes in enzyme activities and phosphorylation of key regulatory proteins. For example, cAMP regulates a transcription factor called **cAMP response element–binding protein (CREB)** by stimulating the phosphorylation of the protein (via protein kinase A). CREB then binds to the promoter of the deoxyribonucleic acid (DNA), where it can act as a transcription factor. CREB is also an example of a Ca^{2+}-regulated protein. Many other transcription factors are activated by cAMP-regulated protein kinase A. Protein kinase C can also regulate gene expression through altering transcription factors. Figure 1-10 illustrates this relationship. The second messenger regulates production or activity of an effector, which can alter the status of one or more transcription factors that can associate with the promoter region of the DNA and influence the regulation of transcription. Proteins such as RNA polymerase (P) bind at the proximal promoter and direct transcription.

Internalization of Protein Hormones After binding to membrane-bound receptors, many HR complexes enter the cell (receptor-mediated endocytosis). Internalization of the HR complex often serves to terminate the response. Frequently the HR unit is transported to lysosomes, where the hormone is degraded. Either the receptor is recycled to the membrane or it is degraded at the lysosome. Receptor internalization is a major mechanism for down regulation of hormones.

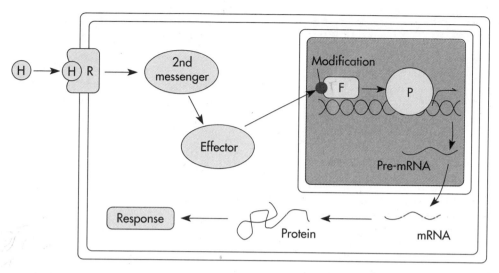

Figure 1-10 ■ Regulation of transcription by hormones not entering cells. *H,* Hormone; *R,* receptor; *F,* transcription factor; *P,* RNA polymerase. (Redrawn from Greenspan FS, Baxter JD: *Basic and clinical endocrinology,* ed 4, Norwalk, Conn, 1994, Appleton & Lange.)

Hormones That Enter the Cell Before Receptor Binding

Steroid and thyroid hormones act through intracellular receptors. These receptors are structurally similar and are members of the superfamily of nuclear receptors that includes steroid, thyroid, vitamin D, and retinoic acid receptors. These receptors act like transcription factors in that they bind to the hormone-responsive elements in the promoter and thereby regulate transcription. These receptors have three domains: the **ligand-binding domain** (that binds the hormone), the **DNA-binding domain,** and an **N-terminal portion.** The DNA-binding domain contains two **zinc fingers,** which often contain cysteine residues complexed with zinc. This region binds to DNA. The receptors in this superfamily have similar DNA-binding domains. The ligand-binding domains regulate the specificity of the hormone binding to the receptor. Hormone binding to this region changes the conformation of the DNA-binding domain and increases the DNA-binding affinity.

Steroids Steroids diffuse across both the plasma and nuclear membranes and bind to nuclear and sometimes cytosolic receptors. Receptors that are not bound to hormone are associated with proteins called **heat shock proteins (HSPs).** HSPs stabilize the receptors and prevent receptor binding to DNA. HR binding changes the conformation of the receptor and stimulates dissociation of HR complex from the HSPs. This dissociation permits the receptors to dimerize. The release of the HSPs increases receptor affinity for specific DNA sequences termed **hormone response elements (HREs).** HSPs are not associated with thyroid hormone, vitamin D, and retinoic acid receptors. The HRE is located in the promoter, which is "upstream" from the hormone–responsive genes. The HR complex is then thought to act as a transcription factor, modulating the transcription rate for steroid hormone–responsive genes

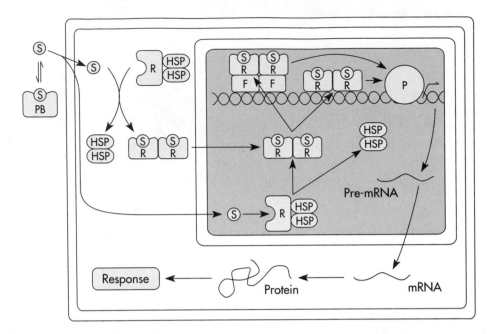

Figure 1-11 ■ **Steroid hormone regulation of transcription.** *S,* Steroid hormone; *PB,* plasma binding protein; *HSP,* heat shock protein; *R,* receptor; *F,* transcription factor; *P,* RNA polymerase. (Redrawn from Greenspan FS, Baxter JD: *Basic and clinical endocrinology,* ed 4, Norwalk, Conn, 1994, Appleton & Lange.)

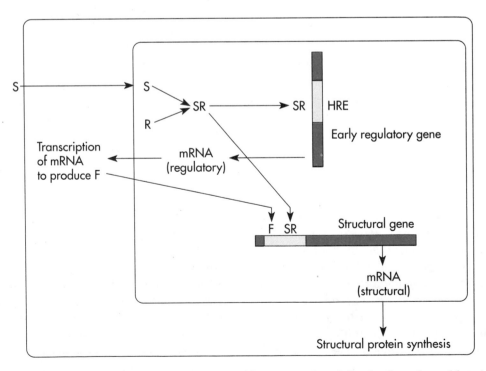

Figure 1-12 ■ **Proposed model for action of steroid hormones involving both early and late genes.** *S,* Steroid; *R,* receptor; *F,* transcription factor; *HRE,* hormone response element.

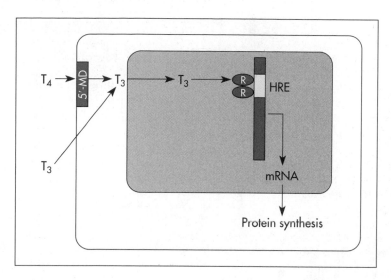

Figure 1-13 ■ **Proposed model for the action of thyroid hormones. 5′-Monodeiodinase** *(5′-MD)* **converts thyroxine** *(T₄)* **to triiodothyronine** *(T₃)*. *R*, **Thyroid hormone receptor;** *HRE*, **hormone response element.**

and in some cases altering posttranscriptional steps, thereby changing the levels of specific messenger RNAs (mRNAs). The mature mRNA then enters the cytoplasm, where its message is translated by ribosomes and the corresponding protein is produced (Figure 1-11).

Steroid hormones can rapidly direct transcription of early regulatory genes such as c-myc, c-fos, and c-jun (growth-regulating or proto-oncogenes). These genes direct synthesis of mRNAs for proteins that are transcription factors or enzymes regulating these factors. Hence, regulation of early regulatory genes can influence transcription of "late" structural genes (Figure 1-12). Whereas the mRNAs from these early proto-oncogenes are seen within minutes after adding steroid, the mRNAs for the "late" structural genes do not become apparent for 1 hour or more after steroid administration.

Thyroid hormones cross the plasmalemma and enter the nucleus to bind to high-affinity, low-capacity nuclear receptors. These receptors typically are bound to DNA at the HRE. When the hormone binds to the ligand-binding domain of the DNA-bound receptor, it can regulate gene transcription of certain mRNAs (Figure 1-13). These receptors function like hormone-dependent gene–regulatory elements. Thyroid hormone receptors have also been proposed for the mitochondria and the plasma membrane. Thyroid hormones can act on mitochondria independent of any nuclear action.

A summary of hormone actions through various mechanisms is listed in Box 1-6.

■ HORMONAL RHYTHMS

Most endocrine secretion show periodicity or rhythms. Frequently there are multiple, superimposed rhythms for a given hormone. The periods of these rhythms range from minutes to months (Figure 1-14).

These rhythms are important for normal endocrine function. Changes in endocrine rhythms are a major factor in the problems asso-

Actions of Hormones Through Various Mechanisms

Hormones Acting Through Cyclic Adenosine Monophosphate (cAMP)

Hormones Acting by Raising cAMP

Catecholamines—β-adrenergic receptors
Glycoprotein hormones
  Luteinizing hormone (LH), follicle-stimulating hormone (FSH), thyroid-stimulating hormone (TSH), human chorionic gonadotropin (hCG)
Glucagon
Parathyroid hormone (PTH), calcitonin
Antidiuretic hormone (ADH) (V_2 receptors)
Adrenocorticotropic hormone (ACTH)

Hormones Acting by Lowering cAMP

Acetylcholine (ACh)
Catecholamine α_2-adrenergic receptors
Somatostatin

Hormones Acting Through Ca^{2+}-Diacylglycerol (DAG)

Acetylcholine (muscarinic)
a_1-Adrenergic receptors
Angiotensin
Gonadotropin-releasing hormone (GnRH)
Antidiuretic hormone (ADH)(V_1 receptors)

Hormones Acting Through Tyrosine Kinase

Insulin
Epidermal growth factor (EGF)
Insulin-like growth factor-I(IGF-I)
Fibroblast growth factor (FGF)
Platelet-derived growth factor (PDGF)

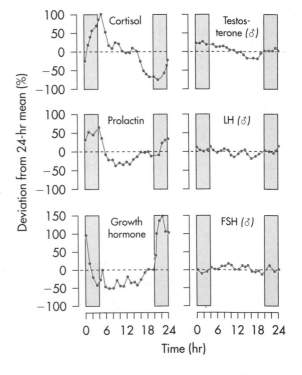

Figure 1-14 ■ **Temporal patterns for plasma hormone levels. Shaded areas represent approximate sleep time.** *LH,* **Luteinizing hormone;** *FSH,* **follicle-stimulating hormone.** (Redrawn from De-Groot LJ, et al: *Endocrinology,* vol 3, New York, 1979, Grune & Stratton.)

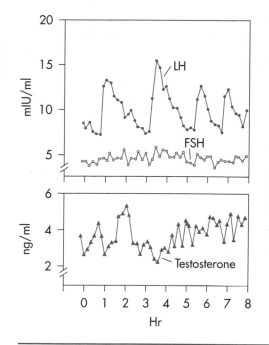

Figure 1-15 ▪ Examples of ultradian rhythms. *LH,* Luteinizing hormone; *FSH,* follicle-stimulating hormone. (Redrawn from Naftolin F, et al: *J Clin Endocrinol Metab* 36:285, 1973.)

opp of nocturnal
not di, le ×2

ciated with jet lag. These rhythms frequently are absent in disease states. The physician must be cognizant of normal endocrine rhythms. Many rhythms have a 24-hour cycle. These rhythms are called **circadian (diurnal) rhythms.** As can be seen in Figure 1-14, the normal serum cortisol, prolactin, or GH levels measured at 5 AM are different from the values obtained at 2 PM.

Pulsatile rhythms (usually a ½- to 2-hour period) frequently are superimposed on these circadian rhythms, and these pulsatile rhythms have functional significance. The role of pulsatile secretion is discussed in Chapters 8 and 9. These rhythms with a periodicity of less than 24 hours are referred to as **ultradian rhythms.** Figure 1-15 illustrates ultradian rhythms for LH, FSH, and testosterone.

Summary

1. Knowledge of the chemical structure of a hormone can facilitate predicting how the hormone will be produced, carried, and act in a physiologic system.
2. Protein/peptide hormones are produced on ribosomes and stored in the endocrine cell in membrane-bound secretory granules. They typically do not readily cross cell membranes and act through membrane-associated receptors.
3. Steroid hormones are not stored in tissues and generally cross cell membranes rela-

tively readily. They act through intracellular receptors.

4. Thyroid hormones are synthesized in the follicular cells and are stored in the follicular colloid as thyroglobulin. They cross cell membranes and associate with intracellular receptors.

5. Catecholamines are synthesized in cytosol and chromaffin granules and do not readily cross cell membranes. They act through cell membrane–associated receptors.

■ KEY WORDS AND CONCEPTS

- Autocrine actions
- Paracrine actions
- Internal milieu
- Steroids
- Protein/peptides
- Amines
- Cyclopentanoperhydrophenanthrene ring
- Signal peptide
- Signal recognition complex
- Docking protein
- Prehormone
- Preprohormone
- Prohormone
- Thyroid hormones
- Catecholamines
- Thyroglobulin
- Eicosanoids
- Prostaglandins
- Leukotrienes
- Thromboxanes
- Prostacyclin
- Spare receptors
- Cyclic adenosine monophosphate (cAMP)
- Adenylyl cyclase
- Protein kinase A
- Transcription factors
- Phosphodiesterase
- Phosphatidylinositol bisphosphate (PIP_2)
- Inositol triphosphate (IP_3)
- Diacylglycerol (DAG)

6. Some hormones act through membrane receptors, with their responses being mediated by G-protein–associated systems (adenylyl cyclase phosphatidylinositol), calcium-calmodulin, or tyrosine kinase–containing receptor or tyrosine kinase–associated systems.

7. Other hormones bind to nuclear receptors and act by directly regulating gene transcription.

8. Hormonal rhythms play a major role in physiologic responses.

- Protein kinase C
- Calmodulin
- Tyrosine kinase
- cAMP response element–binding protein (CREB)
- Internalization of protein hormones
- Ligand-binding domain
- DNA-binding domain
- Zinc fingers
- Heat shock proteins (HSPs)
- Hormone response elements (HREs)
- Circadian (diurnal) rhythms
- Ultradian rhythms

■ SELF-STUDY PROBLEMS

1. What would be the most appropriate route of administration of a protein hormone?

2. In what form are protein hormones typically stored in the endocrine gland?

3. How does binding to serum-transport proteins influence hormone metabolism and hormone action?

4. What is a transcription factor?

5. What is a second messenger?

■ BIBLIOGRAPHY

Berridge MJ: Inositol trisphosphate and calcium signalling, *Nature* 361:351, 1993.

Birnbaumer L: Receptor-to-effector signaling through G proteins: roles for βγ dimers as well as α subunits, *Cell* 71:1069, 1992.

Chin WW: Current concepts of thyroid hormone action: progress notes for the clinician, *Thyroid Today* 15 (3): July/Aug/Sept 1992.

Hadcock JR, Malbon CC: Agonist regulation of gene expression of adrenergic receptors and G proteins, *J Neurochem* 60:1, 1993.

Jones KE, Brubaker JH, Chin WW: Evidence that phosphorylation events participate in thyroid hormone action, *Endocrinology* 134:543, 1994.

Schuchard M, Landers JP, Sandhu NP, Spelsberg TC: Steroid hormone regulation of nuclear proto-oncogenes, *Endocr Rev* 14:659, 1994.

Appendix

■ HORMONAL REGULATION OF GENE EXPRESSION

The typical gene consists of a strand of DNA that contains a promoter on the 5′ flanking region and a transcription unit (Figure 1-16). The cap site is located at the origin of the transcription unit and represents the point at which transcription originates. The transcription unit extends from the cap site and ends approximately 20 bases beyond the signal sequence AATAAA at the end of a poly A addition site. The region between the transcription unit and the 3′ end of the DNA is called the 3′ flanking region of the DNA. The promoter is the 5′ flanking region of the cap site, and it contains the DNA segments that regulate gene expression. It often includes the TATA box (a sequence of TATAA that regulates the point at which transcription begins). The enzyme polymerase II associates with the TATA box; from this location the polymerase II directs transcription. The promoter is the site of action of many transcription factors, including many hormone receptors.

The initial gene transcript contains sequences that are not found in the final mRNA. This precursor mRNA (pre-mRNA) contains **exons** (coding sequences that remain in the mature mRNA) and **introns** (noncoding sequences that are cleaved from the mRNA when pre-mRNA is processed to mature mRNA). mRNA processing occurs before the mRNA leaves the nucleus. During this process, not only are the introns removed but also, with most mRNAs, the 3′ end is cleaved and a chain of adenosine residues is added (the poly A tail). In addition, a "cap" of methylated guanosine is added to the 5′ end of the RNA.

Hormones typically regulate gene expression by regulating the initiation of gene transcription. However, regulation can occur at termination of transcription, processing of pre-mRNA, mRNA degradation, and translation.

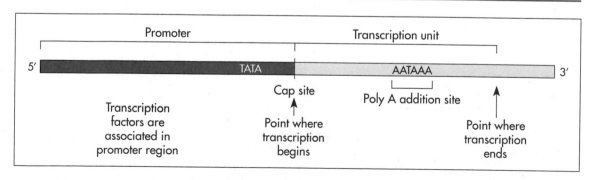

Figure 1-16 ■ Structure of strand of DNA.

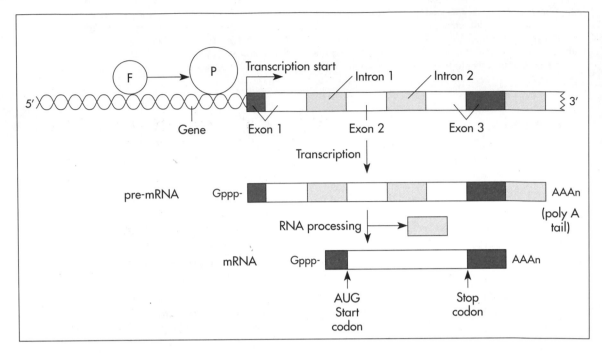

Figure 1-17 ■ **Translational events in synthesis of mRNA.** *F,* Transcription factor; *P,* RNA polymerase. (Redrawn from Greenspan FS, Baxter JD: *Basic and clinical endocrinology,* ed 4, Norwalk, Conn, 1994, Appleton & Lange.)

Hormones acting at the cell surface can alter gene expression by regulating the activity of transcription factors, which thereby can alter gene expression. For example, protein kinase A or C can phosphorylate some transcription factors (e.g., Pit-1, a transcription factor found in pituitary cells that regulates expression of the genes encoding for GH, thyroid-stimulating hormone, and prolactin).

The mature mRNA is transported to the cytoplasm, where it can be translated on the ribosomes to proteins (Figure 1-17).

Transcription factors usually (but not exclusively) bind to the promoter in the region constituting the first 200 base pairs "upstream" (toward the 5' end) of the TATA box. The receptors for the thyroid hormone–steroid hormone–vitamin D–retinoic acid superfamily are DNA-binding transcription factors. Those hormones that act through cell membrane receptors and do not enter the cells can regulate gene expression by regulating transcription factor production.

Anterior Pituitary Gland

Objectives

1. Explain the relationship between the hypothalamus and the anterior pituitary.

2. List the hormones of the anterior pituitary gland.

3. Describe the relationship between pro-opiomelanocortin and the hormones secreted by the corticotropes.

4. Explain why pulsatile secretion of hypothalamic releasing factors is significant.

5. List the major actions of the anterior pituitary hormones.

6. Describe the major regulators of anterior pituitary hormone secretion.

7. Explain the relationship between growth hormone and insulin-like growth factors.

8. Explain the physiologic basis for the major symptoms of anterior pituitary pathologic conditions.

■ ANATOMY

The pituitary gland (Box 2-1) is composed of two lobes—the anterior pituitary (**adenohypophysis**) and the posterior pituitary (**neurohypophysis**) (Figure 2-1). Most animals have a third lobe, the intermediate lobe or pars intermedia. Only rudimentary vestiges of this lobe remain in adult humans. The cell types found in the pars intermedia in other species are distributed throughout the anterior and posterior pituitary in humans.

The pituitary is located in a saddle-shaped cavity in the sphenoid bone called the **sella turcica,** or Turkish saddle (Figure 2-2).

The anterior pituitary consists of the **pars distalis, pars intermedia** (intermediate lobe), and **pars tuberalis.** It is glandular in origin and is derived from **Rathke's pouch.** Rathke's pouch is ectodermal tissue that originates from the primitive oropharynx and migrates to a position adjacent to neural tissue that has evaginated downward from the diencephalon to become the neurohypophysis. The posterior pituitary is discussed in Chapter 3.

BOX 2-1

Overview

Many of the anterior pituitary hormones have another endocrine organ as their primary target organ. Therefore the anterior pituitary gland is often called the *master gland.*

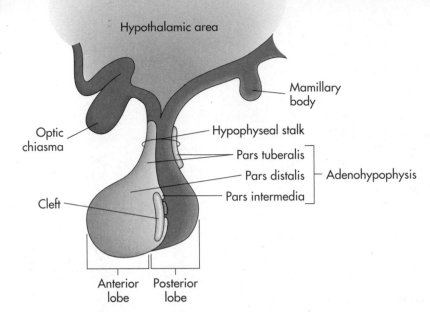

Optic chiasma

Mamillary body

Hypophyseal stalk

Pars tuberalis

Pars distalis — Adenohypophysis

Pars intermedia

Cleft

Anterior lobe

Posterior lobe

Figure 2-1 ■ Anatomy of pituitary gland. (Modified from Genuth SM: The hypothalamus and pituitary gland. In Berne RM, Levy MN, editors: *Physiology,* ed 4, St Louis, 1998, Mosby.)

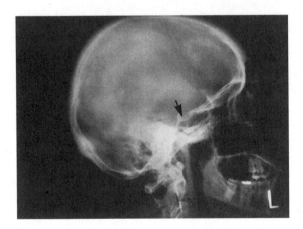

Figure 2-2 ■ Pituitary gland is located in sella turcica *(arrow).* (Courtesy Dr. C. Joe.)

■ HORMONES OF THE ADENOHYPOPHYSIS

The adenohypophysis is where many hormones are synthesized and secreted. It synthesizes **thyroid-stimulating hormone** or **thyrotropin (TSH)** in the thyrotropes, **luteinizing hormone (LH)** and **follicle-stimulating hormone (FSH)** in the gonadotropes, **prolactin (PRL)** in the lactotropes, **growth hormone (GH)** in the somatotropes, and **pro-opio-**

melanocortin (POMC) in the corticotropes (Box 2-2). Pro-opiomelanocortin is the prohormone to **adrenocorticotropic hormone (ACTH), β-lipotrophic hormone (β-LPH), β-endorphin,** and other corticotropin-related hormones.

■ STRUCTURES OF THE ANTERIOR PITUITARY HORMONES

The anterior pituitary hormones LH, FSH, and TSH are glycoprotein hormones. There is a fourth hormone in this family, the placental hormone, **human chorionic gonadotropin (hCG).** All four of these glycoprotein hormones contain an α and a β chain. The α chains are identical for LH, FSH, and TSH and similar for hCG. However, the hormone's specificity is conveyed in the β chain, and all four compounds have different β chains. Glycosylation of these hormones increases the half-life ($t_{1/2}$), and all four of these compounds have relatively long $t_{1/2}$s (20 minutes to 6 hours). Both GH and PRL are proteins, and ACTH is a polypeptide.

■ CONTROL OF THE ADENOHYPOPHYSIS

The synthesis and secretion of the anterior pituitary hormones are regulated by releasing and inhibiting hormones (or factors) that originate in the hypothalamus and are carried to the anterior pituitary by the **hypophyseal portal system.** These releasing and inhibiting hormones are produced in various nuclei in the hypothalamus. High concentrations are found in the median eminence, where they are in close proximity to the first capillary bed of the hypophyseal portal system. This capillary bed is outside the blood-brain barrier. After the releasing and/or inhibiting hormones enter the capillaries, they are carried via a group of hypophyseal portal veins to the second capillary network in the anterior pituitary (Figure 2-3). As is typical of endocrine glands, the anterior pituitary has an exceptionally high blood flow. The releasing and/or inhibiting hormones are released from the capillary bed in close proximity to the hormone-producing cells of the anterior pituitary. The major hypophyseotropic regulators of anterior pituitary function are shown in Figure 2-4. Table 2-1 lists the hypophyseotropic hormones.

When the pituitary is ablated *(hypophysectomy)*, the anterior pituitary hormones are lost. However, unless the hypothalamus is severely damaged, the ability to produce antidiuretic hormone (ADH) and oxytocin is retained (following a recovery period). If instead the hypothalamus is destroyed but the anterior pituitary remains intact, the secretion of all of the anterior pituitary hormones except PRL declines and ADH and oxytocin production is lost. *Prolactin secre-*

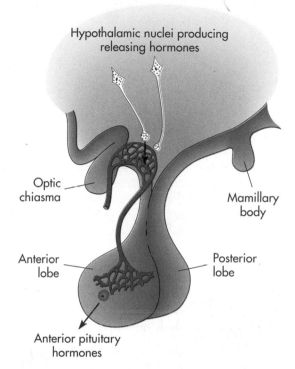

Figure 2-3 ■ Hypophyseotropic hormones are secreted into hypophyseal portal circulation and then transported to anterior pituitary. (Modified from Tyrrell JB, et al: Hypothalamus and pituitary. In Greenspan FS, Strewler GJ, editors: *Basic and clinical endocrinology,* ed 5, Norwalk, Conn, 1997, Appleton & Lange.)

tion rises because the predominant tonic influence on PRL secretion is prolactin-inhibiting hormone (PIH, or dopamine). Following hypothalamic ablation, the lactotrope is released from the suppressive influence of PIH.

Feedback Regulation of the Pituitary-Thyroidal System

There are three types of feedback systems (Figure 2-5).

1. With the **long loop system** (Figure 2-5, *A*), the anterior pituitary hormone acts on the target organ (the adrenal cortex in this

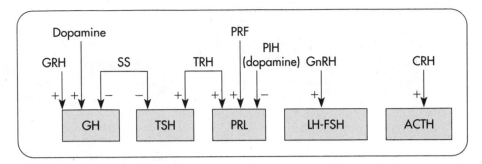

Figure 2-4 ■ Major hypophyseotropic regulators of anterior pituitary function. *GRH,* Growth hormone–releasing hormone; *GH,* growth hormone; *SS,* somatostatin; *TSH,* thyroid-stimulating hormone; *TRH,* thyrotropin-releasing hormone; *PRF,* prolactin-releasing factor; *PRL,* prolactin; *PIH,* prolactin-inhibiting hormone; *GnRH,* gonadotropin-releasing hormone; *LH,* luteinizing hormone; *FSH,* follicle-stimulating hormone; *CRH,* corticotropin-releasing hormone; *ACTH,* adrenocorticotropic hormone.

TABLE 2-1

Hypophyseotropic hormones: hypothalamic releasing or inhibiting hormones (or factors)

Hormone	Action	Molecular structure
Corticotropin-releasing hormone (CRH)	Stimulates ACTH synthesis and release	41–Amino acid peptide
Thyrotropin-releasing hormone (TRH)	Stimulates TSH synthesis and release; also stimulates PRL	3–Amino acid tripeptide
Gonadotropin-releasing hormone (GnRH)	Stimulates LH and FSH synthesis and release	10–Amino acid decapeptide
Growth hormone–releasing hormone (GRH)	Stimulates GH synthesis and release	44–Amino acid peptide
Growth hormone–inhibiting hormone, somatostatin (GIH)	Inhibits GH synthesis and release; also inhibits TSH	14–Amino acid peptide
Prolactin-releasing factor (PRF)	Stimulates PRL release	Not known
Prolactin-inhibiting hormone (PIH)	Inhibits PRL synthesis and release	Dopamine

ACTH, Adrenocorticotropic hormone; *TSH,* thyroid-stimulating hormone; *PRL,* prolactin; *LH,* luteinizing hormone; *FSH,* follicle-stimulating hormone; *GH,* growth hormone.

---

example) to increase the production of hormone (cortisol). The hormone exerts a negative feedback on the hypothalamus and anterior pituitary.

2. With the **short loop system** (Figure 2-5, *B*), the anterior pituitary hormone it-self feeds back on the hypothalamus, exerting a negative feedback.

3. With the **ultrashort loop system** (Figure 2-5, *C*), the releasing hormone acts directly on the hypothalamus to control its own secretion.

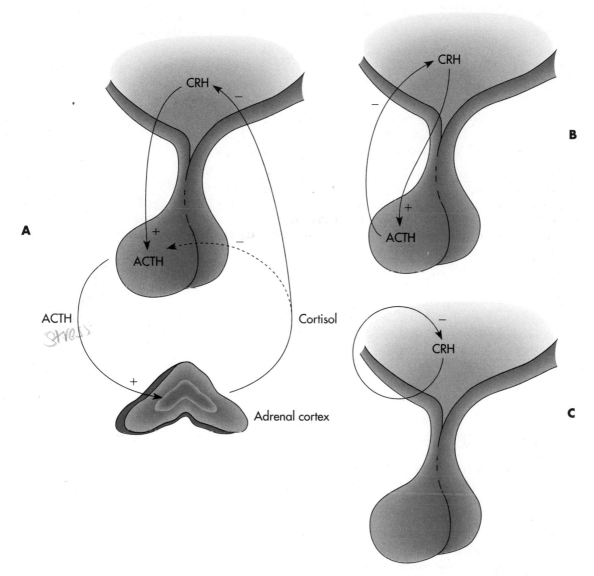

Figure 2-5 ■ Examples of types of endocrine feedback systems. A, **Long loop.** B, **Short loop.** C, **Ultra-short loop.** *CRH,* **Corticotropin-releasing hormone;** *ACTH,* **adrenocorticotropic hormone.**

Pulsatile Secretion of Hypothalamic and Pituitary Hormones

All hypothalamic releasing hormones, and consequently all anterior pituitary hormones, exhibit the phenomenon of **pulsatile episodic secretion,** which consists of short, regular quantal bursts of hormone release. These pulsatile secretions are superimposed on longer rhythms such as circadian rhythms and seasonal rhythms. This pattern of pulsatile secretion, which is thought to be a function of intrinsic neural oscillators within the cells producing the hormones, is absolutely essential for normal hypothalamic-pituitary function. Information appears to be transferred from the hypothalamus to the pituitary by pulse amplitude and frequency. This pulsatile secretion decreases pituitary receptor down regulation. If the pattern of pulsatile secretion is abolished, anterior pituitary hormone secretion is impaired even if hypothalamic releasing hormone levels remain high. Synthetic analogs of gonadotropin-releasing hormone can be used tonically to suppress LH secretion. They have been proposed as a mechanism of birth control. However, if these analogs are given in the appropriate pulsatile manner, they can stimulate LH and FSH secretion. Normal hormonal rhythms are frequently lost in pathologic conditions.

Classification of Endocrine Disorders

Endocrine disorders are classified as primary, secondary, and tertiary. A **primary endocrine disorder** is one in which the target gland itself (e.g., thyroid, adrenal, or ovary) is not functioning normally. A **secondary endocrine disorder** occurs when the initial disorder is in the pituitary and the problem in the target organ is secondary to the pituitary disorder. A **tertiary endocrine disorder** is one in which the problem originates in the hypothalamus.

The physical symptoms of hormonal excess or deficiency ultimately result from problems in the secretion of the releasing or inhibiting hormones. The clinician diagnosing the problem must know the site of the original disorder. If a patient shows symptoms of hyperadrenalism and the clinician orders a bilateral adrenalectomy without ascertaining the initial site of the problem, the patient's condition could deteriorate. This patient could have hypercortisolism because of a functional tumor in the pituitary that results in excess ACTH secretion. This condition is called **Cushing's disease,** which is the most prevalent cause of endogenous hypercortisolism (excessive cortisol produced in the body vs. excessive cortisol resulting from pharmacologic administration). Because the high levels of adrenal corticosteroids partially suppress the pituitary tumor, removing the adrenal glands would cause the pituitary tumor to grow unchecked and increase ACTH secretion even further. The pituitary tumor probably would grow more rapidly, and the patient's skin would darken as a result of the melanocyte-stimulating hormone (MSH)–like activity of ACTH and β-LPH. This condition is called **Nelson's syndrome.** Obviously, the bilateral adrenalectomy would be considered inappropriate and unnecessary surgery. In fact, the patient needed a hypophysectomy, not an adrenalectomy.

In primary *hypothyroidism,* the problem originates in the thyroid, which is unable to produce normal levels of thyroid hormone. Pituitary TSH secretion increases because the negative feedback of T_4 (and T_3) on the pituitary and hypothalamus is lost. The pituitary response to thyrotropin-releasing hormone (TRH) stimulation also increases.

Mechanism of Action of the Releasing Hormones

Hypothalamic releasing hormones act on the anterior pituitary by binding to specific cellular membrane receptors. Although most of these hormones act by stimulating cyclic adenosine monophosphate (cAMP) production, this is not the exclusive mechanism of action.

■ ANTERIOR PITUITARY HORMONES

Luteinizing Hormone

Luteinizing hormone (LH) is thus named because it stimulates the conversion of the ovarian follicle to a corpus luteum. It also acts to maintain the corpus luteum. Its primary target organ is the *ovary* in women and the *Leydig cells* of the testis in men. LH acts on the corpus luteum to stimulate estrogen and progestogen secretion. In the preovulatory follicle it acts on the theca interna cells to stimulate steroidogenesis, and it acts on the granulosa cells late in the follicular phase to stimulate the production of estrogens from androgens produced by thecal cells. The large midcycle LH surge is the stimulus for ovulation. If the LH surge is blocked, ovulation will not occur.

In the male, LH is the predominant regulator of testicular **steroidogenesis** (the production of steroid hormones). It acts on the Leydig cells to stimulate the production of testicular androgens. LH stimulates growth of the testis. If LH secretion is suppressed, as it is following inappropriate use of anabolic steroids for muscle and body building, the testicles atrophy.

Both LH and FSH are secreted from the same anterior pituitary cell—the gonadotrope. Their primary actions are mediated by cAMP. The secretion of LH and FSH is regulated by the hypothalamic releasing hormone, **gonadotropin-releasing hormone (GnRH)**. GnRH is formed in the **arcuate** and **preoptic areas** of the hypothalamus and is transported to the median eminence. It is stored there in membrane-bound granules until transported via the hypophyseal portal system to the anterior pituitary. GnRH-producing neurons are affected by multiple factors, including dopaminergic, serotonergic, noradrenergic, and endorphinergic influences. Dopamine, endorphins, and melatonin inhibit GnRH release, whereas norepinephrine stimulates it. GnRH action is thought to be mediated primarily through phosphatidylinositol turnover and the calcium-calmodulin system. The GnRH receptor is prone to desensitization on prolonged exposure to GnRH.

Follicle-Stimulating Hormone

In the female, follicle-stimulating hormone (FSH) acts on the **ovarian follicle** to stimulate follicular growth and on the granulosa cells to stimulate aromatization of thecal androgens to estrogens. In the male, FSH acts on the **Sertoli cells** to stimulate estrogen formation from androgens and synergizes with testosterone in stimulating the production of **androgen-binding protein.** Androgen-binding protein binds androgens within the testis, maintaining high levels of androgens in the vicinity of the developing germ cells.

Thyroid-Stimulating Hormone

Thyroid-stimulating hormone (TSH) is a large glycoprotein hormone that is similar to LH, FSH, and hCG. Because the four glycoprotein hormones have similar structures, their activities sometimes overlap in pathologic conditions in which hormone secretion is exceptionally high. Like all the anterior pituitary hormones, TSH is stored in membrane-bound secretory granules. Its primary action is to regulate growth and metabolism of the thyroid gland. It stimulates the synthesis and secretion of thyroid hormones. TSH, like LH, FSH, and ACTH, acts by stimulating cAMP production. **Thyrotropin-releasing hormone (TRH)** is a 3–amino acid peptide produced in the hypothalamus and many other areas. Its primary action in the hypothalamus is to stimulate TSH release. Although TRH also stimulates PRL release, its role in the regulation of lactation is debated. TRH acts by the phosphatidylinositol pathway. The thyrotrope is responsive to the level of intracellular T_3. When thyrotrope T_3 is high, TRH receptors decrease; hence, the responsiveness of the thyrotrope to TRH decreases.

Pro-opiomelanocortin

The precursor to ACTH is the prohormone proopiomelanocortin (POMC) (Figure 2-6). This large protein is processed in the anterior lobe to form an N-terminal peptide, whose function is unknown (it may serve as a growth factor), and the compounds β-LPH and ACTH. ACTH, N-terminal peptide, and β-LPH are secreted by the anterior pituitary. The cleavage products of β-LPH, β-endorphin and γ-LPH, also are released into the circulation, and they may play a physiologic role in humans. β-LPH and γ-LPH are lipolytic; however, their physiologic role in fat mobilization in human adipose tissue is unknown. β-LPH's molecular structure contains the compounds γ-LPH and β-endorphin. β-LPH contains the amino acid sequence of **β-melanocyte-stimulating hormone (β-MSH),** and the β-endorphin contains the sequences of **metenkephalin.** Although β-endorphin is found in serum, there is no evidence that β-endorphin is cleaved in the pituitary to form metenkephalin. β-MSH is not thought to be secreted as such in humans, and MSH levels reported in the past in human serum are probably caused by MSH sequences in circulating LPH and ACTH.

In those species containing a prominent pars intermedia, ACTH is cleaved to α-MSH and **corticotropin-like intermediate peptide (CLIP).** The hormones α-MSH and β-MSH cause dispersion of pigmented melanin granules in melanophores of many fish, reptiles, and amphibians, thereby darkening the skin. Whereas humans lack the melanophores of these other

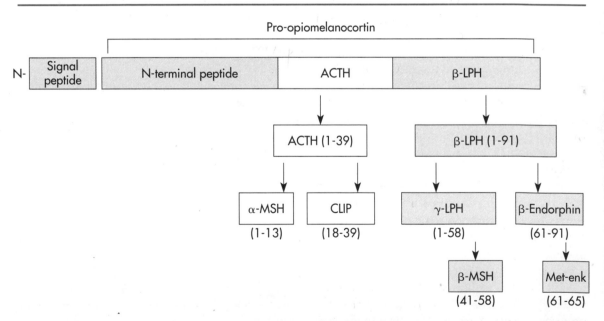

Figure 2-6 ■ **Original gene transcript of pro-opiomelanocortin contains structures of multiple bioactive compounds.** *ACTH,* Adrenocorticotropic hormone; *β-LPH,* β-lipotrophic hormone; *α-MSH,* α-melanocyte-stimulating hormone; *CLIP,* corticotropin-like intermediate peptide; *γ-LPH,* γ-lipotrophic hormone; *β-MSH,* β-melanocyte-stimulating hormone; *Met-enk,* metenkephalin.

species, MSH is capable of causing some skin darkening. The role of CLIP is not known. The human pituitary gland lacks a prominent pars intermedia, and hence processing of ACTH to α-MSH and CLIP does not occur in the human pituitary gland except during fetal development and late in pregnancy.

Adrenocorticotropic Hormone or Corticotropin

Adrenocorticotropic hormone (ACTH) is a 39–amino acid peptide. *Its primary action is to stimulate growth and steroid production in the adrenal cortex.* It acts predominantly on the zona fasciculata and zona reticularis of the adrenal; angiotensin II has the same action on the zona glomerulosa of the adrenal. ACTH acts on the adrenal cortex via cAMP production.

ACTH has extraadrenal actions, one of which is to increase skin pigmentation. The skin darkening that occurs in conditions in which excess ACTH is secreted, such as Addison's disease and Cushing's disease, once were considered to result from high MSH levels. Now this darkening is thought to be caused by high ACTH levels because MSH is not normally present in human serum. Other extraadrenal actions include the stimulation of lipolysis. ACTH is a small molecule and has a short circulating $t_{1/2}$ (7 to 12 minutes).

Control of Secretion ACTH secretion is influenced by many factors (Figure 2-7). **Corticotropin-releasing hormone (CRH)** from the hypothalamus increases ACTH secretion. CRH is co-localized with ADH in the paraventricular nuclei. Both ADH and angiotensin II potentiate the effects of CRH on ACTH release. CRH action is mediated by cAMP.

ACTH secretion shows a pronounced diurnal pattern, with a peak in early morning and a valley in late afternoon (Figure 2-8). In addition, secretion of CRH, and hence secretion of ACTH, is pulsatile. There are multiple regulators of the **hypothalamic-pituitary-adrenal (HPA) axis,**

and many of them are mediated through the central nervous system. Many types of stress stimulate ACTH secretion (Box 2-3). The stress effects are mediated through ADH, angiotensin II, CRH, and the central nervous system. Stressors may be physical, emotional, or chemical. Acute hypoglycemia and hypoxia are effective stimulators. The response to many forms of severe stress can persist despite high cortisol levels. The HPA axis and the immune system are closely coupled, and cytokines—particularly interleukin-1 (IL-1), IL-2, and IL-6—stimulate the HPA axis. Cortisol exerts a negative feedback on the pituitary, where it suppresses ACTH synthesis and secretion, and on the hypothalamus, where it decreases the release of CRH.

Growth Hormone

Growth hormone (GH, somatotropin, STH) is a 191–amino acid protein that is similar to PRL and human placental lactogen (hPL). Whereas PRL is

---

BOX 2-3

Regulators of ACTH Secretion

Stimuli	Inhibitors
CRH	Cortisol
Stress	
Surgery	
Trauma	
Infection	
Hypoxia	
Hypoglycemia	
ADH	
Diurnal pattern:	
peak just	
before awakening	
Anxiety, depression	
α- and β adrenergic	
agonists	

CRH, Corticotropin-releasing hormone; *ADH,* antidiuretic hormone.

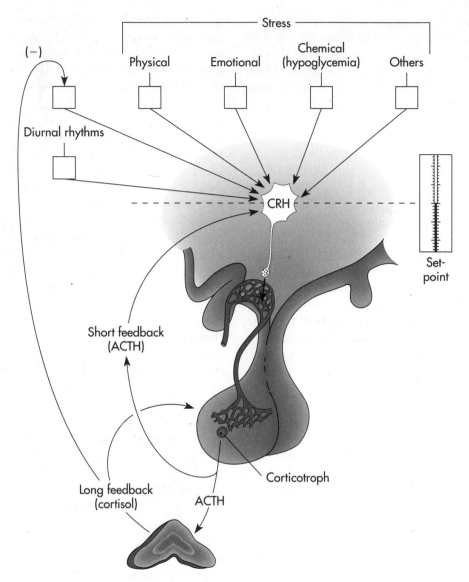

Figure 2-7 ■ Hypothalamic-pituitary-adrenal axis illustrating factors regulating secretion of corticotropin-releasing hormone *(CRH)*. *ACTH,* Adrenocorticotropic hormone. (Modified from Gwinup G, Johnson B: *Metabolism* 24:777, 1975.)

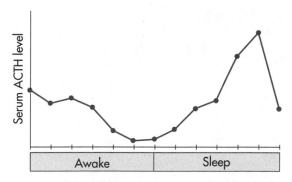

Figure 2-8 ■ Diurnal pattern for serum adreno-corticotropic hormone *(ACTH).*

a 199–amino acid protein, hPL is a 191–amino acid protein (92% homologous with GH), and 161 of these amino acids are identical to those in GH. There is some overlap in activity between GH, hPL, and PRL. Multiple forms of the hormone are seen in serum, thereby constituting a "family of hormones," with the 191–amino acid (22 kd) form representing approximately 75% of the circulating GH. Furthermore, GH in serum is sometimes bound to the N-terminal portion (the extracellular domain) of its receptor (GH-binding protein). Approximately 30% to 40% of the predominant form of GH is thought to be bound to this receptor fragment.

The GH receptor is a member of the cytokine/GH/PRL/erythropoietin receptor family and, as such, acts through receptors associated with cytosolic tyrosine kinase–containing proteins.

Laron dwarfs, who lack normal GH receptors but have normal GH secretion, do not have detectable binding protein in their serum. The exact biologic significance of these binding proteins (receptor fragments) is not yet clear, but GH molecules bound to the protein have much longer $t_{1/2}$s than those not bound.

GH is very species specific, and only primate GH has any significant biologic activity in humans. Unlike the simpler hormone insulin, in which bovine or porcine hormone can be used for hormone replacement in humans (human recombinant insulin is generally used now), GH replacement requires human hormone. At one time, human GH was obtained by the laborious task of extracting it from human cadaver pituitary glands. At least 120 cadaver pituitary glands were needed to obtain enough hormone to treat one GH-deficient child for 1 year. In addition, this therapy was quite expensive. It was discontinued when scientists found that the virus causing the fatal neurologic disorder, Creutzfeldt-Jakob disease, was not destroyed in the extraction procedure. Human-recombinant GH is now commercially available and is the source for GH-replacement therapy in humans. Human GH is biologically active in lower order species, but it is a foreign protein, so long-term use in animals stimulates antibody formation. Because GH is a protein hormone, GH-replacement therapy can be given only by injection.

GH secretion, like that of ACTH, shows prominent diurnal rhythms, with peak secretion occurring in the early morning just before awakening (Figure 2-9). Its secretion is stimulated during deep, slow-wave sleep (stages III and IV). GH secretion is lowest during the day. This rhythm is entrained to sleep-wake patterns rather than light-dark patterns, so a phase shift occurs in people who work night shifts. As is typical of anterior pituitary hormones, GH secretion is pulsatile. The levels of GH in serum vary widely (0 to 30 ng/ml, with most values usually falling between 0 and 3). Because of this marked variation, serum GH values are of minimal clinical value unless the sampling time is known. Frequently, rather than measuring GH, the clinician measures insulin-like growth factor-I (IGF-I) because its secretion is regulated by GH, and IGF-I has a relatively long circulating t½ that buffers pulsatile and diurnal changes in secretion. The circulating $t_{1/2}$ for GH is only about 20 minutes. The liver and kidney are major sites of hormone degradation.

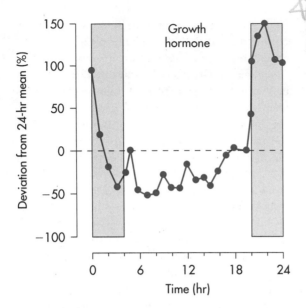

Figure 2-9 ■ Diurnal variation in serum growth hormone. (Redrawn from Krieger DT, Aschoff J: Endocrine and other biological rhythms. In DeGroot LJ et al, editors: *Endocrinology,* vol 3, New York, 1979, Grune & Stratton.)

BOX 2-4

Metabolic Actions of Growth Hormone

Carbohydrates

Increases blood glucose; decreases peripheral insulin sensitivity; increases hepatic output of glucose; administration results in increased serum insulin levels

Proteins

Increases tissue amino acid uptake; increases incorporation into proteins; decreases urea production; produces positive nitrogen balance

Lipids

Is lipolytic; can be ketogenic after long-term administration, particularly if insulin is deficient

Insulin-Like Growth Factor

Stimulates IGF production; stimulates growth; is mitogenic

Actions GH stimulates growth and has metabolic actions. It shifts metabolism to lipid use for energy, thereby conserving carbohydrates and proteins. It stimulates cellular amino acid uptake and protein synthesis.

Metabolic Actions GH has short-term, insulin-like actions; the significance of these actions is not well understood. They may result from the effects of GH fragments. The long-term actions discussed are the metabolic actions that begin at least 1 to 2 hours after GH is administered (Box 2-4).

GH is a **protein anabolic hormone** that increases cellular amino acid uptake and incorporation into protein. Consequently, it produces nitrogen retention (a positive nitrogen balance) and a decreased urea production. The muscle wasting that occurs concomitant with aging has been proposed to be caused, at least in part, by

the decrease in GH secretion that occurs with aging.

GH is a **lipolytic hormone.** It activates hormone-sensitive lipase and therefore mobilizes neutral fats from adipose tissue. As a result, serum fatty acid levels rise after GH administration. More fats are used for energy production. Fatty acid uptake and oxidation increase in skeletal muscle and liver. GH can be ketogenic as a result of the increase in fatty acid oxidation (GH's ketogenic effect is not seen when insulin levels are normal). If insulin is given along with GH, the lipolytic effects of GH are abolished.

GH alters carbohydrate metabolism. Many of its actions may be secondary to the increase in fat mobilization and oxidation. (Remember, an increase in serum free fatty acids inhibits glucose uptake in skeletal muscle and adipose tissue.) Following GH administration, blood glucose rises. The hyperglycemic effects of GH are mild compared with those of glucagon and epinephrine. The increase in blood glucose results in part from decreased glucose uptake and use in skeletal muscle and adipose tissue. Liver glucose output increases, and this is probably not a result of glycogenolysis. In fact, glycogen levels can rise after GH administration. However, the increase in fatty acid oxidation and hence the rise in liver acetyl coenzyme A (acetyl CoA) stimulate reverse glycolysis (gluconeogenesis), followed by increased glucose production from substrates such as lactate and glycerol.

GH antagonizes the action of insulin at the postreceptor level in skeletal muscle and adipose tissue (but not the liver).

Hypophysectomy can improve diabetic management because GH, like cortisol, decreases insulin sensitivity. Because GH produces **insulin insensitivity,** it is considered a **diabetogenic hormone.** When secreted in excess, GH can cause diabetes mellitus, and the insulin level necessary to maintain normal metabolism increases; the excessive pancreatic insulin secretion resulting from the GH excess can damage ("burn out") the pancreatic beta cells. Paradoxically, GH is required for normal pancreatic function and insulin secretion. In the absence of GH, insulin secretion declines.

Actions on Growth GH administration increases skeletal and visceral growth; children without GH show growth stunting or dwarfism. If given in vivo, it results in increased cartilage growth, long-bone length, and periosteal growth. These actions are not generally considered to be direct actions of GH but rather are mediated by a group of hormones called **insulin-like growth factors (IGFs).** These compounds were once called **somatomedins.**

INSULIN-LIKE GROWTH FACTORS The insulin-like growth factors (IGFs) are multifunctional hormones that regulate cellular proliferation, differentiation, and cellular metabolism. These pro-

tein hormones resemble insulin in structure and function. The two hormones in this family, IGF-I and IGF-II, are produced in many tissues and have autocrine, paracrine, and endocrine actions. IGF-I is the major form produced in most adult tissues, and IGF-II is the major form produced in the fetus. Both compounds are structurally similar to proinsulin, with IGF-I having 42% structural homology with proinsulin. IGFs and insulin cross-react with each other's receptors, and IGFs in high concentration mimic the metabolic actions of insulin. Both IGF-I and IGF-II act through type-I IGF receptors, which are similar to insulin and EGF receptors and contain intrinsic tyrosine kinase. However, IGF-II also binds to the type II IGF/mannose-6-phosphate receptor. This receptor does not resemble the insulin receptor and does not have intrinsic tyrosine kinase. Binding to these receptors probably facilitates internalization and degradation of the growth factor. IGFs stimulate glucose and amino acid uptake and protein and DNA synthesis. They were initially called *somatomedins* because they mediate GH (somatotropin) action on cartilage and bone growth. IGFs have many other actions, and GH is not the only regulator of IGF formation. Initially, IGFs were thought to be produced in the liver in response to a GH stimulus. It is now known that IGFs are produced in many tissues, and many actions are autocrine or paracrine. The liver is probably the predominant source of circulation IGFs (Figure 2-10).

TRANSPORT OF INSULIN-LIKE GROWTH FACTORS IN SERUM IGFs are transported in serum bound to **insulin-like growth factor–binding proteins (IGFBPs).** These IGFBPs mediate transport and bioavailability of the IGFs. The liver is the predominant site for IGF degradation. Because IGFs bind to serum proteins, they have long $t_{1/2}$s (up to 12 hours).

CONTROL OF INSULIN-LIKE GROWTH FACTOR PRODUCTION Although GH is an effective stimulator for

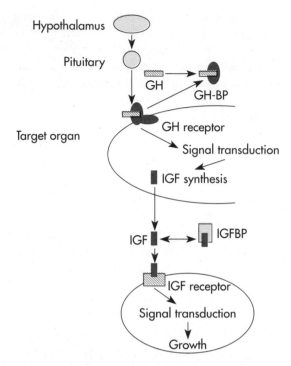

Figure 2-10 ▪ GH-IGF axis. *GH*, Growth hormone; *BP*, binding protein; *IGF*, insulin-like growth factor; *IGFBP*, insulin-like growth factor–binding protein. (Redrawn from Fielder PJ, et al: *Acta Paediatr Scand Suppl* 337:104, 1991.)

IGF production, the correlation between GH and IGF-I is greater than the correlation between GH and IGF-II. During puberty, when GH levels increase, IGF-I levels increase in parallel. Insulin also stimulates IGF production, and GH cannot stimulate IGF production in the absence of insulin. Starvation effectively inhibits IGF secretion, even when GH levels are high. PRL or hPL can increase IGF-II secretion in the fetus, and IGF-II is considered a fetal growth regulator. Although GH is a primary stimulant for liver IGF production, parathormone (PTH) and estradiol are more effective stimuli for osteoblastic IGF-I production. Less is known about the control of bone IGF-II production. IGFs act on the hypothalamus to increase somatostatin secretion and

on the pituitary to inhibit GH secretion, thereby completing the feedback loop.

ACTIONS OF INSULIN-LIKE GROWTH FACTORS IGFs have profound effects on bone and cartilage. They stimulate the growth of bones, cartilage, and soft tissue as well as affect all aspects of the metabolism of the cartilage-forming cells—the chondrocytes. IGFs are mitogenic. Although appositional growth of long bones continues after closure of the epiphyses, growth in length ceases. IGFs stimulate osteoblast replication and collagen and bone matrix synthesis. Serum IGF levels correlate well with growth in children.

The metabolic actions of IGF mimic the metabolic actions of insulin. However, although these effects might be significant at the local (paracrine) level, IGFs are probably not major regulators of intermediary metabolism in the body.

Role of Growth Hormone, Insulin-like Growth Factor, and Insulin in Starvation When ample supplies of nutrients are available, the high serum amino acid levels stimulate GH and insulin secretion and the high serum glucose levels stimulate insulin secretion. The high serum GH, insulin, and nutrient supply stimulate IGF production, and these conditions are appropriate for growth. However, if the diet is high in calories but low in amino acids, the conditions change. Whereas the high carbohydrate availability results in high insulin availability, the low serum amino acid levels inhibit GH and IGF production. These conditions allow dietary carbohydrates and fats to be used, but conditions are unfavorable for tissue growth. On the other hand, during fasting, when nutrient availability decreases, serum GH levels rise and serum insulin levels fall (because of hypoglycemia). IGF production is low, and the conditions are not favorable for growth. Under these circumstances, the rise in GH secretion is beneficial because it promotes fat mobilization while minimizing tissue protein loss. In the absence of insulin, peripheral tissue glucose use decreases, thereby conserving glucose for essential tissues such as brain.

Control of Growth Hormone Release
The hypothalamus regulates pituitary GH synthesis and release via the peptides somatostatin and growth hormone–releasing hormone. **Somatostatin (growth hormone–inhibiting hormone [GIH])** is a cyclic tetradecapeptide that is found in many locations in the body. Somatostatin in the anterior pituitary inhibits GH and TSH release mediated through G_i-associated receptors. Somatostatin is found in many locations in the body and has numerous endocrine and nonendocrine functions. **Growth hormone–releasing hormone (GRH)** is a member of the vasoactive intestinal peptide (VIP)/secretin/glucagon family, and its actions are mediated by cAMP. Dopamine is an effective stimulator of GRH release.

Hypoglycemia is a stimulus for GH secretion, and GH is classified as a **hyperglycemic hormone.** Although its secretion is not regulated by minor variations in serum glucose levels, its release is stimulated by falling glucose levels or by hypoglycemia. Falling blood glucose levels are such an effective stimulus that insulin-induced hypoglycemia is sometimes used as a provocative test of a person's ability to secrete GH. A *rise in certain serum amino acids* also serves as an effective stimulus for GH secretion. Arginine is one of these amino acids, and the GH response to arginine infusion may be used to evaluate GH secretion (Figure 2-11). *Deep or stage III or IV sleep* is an effective stimulator of GH secretion, as are *stress* and *exercise.* GH is classified as one of the **"stress" hormones.** In association with the physiologic response to stress, ADH and glucagon (two other stress hormones) can stimulate GH secretion. Other regulators of GH secretion are listed in Box 2-5.

Pathologic Conditions Involving Growth Hormone GH is necessary for growth before adulthood. Deficiencies can produce dwarfism,

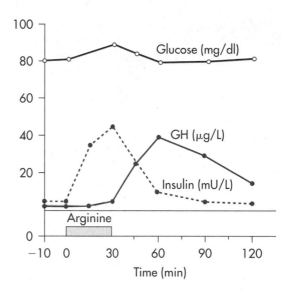

Figure 2-11 ■ Effect of intravenous arginine infusion on plasma growth hormone *(GH)*, **glucose, and insulin concentrations.** (Redrawn from Wilson JD, Foster DW, editors: *Williams' textbook of endocrinology,* ed 8, Philadelphia, 1992, WB Saunders.)

and excesses can produce gigantism. Normal growth requires not only normal levels of GH but also normal levels of thyroid hormones and insulin.

Dwarfism If a GH deficiency occurs before puberty, growth is severely impaired (Figure 2-12). Individuals with this condition are relatively well proportioned and have normal intelligence. If the anterior pituitary deficiency is limited to GH, they can have a normal life span. They are sometimes "pudgy" because they lose GH-induced lipolysis. If they have panhypopituitary dwarfism (all anterior pituitary hormones are deficient) so that gonadotropins are deficient, they may not mature sexually. If the gonadotropins are normal, they are capable of reproduction. People with dwarfism show few metabolic abnormalities other than a tendency toward hypoglycemia, insulinopenia, and increased insulin sensitivity. There are multiple po-

BOX 2-5

Regulators of Growth Hormone Secretion

Factors Stimulating GH Secretion
Metabolic

Decreased serum glucose
Increased serum amino acids, particularly arginine, leucine

Hormonal

GRH
TRH
ADH, glucagon
Dopamine
Uncontrolled diabetes mellitus

Drugs

Dopamine agonists

Other

Exercise
Sleep (stages III and IV)
Stress
Puberty

Factors Inhibiting GH Secretion
Metabolic

Increased blood glucose

Hormonal

Somatostatin
IGF
Hypothyroidism

Drugs

Dopamine antagonists

Other

Emotional deprivation of children
Aging

GH, Growth hormone; *GRH,* growth hormone–releasing hormone; *TRH,* thyrotropin-releasing hormone; *ADH,* antidiuretic hormone; *IGF,* insulin-like growth factor.

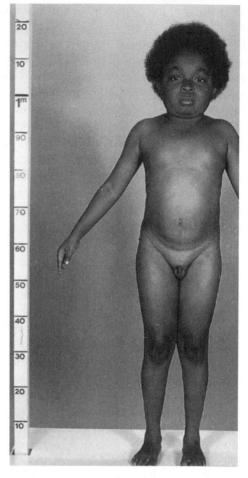

Figure 2-12 ■ **A 17-year-old boy with GH deficiency associated with hypopituitarism. The patient has short stature for his age and underdeveloped genitalia.** (From Besser GM, Thorner MO: *Clinical endocrinology,* London, 1994, Mosby-Wolfe.)

tential sites of impairment. GH secretion may be reduced, GH-stimulated IGF production may decrease, or IGF action may be deficient. **Laron dwarfs** are GH resistant because of a genetic defect in the expression of the GH receptor so that response to GH is impaired. Hence, although the serum GH levels are normal to high, they do not produce IGFs in response to GH; treating them with GH will not correct the growth deficiency.

The **African pigmy** represents another example of abnormal growth. Individuals with this condition have normal serum GH levels, but they do not exhibit the normal rise in IGF that occurs at puberty. They also may have a partial defect in GH receptors because IGF-I levels do not rise normally after GH is administered. However, the IGF-II levels are normal. Unlike the Laron dwarfs, they do not totally lack the IGF response to GH.

Growth Hormone Deficiency in Adults GH deficiency in adults is only currently becoming recognized as a pathologic syndrome. If the GH deficiency occurs after the epiphyses close, growth is not impaired. A GH deficiency is one of many possible causes of hypoglycemia. Recent studies have shown that extended deficiencies of GH lead to body composition changes. The percentage of the body weight that is fat increases, whereas the percentage that is protein decreases. In addition, muscle weakness and early exhaustion are symptoms of GH deficiency.

Because the muscle loss that occurs with aging may result from an age-related decline in GH production, GH is being used experimentally in elderly people to delay the physical decline associated with aging. The efficacy of this treatment in humans has not been established.

Growth Hormone Excess Before Puberty If there is excessive GH production before puberty, gigantism can result. Individuals with this condition can reach heights greater than 8 feet. The GH excess results in an increase in body weight as well as height. Many complications are associated with **gigantism.** These individuals frequently have glucose intolerance and hyperinsulinism. Overt clinical diabetes can develop, but ketoacidosis is rare. They have cardiovascular problems, including cardiac hypertrophy (all viscera increase in size), they are more susceptible to infections than normal,

and they rarely live past their 20s. Hypersecretion of GH generally results from pituitary tumors; tumor growth eventually compresses other components of the anterior pituitary, decreasing secretion of other anterior pituitary hormones.

Figure 2-13 shows Robert Wadlow, the Alton Giant. At 1 year he weighed 62 pounds. His adult size was 8 feet, 11 inches and 475 pounds. Note the long extremities. The androgen deficiency secondary to the gonadotropin deficiency caused delayed puberty, resulting in late closure of the epiphyses.

Acromegaly If excessive GH is secreted after the epiphyses close, the long bones do not grow in length, but appositional growth occurs. Cartilage and membranous bones continue to grow, and gross deformities can result. In addition, soft tissue growth increases and the abdomen protrudes as a result of visceral enlargement. Brain weight increases, with a resultant decrease in ventricular size. There is an increase in the growth of the nose, ears, and mandible, with the mandibular enlargement producing prognathism and widely spaced teeth. The calvarium thickens and the frontal sinuses enlarge, resulting in protrusion of the frontal ridge of the orbit of the eye. The characteristic enlargement of the hands and feet is the basis for the name **acromegaly** (*acro,* end or extremity; *megaly,* enlargement). The excessive bone and cartilage growth can produce carpal tunnel syndrome and joint problems. The voice deepens because of laryngeal growth. Acromegaly usually results from a functional tumor of the somatotropes. As it is generally slow in onset, patients typically do not seek medical help for 13 to 14 years. Unfortunately, by that time they typically have permanent physical deformities. People with gigantism eventually exhibit acromegaly if the condition is not corrected before puberty. A person with untreated acromegaly has a shortened life expectancy (Figure 2-14).

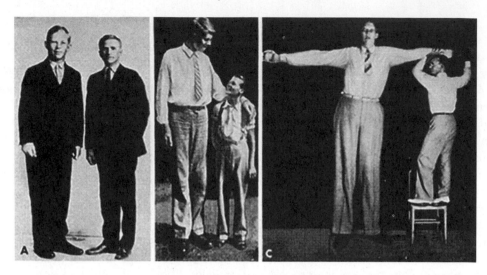

Figure 2-13 ▪ A notable example of growth hormone excess was Robert Wadlow, later known as the "Alton Giant." Although he weighed only 9 pounds at birth, he grew rapidly, and by 6 months of age he weighed 30 pounds. At 1 year of age he weighed 62 pounds. Growth continued throughout his life. Shortly before his death at age 22 from cellulitis of the feet, he was 8 feet, 11 inches tall and weighed 475 pounds. (**A** and **B** from Fadner F: *Biography of Robert Wadlow,* 1944, Bruce Humphreys. **C** courtesy Dr. C.M. Charles and Dr. C.M. MacBryde.)

Extended treatment of adults with GH results in changes in body composition, with the percentage of body protein increasing and the percentage of body fat decreasing.

Tests for Growth Hormone Secretion Normal ability to secrete GH can be tested in several ways: (1) measurement of the GH response to insulin-induced hypoglycemia (hypoglycemia stimulates GH secretion), (2) measurement of the GH response to arginine administration (arginine stimulates GH secretion), (3) measurement of the GH stimulation resulting from dopamine administration (dopamine stimulates GH secretion), and (4) measurement of the GH response to glucagon administration.

Prolactin

Prolactin (PRL) is an 199–amino acid single-chain protein produced in the anterior pituitary lactotropes. PRL, GH, and hPL share some amino acid sequences, and consequently there is overlap in activity among the three hormones. Because the amount of PRL is 1/100 that of GH, it is difficult to obtain enough PRL to study its actions in humans. As is typical of protein hormones, there is heterogeneity of circulating PRL, and the 199–amino acid form represents only 60% to 80% of the PRL measured by radioimmunoassays.

PRL circulates unbound to serum proteins and thus has a relatively short $t_{1/2}$ of about 20 minutes. Normal basal serum concentrations are similar in men and women.

Mechanism of Action The PRL receptor belongs to the cytokine/GH/PRL/erythropoietin receptor superfamily. The exact mechanism of action of the hormone is not known, but the receptors contain intrinsic tyrosine kinase activity

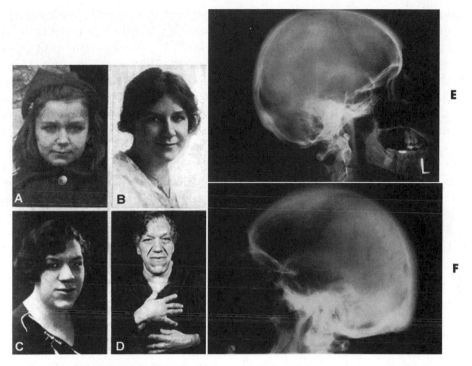

Figure 2-14 ▪ Progression of acromegaly. A, **Normal appearance (age 9).** B, **Possible coarsening of features (age 16).** C, **Well-established acromegaly (age 33).** D, **Severe acromegaly (age 52).** E, **X-ray film of a normal skull.** F, **X-ray film of skull of woman with acromegaly that demonstrates effects of acromegaly on morphologic features of skull. Sella turcica is enlarged as a result of growth of pituitary adenoma. Skull is thicker than normal, and protrusion of frontal ridge with enlargement of frontal sinuses is evident.** (A to D from Clinical Pathological Conference, *Am J Med* 20:133, 1956. E and F courtesy Dr. C. Joe).

and the action might be mediated by increasing calcium entry into the cells through voltage-dependent calcium channels. GH can cross-react with the PRL receptors in humans.

Actions At least 85 different actions have been proposed for PRL, and which actions are seen often depends on the dose of hormone used and the species studied. In humans, the predominant action is the initiation and maintenance of lactation. **Lactation** involves mammogenesis, lactogenesis, and galactopoiesis.

Mammogenesis is the growth and develop-

ment of the mammary gland. This process is stimulated by the actions of multiple hormones. Estrogens and progestogens are the primary hormones involved in mammogenesis, but they exert their actions in concert with PRL. In pregnancy, estrogens, progestogens, PRL, and hPL (placental analog of PRL) act to stimulate the further development of the mammary gland. Although some lactation sometimes occurs during pregnancy, copious lactation does not occur until after parturition because high estrogen and progestogen levels inhibit lactation.

Lactogenesis is the initiation of lactation. Considerable mammary gland development occurs during pregnancy. This growth results from the actions of many hormones including estrogens, progestogens, hPL, GH, insulin, cortisol, and thyroid hormones. However, lactation is inhibited by the high levels of estrogens and progestogens during pregnancy. The fall in serum estrogen and progestogen levels that occurs at delivery allows PRL to stimulate lactation. If PRL secretion is blocked at this time by dopamine administration, lactation will not begin. Cortisol is also important for initiating lactation, and the cortisol surge occurring during delivery facilitates initiation of lactation.

Lactation begins following parturition because PRL acts on mammary glands that have been optimally developed by the actions of estrogens and progestogens during pregnancy. Cortisol is necessary for initiating, but not maintaining, lactation.

Estradiol antagonizes PRL's action on milk synthesis, and either estradiol or prolactin antagonists are sometimes administered to stop lactation. PRL stimulates milk production by stimulating transcription of the mRNA-directing synthesis of milk casein, lactalbumin, and b-lactoglobulin, as well as galactosyltransferase and N-acetyl lactosamine synthetase, enzymes important in lactose synthesis.

Galactopoiesis is the maintenance of milk production. This stage requires PRL and oxytocin. Serum PRL levels initially remain high after parturition in a lactating woman. However, 8 to 10 weeks after a woman gives birth, basal PRL levels decrease and approximate those in a nonlactating woman, with periodic increases continuing to occur, coinciding with and following each period of suckling (Figure 2-15). These intermittent surges stimulate milk synthesis.

Other Actions PRL has behavioral effects in some nonmammalian species. It is responsible for parental behavior in birds and stimulates nest building in mice.

It can have reproductive actions in many species, including humans, and can decrease GnRH release. It alters the pattern of pulsatile GnRH secretion, thereby decreasing LH release in response to GnRH. Excessive PRL secretion in humans inhibits reproductive function in both men and women. In the fetus, PRL and hPL have been proposed as growth stimulators through their effects on fetal IGF-II production. Hyperprolactinemia in humans produces glucose intolerance and hyperinsulinemia. The high hPL levels late in pregnancy are a major cause of the diabetogenicity of pregnancy.

Control of Prolactin Release PRL release is normally under tonic PIH (dopamine) inhibition. If the pituitary is transplanted to below the renal capsule where it can revascularize and resume functioning without the direct influence of hypothalamic releasing and inhibiting hormones, PRL secretion increases markedly whereas the secretion of all other anterior pituitary hormones decreases. The transplanted pituitary eventually contains almost entirely lactotropes. PRL is also controlled through a prolactin releasing factor (PRF). The exact nature of this compound is not known, although many factors, including TRH and hormones in the glucagon family (secretin, glucagon, VIP and gastroinhibitory peptide [GIP]) can stimulate PRL release.

Stimuli for Prolactin Release Nursing and breast stimulation are probably the strongest and most specific stimuli for PRL secretion. This

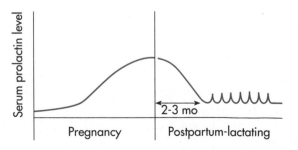

Figure 2-15 ■ **Changes in serum prolactin levels in pregnancy and during lactation.**

response occurs within minutes and is mediated through a neurohormonal reflex. Manipulation of the breast in a nonlactating, cycling woman produces a small PRL response, but manipulating the breast in a man produces no response. PRL is one of the many hormones released in response to *stress*. Surgery, fear, stimuli causing arousal, and exercise are all effective stimuli. As is the case with GH, sleep increases PRL secretion, and PRL has a pronounced sleep-associated diurnal rhythm (Figure 2-16). However, unlike GH, the sleep-associated PRL rise is not associ-

ated with a specific sleep phase. *Estrogen* increases PRL secretion. It acts directly on the lactotropes to increase the number and the size of the lactotropes. This effect is particularly noticeable in pregnancy, when the pituitary enlarges considerably.

TRH can stimulate PRL release as well as TSH release, and hyperprolactinemia sometimes occurs in primary hypothyroidism. As dopamine is PIH, drugs that interfere with dopamine synthesis or action increase PRL secretion. Many commonly prescribed antihypertensive drugs and tricyclic antidepressant drugs are *dopamine inhibitors*. Bromocriptine is a dopamine agonist that can be used to inhibit PRL secretion. Somatostatin, TSH, and GH also inhibit PRL secretion (Box 2-6).

Pathologic Conditions Involving Prolactin

Hyperprolactinemia PRL-secreting tumors account for approximately 70% of all anterior pituitary tumors. Furthermore, many drugs interfere with dopamine production or action and hence increase PRL release. For these reasons, hyperprolactinemia is a common disorder in humans. Hyperprolactinemia in women is associ-

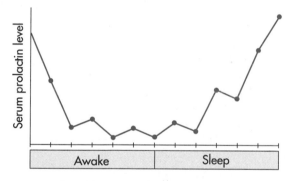

Figure 2-16 ■ Diurnal variation of serum prolactin levels.

BOX 2-6

Regulators of Prolactin Secretion

Stimulators	Inhibitors
Nursing, breast manipulation	
Stress	
Hormones	Hormones
PRF(?)	Somatostatin
Estrogen (or pregnancy)	PIH(dopamine)
VIP, GIP, secretin, glucagon, TRH	
Sleep	
Dopamine antagonists	Dopamine agonists
Chlorpromazine, many antihypertensives,	
tricyclic antidepressives	

PRF, Prolactin releasing factor; *VIP,* vasoactive intestinal peptide; *GIP,* gastrointestinal peptide; *TRH,* thyrotropin-releasing hormone; *PIH,* prolactin-inhibiting hormone.

ated with oligomenorrhea or amenorrhea and infertility. GnRH release, the gonadotrope response to GnRH, and the ovarian response to LH all decrease. In the early stages of the pathologic condition, PRL suppresses follicular maturation, leading to an inadequate corpus luteum and a short luteal phase. As the hyperprolactinemia persists, the preovulatory estrogen peak is lost, thereby lengthening the cycle and leading to oligomenorrhea and anovulatory cycles. Some women experience postpartum amenorrhea during lactation as a result of elevated PRL levels. However, lactation is a poor method of birth control in humans.

Hyperprolactinemia can produce infertility in men. While breast enlargement can occur, true gynecomastia and galactorrhea are rare.

The primary symptoms causing men and postmenopausal women with PRL-secreting tumors to seek medical attention may be those resulting from compression by the pituitary mass. These patients may experience severe headaches or visual disturbances that can include bitemporal hemianopia. Both men and women may complain of decreased libido and signs of hypogonadism.

Prolactin Deficiency The only pathologic problem known to be associated with a deficiency in PRL secretion is the inability to initiate postpartum lactation.

■ HYPOPITUITARISM
Panhypopituitarism

There are many causes of hypopituitarism, which can involve either hypothalamic or pituitary problems. The deficiencies can be variable for the different anterior pituitary hormones. The symptoms of hypopituitarism are slow in onset and are reflected in deficiencies in the target organs of the anterior pituitary. Hypogonadism, hypothyroidism, hypoadrenalism, and growth impairment (in children) may be present. People with panhypopituitarism tend to have sallow

complexions because of the ACTH deficiency, and they become particularly sensitive to the actions of insulin because of the decreased secretion of the insulin antagonists, GH and cortisol. They are prone to develop hypoglycemia, particularly when stressed. Hypogonadism is manifested by amenorrhea in women, impotence in men, and loss of libido in both men and women. Some of the clinical manifestations of hypothyroidism are cold, dry skin, constipation, hoarseness, and bradycardia. The myxedema (nonpitting edema) associated with severe hypothyroidism is rare. Adrenal insufficiency caused by the ACTH deficiency can result in weakness, mild postural hypotension, hypoglycemia, and a loss in pubic and axillary hair. The only symptom associated with the PRL deficiency is the incapacity for postpartum lactation. Finely wrinkled skin is characteristic of a deficiency of both gonadotropin and GH. The GH deficiency can also lead to fasting hypoglycemia in adults and children. In children, growth is impaired and the relative increase in adipose tissue and decrease in muscle mass may produce a "chubby" appearance. The symptoms of the endocrine deficiencies are not as severe as they are in primary thyroid, adrenal, and gonadal deficiencies.

Pituitary Apoplexy

Pituitary apoplexy results from acute infarction of the pituitary gland. There are multiple potential causes for hemorrhagic infarction of the pituitary, including tumor, trauma, bleeding disorder, and postpartum necrosis **(Sheehan's syndrome).** Sheehan's syndrome occurs when excessive blood is lost during and following delivery, resulting in ischemia of the enlarged pituitary of pregnancy. Damage to the pituitary can result in impaired secretion of some or all of the anterior pituitary hormones. The severity of the loss is variable, and most individuals show relatively normal secretion of the posterior pituitary hormones.

Empty Sella Syndrome

Empty sella syndrome occurs when the subarachnoid space extends into the sella turcica, thereby partially filling it with cerebrospinal fluid. This compresses the pituitary and enlarges the sella (Figure 2-17). The flattened pituitary may continue to function, sometimes even normally. There are may different causes of empty sella syndrome, which can be either congenital or acquired. It is relatively common and represents a major cause of sellar enlargement.

■ GROWTH

Normal growth is a complex process that requires normal endocrine function. There are definitive patterns for normal growth. The most rapid growth occurs during fetal development, and the exact fetal growth regulators have not yet been well established. Although GH is not thought to regulate fetal growth, insulin, PRL, and hPL might be growth regulators. Postnatally, the most rapid growth occurs in the neonate. The next period of rapid growth occurs at puberty. It is during puberty that the rising an-

drogen levels act to stimulate closure of the epiphyses and hence cause the termination of long-bone growth.

The role of GH in growth regulation has been discussed. However, appropriate levels of thyroid hormones, insulin, and cortisol are also required for normal growth. The growth deficiencies associated with hypothyroidism are discussed in Chapter 4. Causes of retarded growth in children are listed in Box 2-7. In the absence of normal insulin levels, intermediary metabolism is impaired and IGF production decreases. Both of these hormones are important for normal growth. Whereas a cortisol deficiency is not typically associated with growth impairment, hypercortisolism is. Gonadal steroids are potent growth stimulators in puberty, but they also terminate long-bone growth by stimulating closure of the epiphyses. Growth is stunted if nutrition is not adequate. In either starvation or malnutrition, IGF-I production is low and growth is slowed.

Another cause of growth impairment is psychosocial growth retardation. Infants who are

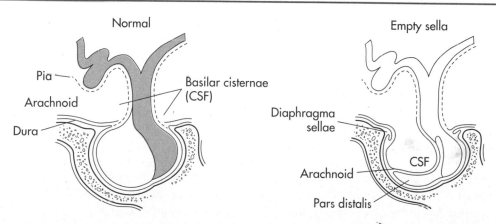

Figure 2-17 ■ Representation of normal relationship of meninges to pituitary gland *(left)* and findings in empty sella *(right)* as arachnoid membrane herniates through incompetent diaphragma sellae. *CSF,* Cerebrospinal fluid. (Redrawn from Jordan RM, Kendall JW, Kerber CW: *Am J Med* 62:569, 1977.)

BOX 2-7

Causes of Retarded Growth in Children

GH deficiency
   IGF-I deficiency
   Impaired IGF-I action
Thyroid deficiency
Insulin deficiency
Cortisol excess
Malnutrition/undernutrition
Psychosocial growth retardation
Constitutional delay
Chronic disease
Genetic disorders characterized by short
   stature

GH, Growth hormone; *IGF-I,* insulin-like growth factor-I.

not stimulated and nurtured or children developing in a hostile environment can demonstrate growth retardation. These children have an immature appearance and often have unusual eating and drinking habits. Pituitary function in these children is suppressed. However, when such children are removed from the poor environment, normal pituitary function resumes and growth resumes.

In many cases, deficient growth is merely a result of constitutional delay. This is not a pathologic condition but a genetic variation from the average. Chronic illnesses also impair growth. Genetic syndromes characterized by short stature such as Turner's syndrome (45,X gonadal dysgenesis) and skeletal dysplasias are not discussed in this section.

Summary

1. The predominant control exerted by the hypothalamus on the anterior pituitary is mediated by releasing and inhibiting hormones. These small peptides are carried via the hypophyseal portal system to the anterior pituitary where they control synthesis and release of the pituitary hormones GH, PRL, TSH, FSH, LH, and POMC.

2. GH stimulates growth primarily through the regulation of the growth-promoting hormones IGF-I and IGF-II. GH also has metabolic actions. It raises blood glucose by decreasing peripheral tissue utilization. It is protein anabolic and lipolytic.

3. The predominant action of PRL in humans is the initiation and maintenance of lactation.

4. Normal growth is a complex process that requires normal endocrine function. Consequently, growth deficiencies are associated with many endocrine disorders in children.

■ KEY WORDS AND CONCEPTS

- Adenohypophysis
- Neurohyophysis
- Sella turcica
- Pars distalis
- Pars intermedia
- Pars tuberalis
- Rathke's pouch

- Thyroid-stimulating hormone or thyrotropin (TSH)
- Luteinizing hormone (LH)
- Follicle-stimulating hormone (FSH)
- Prolactin (PRL)
- Growth hormone (GH)
- Pro-opiomelanocortin (POMC)
- Adrenocorticotropic hormone (ACTH)

- β-Lipotrophic hormone (β-LPH)
- β-Endorphin
- Hypophyseal portal system
- Pulsatile episodic secretion
- Primary endocrine disorder
- Secondary endocrine disorder
- Tertiary endocrine disorder
- Cushing's disease
- Nelson's syndrome
- Thyrotropin-releasing hormone (TRH)
- Gonadotropin-releasing hormone (GnRH)
- Arcuate area
- Preoptic area
- Ovarian follicle
- Sertoli cells
- Androgen-binding protein
- Metenkephalin
- Corticotropin-like intermediate peptide (CLIP)
- Corticotropin-releasing hormone (CRH)
- Insulin insensitivity
- Diabetogenic hormone
- Insulin-like growth factors (IGFs)
- Somatomedins
- Somatostatin (growth hormone–inhibiting hormone, GIH)
- Growth hormone–releasing hormone(GRH)
- Hyperglycemic hormone
- "Stress" hormones
- Dwarfism
- Laron dwarf
- African pigmy
- Gigantism
- Acromegaly
- Lactation
- Mammogenesis
- Lactogenesis
- Galactopoiesis
- Hyperprolactinemia
- Panhypopituitarism
- Pituitary apoplexy
- Sheehan's syndrome
- Empty sella syndrome

■ SELF-STUDY PROBLEMS

1. What is the relationship between GH and PRL?
2. How are anterior pituitary hormones regulated?
3. Cushing's disease is hypercortisolism of pituitary origin. Is this a primary, secondary, or a tertiary endocrine disorder?
4. What is the relationship between GH and IGFs?
5. In gigantism, overt clinical diabetes can develop but ketoacidosis is rare. Why?
6. In hypothyroidism resulting from panhypopituitarism, a goiter does not develop. Why?
7. Why might bilateral hemianopia occur with hyperprolactinemia?
8. Why are primary endocrine deficiencies typically more severe than secondary deficiencies?

■ BIBLIOGRAPHY

DeBoer H, Blok G, Van der Veen EA: Clinical aspects of growth hormone deficiency in adults, *Endocr Rev* 16:63, 1995.

De Feo P, Perriello G, Torlone E, Ventura MM, Santeusanio F, Brunetti P, Gerich JE, Bolli GB: Demonstration of a role for growth hormone in glucose counterregulation, *Am J Physiol* 256 (*Endocrinol Metab* 19): E835, 1989.

Feld S, Hirschberg R: Growth hormone, the insulin-like growth factor system, and the kidney, *Endocr Rev* 17:423, 1996.

Ohlsson C, Bengtsson B, Isaksson O, Andreassen T, Slootweg M: Growth hormone and bone, *Endocr Rev* 19:55, 1998.

Rosenfeld RG, Rosenbloom AL, Guevara-Aguirre J: Growth hormone (GH) insensitivity due to primary GH receptor deficiency, *Endocr Rev* 15:369, 1994.

Sotiropoulos A, Perrot-Applanat M, Dinerstein H, Pallier A, Postel-Vinay M, Finidori J, Kelly PA: Distinct cytoplasmic regions of the growth hormone receptor are required for activation of JAK2, mitogen-activated protein kinase, and transcription, *Endocrinology* 135:1292, 1994.

Thorner MO, Vance ML, Horvath E, Kovacs K: The anterior pituitary. In Wilson JD, Foster DW, editors: *Williams' textbook of endocrinology*, Philadelphia, 1992, WB Saunders, p 221.

Appendix

■ PEPTIDE GROWTH FACTORS

Growth factors are polypeptides that often regulate cellular proliferation (mitogenic activity) and/or differentiation. These compounds are typically produced in multiple tissues and frequently exert their most significant effects through paracrine or autocrine actions. The IGFs are discussed earlier in this chapter and in Chapters 5 and 6. There are, however, many other growth factors. These growth factors include the following peptides.

Platelet-Derived Growth Factor

Platelet-derived growth factor (PDGF) is a polypeptide found in many tissues that acts as an autocrine or paracrine regulator of cell growth. This compound was initially detected in platelets and is released when platelets are lysed in injury. It is a major mitogen for cells of mesenchymal origin, stimulating the cellular proliferation necessary for wound healing and serving as a chemotaxic agent to attract macrophages to the site of the wound. Both PDGF and fibroblast growth factor (FGF) receptors belong to the tyrosine kinase super family.

Fibroblast Growth Factor

Fibroblast growth factor (FGF) is a polypeptide mitogen that was first seen in the CNS but has now been found in many tissues, including bone. It is not thought to be secreted because its original gene transcript lacks an N-signal peptide. This leader sequence is considered essential for entry into the endoplasmic reticulum and subsequent cell packaging for secretion. FGF is therefore thought to be released from cells on lysis. Its name is derived from its mitogenic action on fibroblasts. In bone, it stimulates bone cell proliferation and collagen synthesis. It is a potent mitogen for vascular endothelial cells and is important in neovascularization during fe-

tal growth and wound healing. Its actions are similar to those of PDGF, and it can be substituted for PDGF in cell culture systems.

Epidermal Growth Factor

Epidermal growth factor (EGF) is a polypeptide with well-characterized mitogenic activity. It was originally detected in extracts of mouse salivary glands and was found to accelerate tooth eruption and eye-opening in newborn mice. It stimulates proliferation of various epidermal and epithelial cell types. Its receptor resembles that of insulin, IGF, and TGF, and the receptor has intrinsic tyrosine kinase activity.

Inhibins/Activins

Inhibins are dimers that contain a glycosylated peptide α subunit and one of two possible nonglycosylated peptide β subunits (β_A or β_B) (Figure 2-18). The α and β chains are connected by two disulfide bridges. Activins lack α chains but are composed of two β chains. Therefore they are either homodimers composed of two β_A or

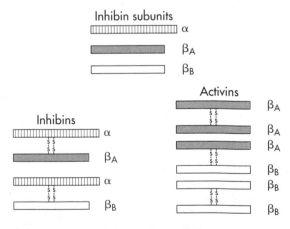

Figure 2-18 ■ Inhibin is formed from one α and one β subunit, and activin is formed from two β subunits.

two β_B subunits or heterodimers of one β_A and one β_B subunit identical to those found in inhibins. Both inhibins and activins are synthesized in the ovaries, testes, and pituitary, and probably other tissues. Inhibins are effective inhibitors of pituitary FSH secretion, whereas activins are stimulators. The actions of inhibins and activins on the gonads are the opposite of those on the pituitary, with inhibins stimulating gonadotropin-stimulated steroidogenesis and cellular proliferation and activins inhibiting them. Inhibins and activins are a part of a family of polypeptide growth factors that include transforming growth factor-β (TGF-β) and müllerian-inhibiting substance (MIS).

Transforming Growth Factors

Transforming growth factors (TGFs) are polypeptides found in both normal and neoplastic tissues. This group of compounds shows considerable homology with EGF, and there is some cross reaction with EGF receptors. TGF-α is a relatively small growth factor that shares homology with epidermal EGF. TGF-βs are larger compounds and resemble PDGF. This group of compounds has the ability to both stimulate and inhibit cell proliferation, depending on the tissue and circumstances involved. They stimulate proliferation of mesenchymally derived cells such as osteoblasts and fibroblasts.

Nerve Growth Factor

Nerve growth factor (NGF) is present in large quantities in mouse salivary glands as is EGF. NGF is important in maintaining viability and promoting differentiation and synaptic outgrowth from sensory and sympathetic ganglionic neurons. It has more recently been shown to be present in brain tissue and may play an important role in central nervous system neuronal outgrowth and synapse formation.

Erythropoietin

Erythropoietin is a protein hormone that is produced predominately in the kidney of the adult in response to hypoxemia. This compound stimulates red blood cell production. Synthesis of this hormone is also stimulated by androgens, and this regulation explains the higher hematocrit values seen in men than in women.

The role of many of these compounds in bone physiology is discussed in Chapter 6.

CHAPTER 3

Posterior Pituitary Gland

Objectives

1. Explain the relationship between the anterior and the posterior pituitary.

2. Explain the relationship between the hypothalamus and the posterior pituitary.

3. List the structures comprising the neurohypophysis.

4. List the major stimuli for the release of antidiuretic hormone and oxytocin.

5. List the major actions for antidiuretic hormone and oxytocin.

6. Distinguish between neurogenic, nephrogenic, and psychogenic diabetes insipidus.

■ ANATOMY

The pituitary gland is composed of two lobes—the anterior pituitary (adenohypophysis) and the posterior pituitary (neurohypophysis).

The posterior pituitary forms as a projection from the ventral surface of the diencephalon, and it retains its neural characteristics (Figure 3-1). It is composed of the neural tracts from two major hypothalamic nuclei—the **supraoptic** and **paraventricular nuclei.** In addition to the processes from these nuclei, there are capillaries and glial-like supportive cells called **pituicytes.** As is typical of endocrine organs, the posterior pituitary is extensively vascularized and the capillaries are fenestrated, thereby facilitating diffusion of hormones into the vasculature. The tracts from these nuclei,

their peripheral terminals, and the lowermost projection of the hypothalamus—the median eminence—constitute the **neurohypophysis.** The neurohypophysis includes the **median eminence,** the **infundibular stem,** and the **infundibular process** (pars nervosa). The neurohypophysis contains the peripheral processes of the magnicellular neurons of the supraoptic and paraventricular nuclei in the hypothalamus. Their axons constitute the **hypothalamohypophyseal tract** that makes up the infundibular stem, and their peripheral terminals are located in the infundibular process or **pars nervosa.**

Some neurons in the paraventricular nuclei have smaller cell bodies, and their axons project to the median eminence rather than to the pos-

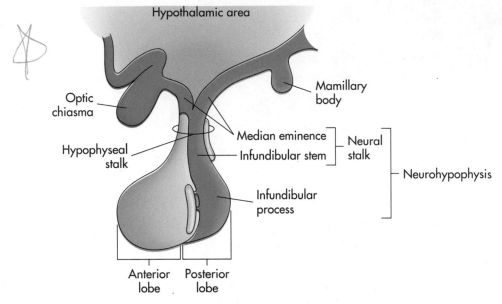

Hypothalamic area

Optic chiasma

Mamillary body

Hypophyseal stalk

Median eminence
Infundibular stem

Neural stalk

Neurohypophysis

Infundibular process

Anterior lobe   Posterior lobe

Figure 3-1 ▪ Anatomy of pituitary gland.

terior pituitary. These neurons are called **parvicellular neurons;** they are responsible for the high levels of **antidiuretic hormone (ADH)** and **oxytocin** found in the median eminence and therefore the hypophyseal portal blood (Box 3-1).

Magnicellular and parvicellular neurons produce hormones that are true neurosecretions. They produce the hormones ADH (or arginine vasopressin [AVP]) and oxytocin. Both the supraoptic and paraventricular nuclei have cells producing these hormones.

The pars nervosa (Figure 3-2) contains the specialized nerve terminals of these magnicellular neurons, along with glial-like supportive cells or pituicytes. The pituitary is exceptionally well vascularized, and the hormones produced in the supraoptic and paraventricular nuclei are stored in the posterior pituitary.

The median eminence is the termination site of neurons from many hormone-producing nu-

BOX 3-1

Overview

The posterior pituitary hormones are ADH and oxytocin. They are synthesized in the hypothalamus and secreted from the posterior pituitary. ADH acts to increase water permeability of the distal nephron, and as such it can decrease free water clearance. The predominant action for oxytocin is stimulation of myoepithelial cell contraction as a part of the milk ejection reflex.

clei in the hypothalamus. Consequently, the median eminence contains high levels of releasing and inhibiting hormones. It also is the site of the first capillary bed constituting the **hypophyseal portal system,** the vascular link responsible for transporting the releasing hormones to the anterior pituitary.

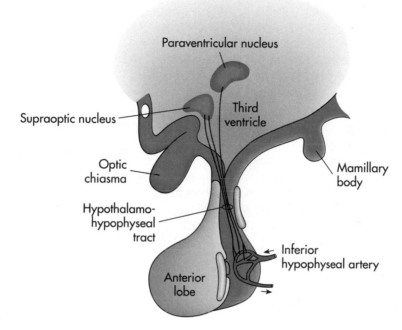

Figure 3-2 ■ Neurohypophysis.

■ SYNTHESIS OF POSTERIOR PITUITARY HORMONES

Posterior pituitary hormones are synthesized in the supraoptic and paraventricular nuclei of the hypothalamus. The supraoptic nuclei produce primarily ADH, and the paraventricular nuclei produce primarily oxytocin. The neurons of these nuclei conduct action potentials, have axons and dendrites, and have synapses as do other neurons. They serve as a link between the nervous system and the endocrine system. They receive input from higher nerve centers, blood, and cerebrospinal fluid–borne chemicals. Many of the axons of these neurons pass through the infundibular stem as the hypothalamohypophyseal tract to the posterior pituitary. These hormones are stored as membrane-bound granules in the terminals of these neurons in the posterior pituitary. Action potentials carried over the

hypophyseal tract to these terminals increase calcium permeability, thereby increasing the inward calcium current; this results in migration of hormone-containing vesicles to the surface of the cell, where the hormones are released by exocytosis. The contents of the secretory vacuoles enter the capillaries served by the inferior hypophyseal artery.

As is typical of protein hormones, ADH and oxytocin are synthesized as preprohormones; the prohormone formed contains segments called neurophysin, which are cleaved during passage to the posterior pituitary. ADH is associated with **neurophysin II** and oxytocin with **neurophysin I.** The N-signal peptide is cleaved as the peptide is transported into the endoplasmic reticulum. The prohormone is packaged in a membrane-bound secretory granule and transported from the cell body to the posterior pituitary. Subsequent cleavage of the prohormone to neurophysin I and oxytocin or neurophysin II and ADH occurs as the secretory granule is transported between the cell bodies of the magnicellular neurons and the terminals in the posterior pituitary. When secretion of the hormones occurs, the contents of the secretory vesicles are released; these vesicles contain equimolar amounts of the hormone and the corresponding neurophysin. No physiologic role for circulating neurophysins has been shown.

Because posterior pituitary hormones are synthesized in the hypothalamus rather than the pituitary, hypophysectomy (pituitary removal) does not necessarily permanently disrupt synthesis and secretion of these hormones. Immediately after hypophysectomy, secretion of the hormones decreases; however, over a period of weeks, the severed proximal end of the tract will show histologic modification and pituicytes will form around the neuron terminals. Secretory vacuoles are seen, and secretion of hormone resumes from this proximal end. Secretion of hormone can even potentially return to normal levels.

■ HORMONE STRUCTURE

ADH and oxytocin are nonapeptides (9 amino acids) and are similar in structure, differing in only two amino acids. They show overlapping activity.

■ ANTIDIURETIC HORMONE

Actions

The primary action of antidiuretic hormone (ADH) is to increase the permeability of the distal nephron to water. Its vasoconstrictive action is the basis for the alternate name—vasopressin (arginine vasopressin or AVP). Other actions of ADH include stimulating renal mesangial cell contraction, inhibiting renin secretion, stimulating adrenocorticotropic hormone (ACTH) secretion, and possibly influencing behavior, learning, and memory.

Renal Actions ADH acts on the kidney to increase water permeability of the luminal surface of the collecting tubules and collecting ducts. In the absence of ADH, water permeability of these membranes is low. ADH acts in these regions by increasing cyclic adenosine monophosphate (cAMP), which stimulates a microtubule-dependent increase in the number of aqueous channels in the membrane, thereby enhancing the water diffusion coefficient. These channels are translocated from a vesicular storage pool in a hormone-dependent manner. ADH also increases urea permeability of the papillary collecting duct. Therefore in the presence of ADH, urine flow decreases and urine osmolality approaches that of the medullary epithelium (about 1200 mOsm/kg). In the absence of ADH, urine flow increases and urine osmolality decreases. Urine osmolality can approach 30 mOsm/kg. ADH is also thought to increase the rate of sodium chloride reabsorption in the thick ascending limb of the loop of Henle.

ADH increases mesangial cell contraction, which lowers the filtration coefficient of the glomerular membrane and therefore decreases the glomerular filtration rate. This action will further decrease the volume of urine flow. ADH inhibits renin release, a response that could be beneficial in compensation for an increase in extracellular fluid osmolality.

Cardiovascular Actions High concentrations of ADH stimulate arteriolar constriction.

Actions on Adrenal-Pituitary Axis ADH produced in parvicellular cells is present in high concentrations in the median eminence. It is transported to the pituitary in the hypophyseal portal system, where it stimulates ACTH secretion, both directly and indirectly, by increasing corticotrope sensitivity to corticotropin-releasing hormone (CRH). ADH is one of many hormones released in response to stress, and its role in pituitary-adrenal cortical activation may become important in times of stress.

Mechanism of Action

There are multiple types of receptors for ADH. The primary actions are mediated through V_{1a}, and V_2 **receptor types.** V_{1a} receptors mediate the vasoconstrictive actions of ADH and act through Gq proteins and cAMP. V_2 receptors are the predominant renal receptors; they act through Gq proteins, inositol triphosphate (IP_3) and diacylglycerol (DAG). These receptors appear to be solely responsible for water transport.

Control of Secretion

ADH is released in response to increased extracellular fluid osmolality (Figure 3-3). Although osmoreceptors have been demonstrated in the medial hypothalamus, the exact location of the osmoreceptors regulating ADH secretion is still debated. Many of these receptors are probably located outside the blood-brain barrier. The actual cells synthesizing ADH are not thought to be the osmoreceptors. However, the magnicellular cells are in close communication with the osmoreceptors. When extracellular fluid osmolality is high, fluid shifts out of the osmoreceptor cells. This resultant cellular dehydration is a stimulus for the osmoreceptors. The magnicellular cells are stimulated, and action potential frequency increases in the neuronal axons constituting the hypothalamohypophyseal tract, with a resultant increase in posterior pituitary ADH release. Because the actual stimulus is cellular dehydration, the response to the hyperosmolality depends on the nature of the solutes. Solutes such as sodium, sucrose, and mannitol that do not readily enter the osmoreceptor cells are effective stimulators, whereas urea, to which the cells are more permeable, has about one third the potency of sodium. These effects may be demonstrated with the following relationship:

$$\uparrow \text{ ECF osmolality} \rightarrow \uparrow \text{ ADH} \rightarrow \uparrow \text{ Renal water}$$

$$\text{reabsorption} \rightarrow \downarrow \text{ ECF osmolality}$$

The regulatory system is sensitive to *serum osmolality* changes in the range between 280 and 295 mOsm/kg. Within this range, a rise as little as 1% in serum osmolality will stimulate a measurable increase in ADH secretion.

ADH release can also be stimulated by a *drop in effective blood volume* (Figure 3-4). The receptors for this stimulus are the cardiovascular volume receptors, including low-pressure receptors in the atria of the heart, great veins, and pulmonary vasculature and high-pressure receptors in the aortic arch and carotid sinus baroreceptors. Although all of these volume receptors are capable of regulating ADH secretion, the predominant regulator appears to be the atrial volume receptors. The sensitivity of the system to volume change is low at small volume changes.

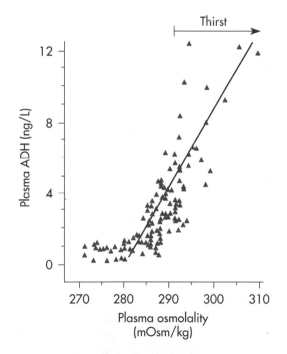

Figure 3-3 ■ Relationship between plasma osmolality and plasma antidiuretic hormone (ADH). (Redrawn from Wilson JD, Foster DW, Kronenberg HM, Larsen PR, editors: *Williams' textbook of endocrinology,* ed 9, Philadelphia, 1998, WB Saunders.)

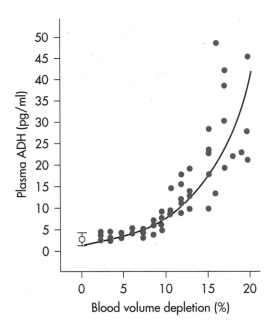

Figure 3-4 ■ **Relationship between blood volume and plasma antidiuretic hormone (ADH).** (Redrawn from Greenspan FS, Strewler GJ: *Basic and clinical endocrinology,* ed 5, Norwalk, Conn, 1997, Appleton & Lange.)

However, volume change does become a significant stimulus when circulating blood volume decreases 8% to 10% or more. This becomes the only mechanism of ADH stimulation during hemorrhage. A decrease in effective blood volume increases the sensitivity of ADH secretion to an increase in extracellular fluid osmolality.

Relationship Between Osmotic Stimuli and Volume Stimuli Vascular volume influences the sensitivity of the system to osmotic stimuli. At lower vascular volumes, the system becomes more sensitive to a rise in serum osmolality. In turn, as vascular volume increases, the sensitivity of ADH release to osmotic stimuli decreases.

Other Factors Altering Secretion Alcohol is an effective suppressor of ADH secretion. For this reason, consumption of alcoholic beverages

can lead to dehydration rather than volume expansion.

Regulation of Thirst

The regulation of thirst and drinking behavior is an important component of body fluid balance regulation. Thirst is regulated by many of the same factors that regulate ADH secretion. Increased serum osmolality, decreased vascular volume, and ADH secretion are effective stimuli for thirst. The osmoreceptors regulating thirst involve medial hypothalamic regions that approximate the osmoreceptors regulating ADH secretion. Angiotensin II is also thought to play a major role in the regulation of thirst. There are many components to the regulation of drinking, which include, in humans, chemical factors, social factors, and pharyngeal and gastrointestinal factors.

Degradation

ADH is predominantly destroyed by proteolysis in the kidney and liver. The circulating t½ of ADH is approximately 15 to 20 minutes.

Pathologic Conditions Involving Antidiuretic Hormone

A deficiency in ADH production results in **diabetes insipidus** (Table 3-1). People with diabetes insipidus are unable to concentrate urine normally and therefore excrete a large volume of urine. These individuals can have urinary flow rates as high as 25 L/day. Thirst increases as a result of the dehydration caused by the high urinary flow.

Diabetes Insipidus

Neurogenic (Pituitary-Hypothalamic) Diabetes Insipidus People with neurogenic diabetes insipidus have a high urine volume and a low urinary osmolality (Figure 3-5). If fluids are withheld, these patients continue to produce an excessive urinary volume and a dilute urine. If ADH is administered to people with this

TABLE 3-1			
Analysis of various types of diabetes insipidus			
	Neurogenic	Nephrogenic	Psychogenic
Plasma osmolality	↑	↑	↓
Urine osmolality	↓	↓	↓
Plasma ADH	Low	Normal to high	Low
Urine osmolality after mild water deprivation	No change	No change	↑
Plasma ADH after water deprivation	No change	↑	↑
Urine osmolality after administration of ADH	↑	No change	↑

ADH, Antidiuretic hormone.

condition, they respond with a decrease in urinary volume and an increase in urinary osmolality.

Nephrogenic Diabetes Insipidus Those with nephrogenic diabetes insipidus have normal ADH production but lack a normal renal ADH response. If ADH is administered, the urinary flow rate does not decrease.

Psychogenic Diabetes Insipidus Those with psychogenic diabetes insipidus are compulsive water drinkers. If water is withheld, the ADH secretion increases and urinary flow decreases while osmolality increases. Individuals with this disorder respond to treatment with ADH.

• • •

Diabetes insipidus differs from osmotic diuresis in that in the former the urinary osmolality (or specific gravity) is much lower than plasma, whereas in the latter the urinary osmolality approaches that of plasma.

Syndrome of Inappropriate Secretion of Antidiuretic Hormone Many disorders can produce inappropriately high ADH concentrations relative to plasma osmolality. Some neoplasms produce ADH and release it into plasma. This is particularly common with pulmonary carcinomas, but it can occur in other types of tu-

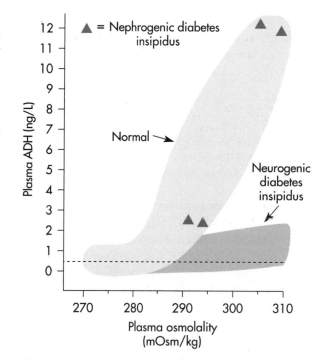

Figure 3-5 ▪ Relationship between antidiuretic hormone *(ADH)* levels and serum osmolality in normal patients, those with neurogenic diabetes insipidus, and those with nephrogenic diabetes insipidus. (Modified from Robertson GL, et al: *J Clin Invest* 52:2340, 1973; and Robertson GL: *Ann Rev Med* 25:315, 1974. Reprinted, with permission, from the *Annual Review of Medicine,* Volume 25 © 1974 by Annual Reviews www.AnnualReviews.org.)

mors, including nonmalignant tumors. In addition, there are many other causes of the syndrome of inappropriate secretion of antidiuretic hormone (SIADH). Pulmonary tuberculosis is often associated with SIADH, as are trauma, anesthesia, and pain. SIADH is similar to the situation seen in Graves' disease in which the hormones are produced without a functional mechanism of regulation of the secretion. In Graves' disease (the most prevalent form of hyperthyroidism), the thyroid is stimulated by abnormal antibodies that are agonists to thyroid-stimulating hormone (TSH); production of these antibodies is not regulated by serum thyroid hormone levels, and consequently the normal mechanism for feedback control of TSH secretion is lost. In SIADH, falling serum osmolality does not inhibit ADH secretion because control of ADH secretion is no longer linked to the normal regulatory mechanisms.

If the person with SIADH has a normal water consumption, water is retained because of the inappropriately high ADH levels. The resultant increase in blood volume and hence blood pressure increases renal glomerular filtration and therefore increases the loss of sodium in the urine. Furthermore, the hypervolemia stimulates release of atrial natriuretic peptide (ANP), which promotes renal sodium loss. The person consequently becomes hyponatremic and has a low serum osmolality. The urine osmolality is inappropriately high (the free water clearance decreases). If water is restricted in an individual with this condition, serum sodium and osmolality will return to normal.

■ OXYTOCIN

The nonapeptide oxytocin is structurally similar to ADH, and there is some overlap in biologic activity. Although the major actions of oxytocin are on uterine motility and milk release, many other biologic actions have been proposed.

BOX 3-2

Major Actions of Oxytocin

Contraction of myoepithelial cells
Uterine contraction

Actions (Box 3-2)

Oxytocin and Uterine Motility Oxytocin stimulates contraction of the uterine myometrium. The magnitude of the oxytocin action depends on the phase of the menstrual cycle (estrus cycle). Estrogens increase the uterine reponse to oxytocin, and progestogens decrease the response. Although uterine responsiveness to oxytocin increases around the time of parturition, oxytocin is not thought to be a factor initiating labor. Oxytocin secretion does not increase until after labor has begun. Once labor begins, the stretching of the vagina and cervix stimulates oxytocin release, which facilitates labor. Although oxytocin is not thought to be a factor initiating labor in normal deliveries, oxytocin administration can initiate labor, and it is used therapeutically to induce labor and decrease postpartum uterine bleeding. Women with diabetes insipidus and the accompanying oxytocin deficiency are capable of a relatively normal labor.

Sexual intercourse can stimulate oxytocin release in both men and women. Although the exact role of oxytocin in men is not entirely understood, the increased release of oxytocin during intercourse in women may aid in sperm transport in the female reproductive tract by stimulating uterine motility.

Oxytocin and Milk "Let-Down" Oxytocin stimulates contraction of the myoepithelial cells surrounding the mammary gland alveoli. Contraction of these cells expels milk from deep in the mammary gland into the larger ducts and sinuses of the gland, where it can be removed more readily by the suckling infant. This process is referred to as **milk ejection** or **let-down of milk.** The release of oxytocin is mediated by a neurohormonal reflex. Suckling or tactile stimulation activates sensory receptors located in the nipple and areola of the breast. These sensory fibers ultimately terminate on hypothalamic magnicellular neurons, producing oxytocin. Stimulation of the magnicellular cells results in an increase in the frequency of transmission of action potentials along the axons from these cells extending to the posterior pituitary, which increases oxytocin secretion. ADH secretion and oxytocin secretion are independently controlled. This reflex can be triggered through a conditioned response; the sight or sound of the hungry infant is adequate to stimulate oxytocin secretion. Oxytocin secretion can be blocked by pain, fear, or stress.

Other Actions Oxytocin stimulates sodium retention and antidiuresis.

Metabolism

Like ADH, oxytocin circulates unbound. It has a relatively short t½ of 3 to 5 minutes. Its degradation occurs primarily in the liver and kidney. However, it can also be degraded in other tissues, including the mammary glands and uterus.

Pathologic Conditions Involving Oxytocin

No known pathologic problems are associated with excess oxytocin. Although a deficiency of oxytocin does not cause major problems, it can, in some individuals, prolong labor and produce lactational difficulties as a result of poor milk ejection.

Summary

1. The hormones of the posterior pituitary are ADH and oxytocin. These compounds are synthesized in the supraoptic and paraventricular nuclei of the hypothalamus and transported within the hypothalamohypophyseal tract to the posterior pituitary where they are stored in the terminals of the same neurons in which they were produced.
2. The hormones are released from the posterior pituitary in response to action potentials carried along the neurons to these terminals.

3. ADH acts to increase water and urea permeability in the collecting tubules and collecting duct. It stimulates mesangial cell contraction and arteriolar constriction and stimulates the adrenal-pituitary axis.
4. Oxytocin stimulates contraction of myoepithelial cells in the mammary gland and myometrial contraction in the uterus.

■ KEY WORDS AND CONCEPTS

- Supraoptic nuclei
- Paraventricular nuclei
- Pituicytes
- Adenohypophysis
- Neurohypophysis

- Median eminence
- Infundibular stem
- Infundibular process
- Magnicellular neurons
- Hypothalamohypophyseal tract

- Pars nervosa
- Parvicellular neurons
- Antidiuretic hormone (ADH)
- Oxytocin
- Hypophyseal portal system
- Neurophysin I
- Neurophysin II
- V_2 receptors
- V_{1a} receptors
- Neurogenic diabetes insipidus
- Nephrogenic diabetes insipidus
- Psychogenic diabetes insipidus
- Syndrome of inappropriate secretion of antidiuretic hormone (SIADH)
- Milk ejection (let-down of milk)

■ SELF-STUDY PROBLEMS

1. Why does hypophysectomy not necessarily permanently disrupt the secretion of ADH?

2. How can ADH, a posterior pituitary hormone, regulate ACTH secretion?

3. How can SIADH result in hyponatremia?

4. How is psychogenic diabetes insipidus distinguished from neurogenic diabetes insipidus?

■ BIBLIOGRAPHY

Aron DC, Findling JW, Tyrrell JB: Hypothalamus and pituitary. In Greenspan FS, Strewler GJ, editors: *Basic and clinical endocrinology,* ed 5, Norwalk, Conn, 1997, Appleton & Lange.

Dibas AI, Mia AJ, Yorio T: Aquaporins (water channels): role in vasopressin-activated water transport, *PSEBM* 219:183-199, 1998.

Reeves WB, Bichet DG, Andreoli TE: The posterior pituitary and water metabolism. In Wilson JD, Foster DW, Kronenberg HM, Larsen PR, editors: *Williams' textbook of endocrinology,* ed 9, Philadelphia, 1998, WB Saunders.

CHAPTER 4

Thyroid Gland

Objectives

1. Explain the mechanism of synthesis of the thyroid hormones.

2. Describe the regulation of thyroid function.

3. Compare and contrast the functions of thyroxine and triiodothyronine.

4. Describe the actions of thyroid hormones.

5. Draw the regulatory feedback loop for the regulation of thyroid function.

6. Describe the etiology, major symptoms, and pathophysiology of those symptoms for Graves' disease, Hashimoto's thyroiditis, sporadic congenital hypothyroidism, and cretinism.

■ ANATOMY AND HISTOLOGY OF THE THYROID

The thyroid is a bilobed structure connected by an isthmus that extends across the ventral surface of the trachea below the larynx (Figure 4-1). As is common with endocrine glands, the thyroid has a sizable blood flow. In fact, when expressed on a tissue weight basis, its blood flow exceeds that of the kidney. In goiters, this flow can increase markedly, and this increased flow can produce an audible **bruit** over the gland. The gland is innervated by adrenergic fibers from the cervical ganglia and by cholinergic fibers from the vagus nerve. This autonomic innervation serves to regulate blood flow (adrenergic increases blood flow, and cholinergic decreases it). Some have proposed that there

might also be some neuronal regulation of hormone synthesis and secretion (adrenergic increases hormone synthesis and secretion, and cholinergic decreases it).

The gland contains follicles formed by epithelial cells called **follicular cells** (Figure 4-2). These cells are cuboidal in a normal gland, columnar in a highly stimulated gland, and squamous in an inactive gland. A clear viscous material called **colloid** is found in the lumen. Colloid is the glycoprotein **thyroglobulin (TG),** which contains the molecular structure of the thyroid hormones (see Figure 4-2). In the stroma around the follicles are the "light" or "C" cells that produce calcitonin. (Calcitonin is discussed in Chapter 6.)

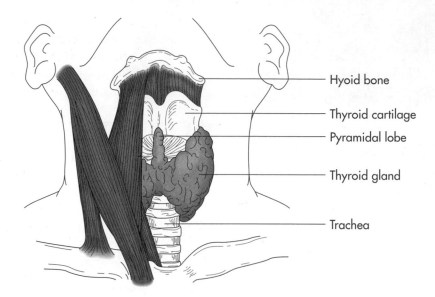

Hyoid bone

Thyroid cartilage

Pyramidal lobe

Thyroid gland

Trachea

Figure 4-1 ■ Anatomy of thyroid. (Redrawn from Greenspan FS, Strewler GJ, editors: *Basic and clinical endocrinology,* ed 5, Norwalk, Conn, 1997, Appleton & Lange.)

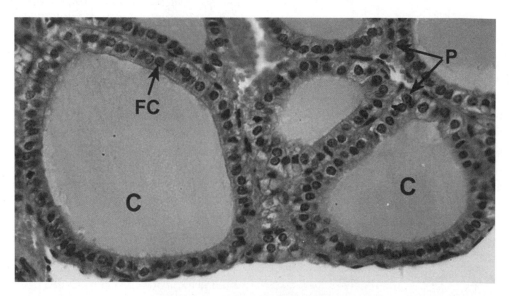

Figure 4-2 ■ Normal rat thyroid. Single layer of cuboidal epithelial cells (follicular cells *[FC]*) surrounds colloid *(C)*. Parafollicular cells *(P)* produce calcitonin.

Overview

The thyroid hormones have widespread actions. They are a major regulator of the body's energy metabolism and regulate many aspects of development. Their actions include regulating neurologic, cardiovascular, musculoskeletal, and reproductive function.

■ THYROID HORMONES (Box 4-1)

The thyroid hormones are **iodothyronines,** compounds formed by coupling two iodinated tyrosine molecules in an ether linkage. The predominant hormones include the following:

1. **Thyroxine (T_4),** or 3,5,3′,5′-tetraiodothyronine, constitutes about 90% of the thyroid hormone secreted by the gland.
2. **Triiodothyronine (T_3),** or 3,5,3′-triiodothyronine, constitutes about 9% of the hormone secreted from the gland. T_4 is sometimes considered the prohormone for T_3.
3. **Reverse T_3** (rT_3), or 3,3′,5′-triiodothyronine, represents about 1% of the hormone secreted from the gland and is not thought to be biologically active.

When tyrosine molecules are iodinated, **monoiodotyrosine (MIT)** and **diiodotyrosine (DIT)** are formed (Figure 4-3). These iodotyrosines are not biologically active.

Synthesis of Thyroid Hormones

Iodide Transport Because iodine is a trace element, an effective mechanism is present for selectively trapping iodide in the thyroid follicular cell. Iodine is taken up as inorganic iodide; this active transport system is referred to as the **iodide trap** (Figure 4-4). The effectiveness of iodide trapping is sometimes assessed by the thyroid/serum **(T/S) ratio.** The T/S [I^-] is generally measured with radioactive iodide. The ability of the thyroid to accumulate iodide is remarkable; values as high as 400 have been reported. The normal T/S [I^-] in a euthyroid person is approximately 30 (the iodide concentration in the follicular cell is 30 times the concentration in the serum). Iodide is concentrated against both its electrical and concentration gradients. The carrier, which is located in the basilar membrane (near extracellular fluids) of the follicular cell, is capable also of transporting other, strongly basic anions, and its affinities for perchlorate and for thiocyanate are actually greater than its affinity for I^-. **Thyrotropin (thyroid-stimulating hormone [TSH])** regulates the T/S ratio for iodide. When the TSH levels drop after hypophysectomy, the T/S ratio drops. If TSH levels are high, as they are in secondary (pituitary) hyperthyroidism, the T/S ratio is high. The salivary glands, mammary glands, gastric mucosa, choroid plexus, placenta, skin, and ovaries are also capable of iodide accumulation. The thyroidal iodide trap is used clinically in several ways; the thyroid gland can be selectively destroyed by oral administration of radioactive iodide [^{131}I] because the isotope is accumulated in the gland, incorporated into TG, and retained there for a prolonged period of time. The beta emissions of the isotope destroy the follicular cells.

The thyroid may be scanned by administering radioactive iodide, allowing time for uptake, and then imaging the gland. Because the radioisotope pertechnetate (TcO_4^-) has a much shorter half-life ($t_{1/2}$) (6 hours) than [^{131}I] (8 days), it is a safer isotope to use for this purpose. It is possible to use [^{123}I] to measure the **radioactive iodide uptake (RAIU)** of the thyroid and hence assess its ability to take up serum iodine (Figure 4-5). An actively functioning gland will have a faster uptake than a poorly functioning gland.

Thyroglobulin Synthesis TG is the precursor of all thyroid hormones. It is a large glyco-

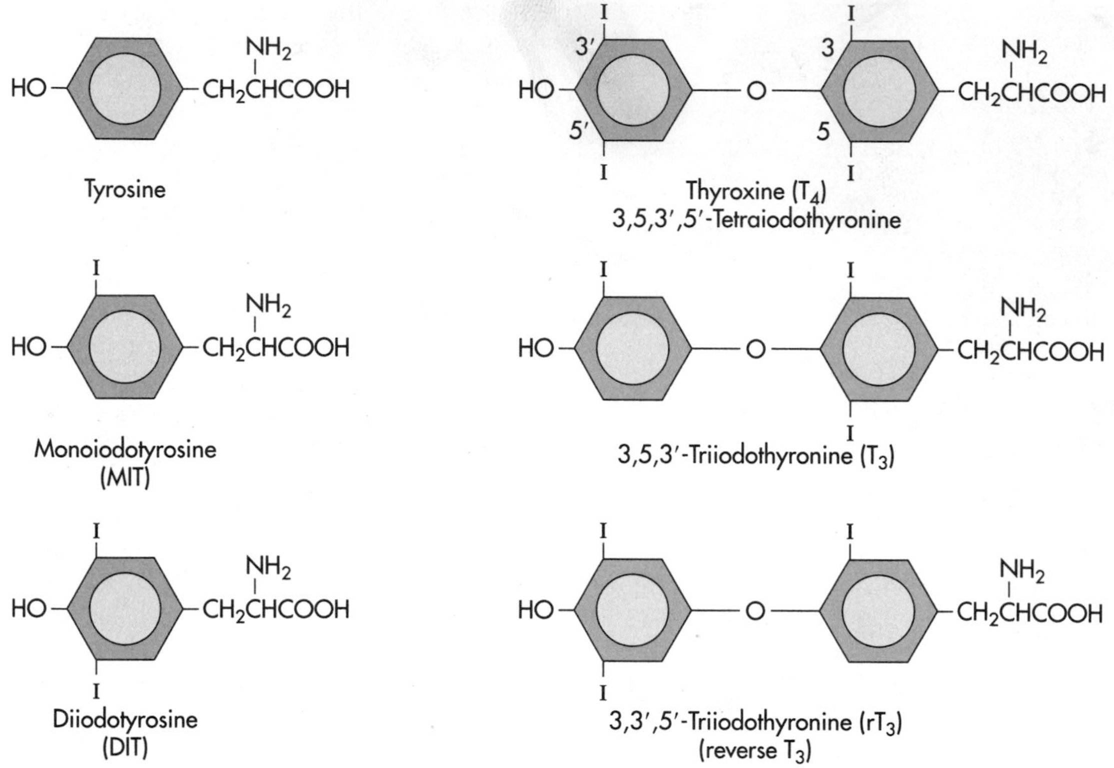

Tyrosine
Thyroxine (T_4)
3,5,3′,5′-Tetraiodothyronine
Monoiodotyrosine
(MIT)
3,5,3′-Triiodothyronine (T_3)
Diiodotyrosine
(DIT)
3,3′,5′-Triiodothyronine (rT_3)
(reverse T_3)

Figure 4-3 ▪ Tyrosine and some of its iodinated derivatives.

protein. The most prevalent form has a molecular weight of 660 kd. TG does not have an unusually high concentration of tyrosine molecules. In fact, this large molecule only has 140 tyrosine residues. These residues are iodinated and coupled to form the active thyroid hormones. Like other proteins in the cell, TG is synthesized on the rough endoplasmic reticulum of the follicular cell, and the glycosylation occurs in the Golgi apparatus. TG is then packaged in exocytotic vesicles and extruded into the lumen of the follicle (Figure 4-6).

Oxidation of Iodide Once within the follicular cell, the iodide is oxidized into an active

Extracellular
fluids
I^-
I^-
Lumen
Follicular cell

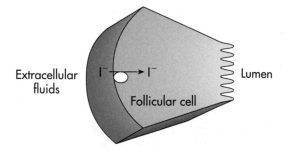

Figure 4-4 ▪ Iodide *(I^-)* is actively transported into follicular cell.

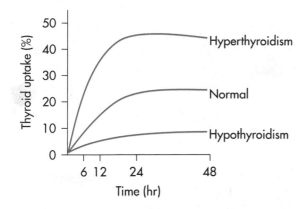

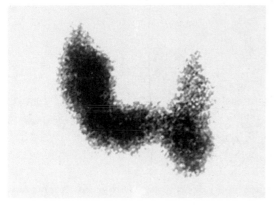

Figure 4-5 ■ A, **Radioactive iodine uptake over 48 hours in patients with normal and abnormal thyroid function. B, Scan of thyroid gland after** ^{123}I **administration.**

intermediate. The reaction is catalyzed by **thyroid peroxidase (TPO)**; hydrogen peroxide (H_2O_2) is the oxidizing agent. TPO is a membrane-bound enzyme found on the apical surface (near the lumen) of the follicular cell. The exact state of this active intermediate is not known. It could be the free radical of iodide. In the latter case, the reaction could be expressed as follows:

$$I^- + H_2O_2 \rightarrow 2\ HO^- + E - I\bullet$$
$$\text{(TPO)} \quad \text{(Active iodide)}$$

Where E = enzyme.

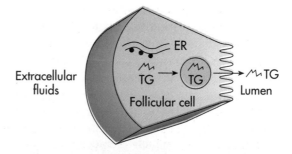

Figure 4-6 ■ **Synthesis of thyroglobulin** *(TG)*. **TG is synthesized on polyribosome of endoplasmic reticulum** *(ER)*, **packaged in membrane-bound secretory vesicle in Golgi apparatus, and secreted into lumen.**

Iodide must be oxidized before organification of iodine can occur.

Organification (Iodination) Iodination is also catalyzed by TPO. "Active iodide" is probably added to the tyrosyl residue after the incorporation of tyrosine into TG. Organification of the iodine produces MIT and DIT residues in the TG molecule.

Coupling Two DITs are coupled to form T_4, or one MIT and one DIT are coupled to form T_3. Such coupling occurs while the DIT and MIT are part of the TG molecule. Both intramolecular and intermolecular coupling occurs. TPO catalyzes this reaction also. TG contains only about three residues of T_4 or T_3 per molecule of TG. There is about 10 times more T_4 than T_3 in TG, and there is very little rT_3 (Figure 4-7).

Storage The thyroid hormones are stored as a part of the TG molecule in the lumen of the follicle. This TG is referred to as colloid.

Thyroid Hormone Secretion

TSH stimulates endocytosis of colloid droplets into the follicular cell (Figure 4-8). Pseudopodia from the follicular cell engulf the droplet, forming a membrane-bound droplet in the interior of the follicular cell rather than in the lumen. This droplet then fuses with a lysosome to form a **phagosome (endosome).** The proteolytic enzymes **(proteases)** within the phagosome hydrolyze TG to the constituent amino acids and T_4, T_3, rT_3, and MIT and DIT. Because MIT and DIT are not biologically active, their secretion into plasma would be inefficient use of the scarce mineral iodine. However, the follicular cells contain **thyroid deiodinase,** which is specific for iodotyrosines and not iodothyronines. This enzyme releases iodine from these iodotyrosines so that it can be reused in the iodination of new TG. The iodothyronines then leave the follicular cell. Although the exact mechanism for transporting the hormones out of the cell is

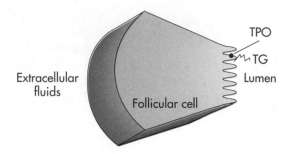

Figure 4-7 ■ Organification and coupling. Thyroid peroxidase *(TPO)* at apical surface of follicular cell catalyzes organification and coupling of thyroglobulin *(TG)*.

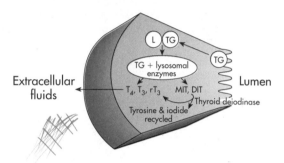

Figure 4-8 ■ Secretion of thyroid hormones. Thyroglobulin *(TG)* is endocytosed and merges with lysosome *(L)* that contains proteolytic enzymes that hydrolyze TG to release hormones. Iodinated tyrosines *(MIT and DIT)* are deiodinated by thyroid deiodinase.

not known, many investigators think it is by simple diffusion.

Extrathyroidal Pools There are large extrathyroidal pools of thyroid hormones. About one third of the body's T_4 is in the liver and kidney. The T_4 pool is larger (20 times greater than the T_3 pool) and slower in turnover (10% per day) than the T_3 pool (70% per day). Because the size of this pool is large relative to the secretion rate, it can serve to "buffer" acute changes in hormone secretion rate. If thyroidal T_4 secretion doubles in a 24-hour period, it only increases serum T_4 levels approximately 5%. Because of this effect, T_4 may be administered orally once a day and serum hormone levels will not change appreciably over the 24-hour period. However, because the pool for T_3 is much smaller, serum concentrations would be more variable if T_3, rather than T_4, were administered. Although it was once thought that T_3 was the best form to use for treating hypothyroidism because it is the more potent form, T_4 is now considered the more appropriate compound for replacement therapy.

Wolff-Chaikoff Effect Excess iodine given to a person with a normal thyroid gland inhibits organification and hormone synthesis. This blockage is temporary, and "escape" generally occurs within several days despite continued high dietary iodine. Exactly how this effect occurs is not known.

Compounds Altering Thyroid Hormone Synthesis

Goitrogens are substances that can block thyroid hormone production and therefore produce goiters. The **thioureas,** like **propylthiouracil (PTU),** act at several points. They inhibit TPO and block oxidation of iodide and organification. They act also on the peripheral tissues to inhibit the enzyme 5'-monodeiodinase, which converts T_4 to the more active compound T_3. *Methimazole* is another commonly used goitrogen. It inhibits organification but does not affect peripheral deiodination. Other compounds act as competitive inhibitors of iodide uptake. These include perchlorate and thiocyanate. The latter is found in cabbage and cassava.

Thyroid Hormone Transport

Protein Binding When thyroid hormones are secreted into the blood, they bind reversibly to serum carrier proteins. Bound and free hormones are in equilibrium; as the levels of free hormones change, the levels of bound hormones also change in accordance with the law

> **BOX 4-2**
>
> *Protein Binding of Thyroid Hormone*
>
> $$T_4 + TBG \leftrightarrow [T_4 \cdot TBG]$$
> $$K = \frac{[T_4] \, [TBG]]}{[T_4 \cdot TBG]}$$

of mass action. The protein with the highest affinity for T_4 and T_3 is **thyroxine-binding globulin (TBG)** (Box 4-2). Although the affinity is high, the capacity (quantity available) is low. This compound binds the largest portion of the circulating thyroid hormones. In fact, 77% of the bound T_4 is bound to TBG. The second highest quantity is bound to **transthyretin (TTR;** also called **thyroxine-binding prealbumin).** This compound's affinity for T_4 is less than that of TBG, and the quantity in the blood is higher (higher capacity). TTR does not effectively bind T_3. Albumin binds a small portion of the circulating thyroid hormones. Although the quantity of circulating albumin is high relative to the other two proteins (high capacity), the affinity of albumins for thyroid hormones is relatively low. Many drugs, such as salicylates and phenytoin, decrease TBG's binding affinity to thyroid hormones (Box 4-3).

Thyroid hormones have an exceptionally high binding affinity for these proteins. Serum T_4 is approximately 99.96% bound and 0.04% free (Figure 4-9). Because T_3 has a lower affinity for these proteins, about 99.6% of serum T_3 is bound and 0.4% is free. These binding proteins play multiple roles. Most think that only the free form of the hormone can enter cells and exert a biologic effect. (This theory has been questioned.) Because there is a simple equilibrium between bound and free forms of the hormone, the bound hormone serves as a reservoir for the hormone (a significant portion of the "nonthyroidal pool") and therefore buffers short-term

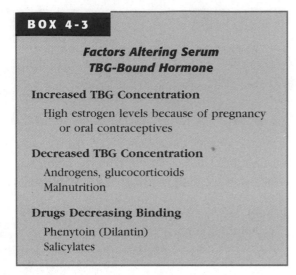

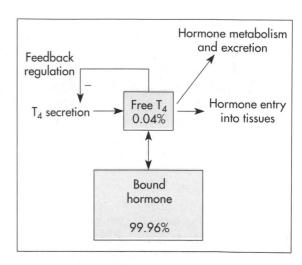

Figure 4-9 ■ Binding of T$_4$. Free serum T$_4$ is in equilibrium with bound hormone. Free form is generally considered to be the biologically active form.

changes in hormone secretion rate. Homeostatic regulation of thyroid hormone levels controls the serum free T$_4$ (T$_3$) and not the total hormone. Thyroid hormones are only sparingly soluble in blood; hence, without the binding proteins, the quantity of hormone that could be transported would be extremely small. Furthermore, binding to the large proteins decreases renal filtration of thyroid hormones. Because protein binding may limit cellular transport of thyroid hormones, it decreases metabolic clearance of the hormones.

Standard radioimmunoassays (RIAs) of the thyroid hormones measure total T$_4$ (or T$_3$) and hence measure both bound and free forms. However, it may be the free hormone that has the greatest clinical significance. Estrogens nonspecifically stimulate the synthesis of liver-binding proteins, including TBG. During pregnancy, TBG levels can increase to the extent that serum total T$_4$ is about twice what it is in the nonpregnant state. However, the woman is not clinically hyperthyroid, and her free T$_4$ level remains within the upper normal range. Obviously, if physicians do not acknowledge the effect of estrogen on

TBG levels, they could erroneously conclude that the woman is hyperthyroid.

There are other disorders or drugs that can alter binding protein levels or affinity. The clinician must be alert to this possibility and understand the significance of such changes. It is now possible to measure free T$_4$ and free T$_3$ levels by RIA, but the assays are not yet completely reliable under all of the conditions that can alter TBG levels.

Metabolism of Thyroid Hormones

T$_4$ is the major secretory product of the thyroid. The predominant pathway for its metabolism is progressive deiodination (Figure 4-10). T$_4$ is initially deiodinated either in the outer ring by **5'-monodeiodinase** to form the more potent compound T$_3$ or deiodinated in the inner ring by **5-monodeiodinase** to form the inactive compound rT$_3$. Triiodothyronines can be progressively deiodinated to **T$_2$, T$_1$,** and **T$_0$.** None of these compounds has biologic activity. Because the thyroid secretes very little T$_3$, 80% of the cir-

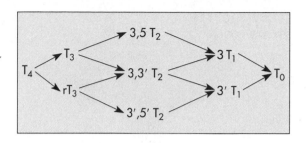

Figure 4-10 ■ Deiodination of iodothyronines by 5-monodeiodinase *(down arrows)* and 5'-monodeiodinase *(up arrows).*

culating T_3 is produced by peripheral deiodination of T_4. Most of the circulating rT_3 is produced by peripheral deiodination of T_4. Because the initial monodeiodination of T_4 produces either a more potent compound or an inactive compound, this is an important step in determining the biologic activity of the thyroid hormones. During starvation and debilitating illnesses, the activity of 5'-monodeiodinase is decreased and hence the production of T_3 is decreased. Because 5'-monodeiodinase is also the enzyme that deiodinates rT_3 to T_2, the levels of rT_3 in serum rise. Some authors have proposed that this is an important control mechanism that serves to decrease the basal metabolic rate under these circumstances.

Other, less important pathways for the thyroid hormone metabolism include (1) conjugation with sulfate or glucuronate and secretion in the bile, (2) decarboxylation and deamination to **triac** and **tetrac,** and (3) decarboxylation to **T_3-amine** or **T_4-amine.**

■ CONTROL OF THYROID FUNCTION

Thyroid-stimulating hormone (TSH) or thyrotropin is a glycoprotein hormone produced in the thyrotropes of the anterior pituitary. The hormone consists of two polypeptide chains. TSH stimulates growth and vascularity of the thyroid gland and the synthesis and secretion of the thyroid hormones. It affects every step in the pathway for hormone synthesis and secretion. It increases iodide uptake, oxidation of io-

dide, organification, and coupling. When TSH levels increase, the follicular cell becomes more columnar in shape, endocytosis of colloid increases, and TG proteolysis increases.

Control Mechanisms

TSH secretion is inhibited by high serum T_4 levels and to a lesser extent by T_3 levels (Figure 4-11). The actual control within the thyrotrope is a function of the intracellular T_3 levels; these levels are determined by the transport of T_4 into the cell from serum and the deiodination of this T_4 to T_3. Approximately 80% of pituitary intracellular T_3 comes from in situ deiodination of T_4, whereas 20% comes from serum T_3. For this reason, regulation of intracellular 5'-monodeiodinase levels can control the sensitivity of the pituitary to feedback inhibition. TSH secretion can be modulated by **thyrotropin-releasing hormone (TRH).** TRH increases the level of the set-point ("thermostat") for the regulatory feedback loop. This compound is a 3–amino acid peptide produced in the hypothalamus (and other regions of the brain) that acts on the pituitary to stimulate TSH synthesis and secretion.

The sensitivity of the pituitary to TRH depends on intrapituitary T_3 levels. When intracellular T_3 is high, there is down regulation of TRH receptors and the pituitary response to TRH decreases. However, if serum T_4 levels are low, intracellular T_3 levels drop and the concentration of thyrotrope TRH receptors increases. As a re-

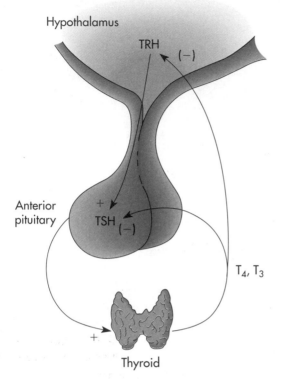

Hypothalamus

TRH

(−)

Anterior
pituitary

+

TSH
(−)

T_4, T_3

+

Thyroid

Figure 4-11 ■ **Hypothalamic-hypophyseal-thyroid axis. Thyrotropin-releasing hormone *(TRH)* produced in hypothalamus reaches the thyrotropes by hypothalamic-hypophyseal portal system and enhances secretion of thyroid-stimulating hormone *(TSH)* by altering the setpoint of T_3 inhibition of TSH secretion.**

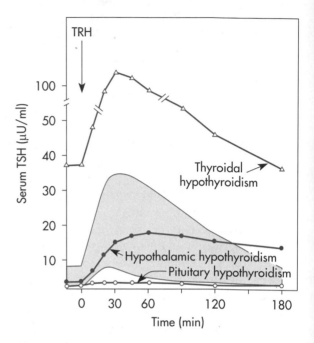

Figure 4-12 ■ **TSH responses to thyrotropin-releasing hormone *(TRH)* in patients with primary, secondary, and tertiary hypothyroidism. The shaded area represents the normal range.** (Redrawn from Utiger RD: Tests of thyroregulatory mechanisms. In Werner SC, Ingbar SM, editors: *The thyroid,* ed 5, Philadelphia, 1986, Lippincott.)

sult of this change, the pituitary sensitivity to TRH stimulation increases. Clinical use has been made of this concept (Figure 4-12). After a bolus injection of TRH, serum TSH levels rise rapidly to reach a peak within 30 minutes in the normal person and then fall to basal levels within 3 hours. If the person is **hypothyroid,** basal serum TSH levels would be higher and the rise in serum TSH in response to the TRH would be greater. If the person has high serum T_4 levels, as in Graves' disease (thyroid hyperplasia not of pituitary or hypothalamic origin), the sensitivity of the pituitary to TRH can

become so low that there is little or no TSH secretion in response to the TRH. If the patient has hypothalamic (tertiary) hypothyroidism, the pituitary can respond to TRH. However, it does not show the exaggerated response that would be expected in a hypothyroid person. This is probably because the pituitary has not been previously exposed to TRH regulation. The most common response is a rise in TSH secretion that is similar in magnitude to that of a euthyroid person, but the response is slower to develop and lasts longer. Although these tests were once used to distinguish hypotha-

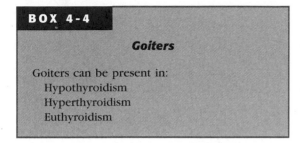

BOX 4-4

Goiters

Goiters can be present in:
Hypothyroidism
Hyperthyroidism
Euthyroidism

lamic from pituitary hypothyroidism, they often are unnecessary now because of the availability of ultrasensitive TSH assays.

Perturbations of Control System

A **goiter** is an enlargement of the thyroid gland; the size of the gland depends on the level of TSH stimulation. However, gland size does not indicate the level of thyroid function. It is possible to have a goiter and be **hypothyroid, euthyroid** (normal thyroid function), or **hyperthyroid** (Box 4-4). To demonstrate this relationship, the role of iodine availability and thyroid function is evaluated. If there is a dietary iodine deficiency, the synthesis of thyroid hormones could be decreased. As glandular T_4 (T_3) secretion decreases, pituitary TSH synthesis and secretion will increase (Figure 4-13). TSH stimulates growth and vascularity of the thyroid. Consequently, the gland will enlarge. However, TSH also stimulates the uptake of the remaining iodide and the synthesis and secretion of hormone. The T/S ratio increases as the "trapping" efficiency of the gland improves. If the iodine deficiency is not too great, the gland can compensate and return serum T_4 to normal levels. However, it took a hypertrophied gland to produce this compensation. Consequently, the patient has a goiter yet is euthyroid. (In long-term iodine-deficient states, the thyroid becomes more sensitive to TSH, and frequently serum TSH levels will be within the normal range but the gland will be enlarged.) If there is insufficient iodide avail-

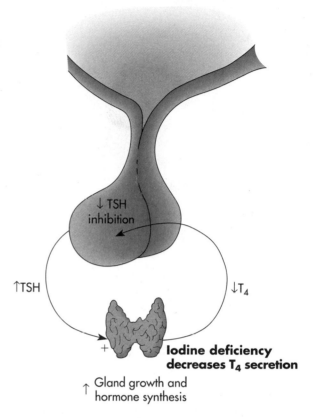

↓ TSH
inhibition

↑TSH   ↓T_4

+   **Iodine deficiency
decreases T_4 secretion**

↑ Gland growth and
hormone synthesis

Figure 4-13 ■ Iodide deficiency decreases hormone synthesis, which can increase thyroid-stimulating hormone *(TSH)* secretion and hence glandular growth.

ability, even with intense TSH stimulation, the patient will be hypothyroid and will have a goiter.

On the other hand, in **Graves' disease,** the thyroid is stimulated by an abnormal immunoglobulin **(thyroid-stimulating immunoglobulins [TSI]** or **thyroid-stimulating antibodies [TSAb]),** which is not regulated by the hypothalamus-pituitary (Figure 4-14). The gland hypertrophies because TSI binds to the TSH receptors on the follicular cell and mimics the action of TSH. TSI, like TSH, can stimulate the synthesis and secretion of T_4 (T_3); consequently, the person is hyperthyroid and has a goiter (Fig-

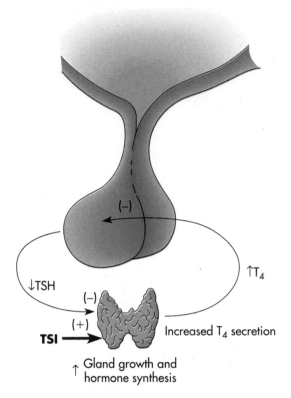

Figure 4-14 ■ Gland growth and function in Graves' disease are stimulated by thyroid-stimulating immunoglobulins (TSI). TSH, Thyroid-stimulating hormone.

ure 4-14). Serum TSH levels in these patients are low to nonmeasurable.

■ MECHANISMS OF HORMONE ACTION
Thyroid Hormone Receptors

Thyroid hormones enter the cell by carrier-mediated transport systems and bind to high-affinity, low-capacity nuclear receptors (Figure 4-15) that are bound to the **thyroid-responsive element** of DNA. When the hormone binds to the ligand-binding domain of the DNA-bound receptor, the hormone-bound receptor can act as a transcription factor to regulate gene transcription of certain mRNAs. There is considerable ho-

mology between the DNA-binding region of this receptor and those for estrogen and retinoic acid. There is some homology with those for glucocorticoid, mineralocorticoid, progesterone, and androgen receptors. These receptors function like hormone-dependent transcription factors. The affinity of the receptor for T_3 is approximately 10 times that for T_4.

Thyroid hormone receptors have also been identified in mitochondria and on the plasma membrane. There are also cytosolic-binding proteins. Thyroid hormones act on mitochondria independent of any nuclear action. They increase the number and size of the mitochondria and increase mitochondrial oxygen consumption (Q_{O_2}) and protein synthesis in vitro. They also increase plasmalemma transport of ions, amino acids, and glucose; one proposed mechanism is interaction with membrane receptors. Some have proposed that the high-affinity receptors in the plasma membrane are the carrier proteins for membrane transport of the thyroid hormones. There does not appear to be a correlation between the extent of hormone binding to cytosolic-binding proteins and the biologic response to thyroid hormones. Consequently, these high-affinity binding proteins are probably not receptors but serve to maintain high intracellular levels of T_3, as TBG does in plasma.

Thyroid-Stimulating Hormone Receptor

TSH receptors are present on the surface of the thyroid follicular cell (type 1). TSH predominantly acts on the thyroid follicular cell by stimulating cyclic adenosine monophosphate (cAMP) production. TSH receptors have been found on nonthyroidal tissues. Although adipocytes, lymphocytes, fibroblasts, and gonads have TSH receptors (type 2), the role of TSH receptors in these tissues is not yet known. However, TSH does stimulate adipocyte lipolysis. Furthermore, in Graves' disease—an autoimmune disease involving the TSH receptor—

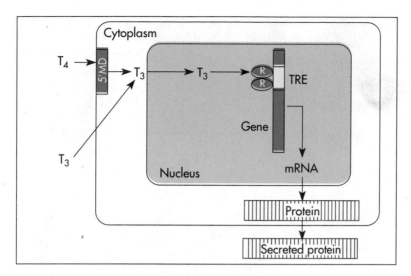

Figure 4-15 ■ **Mechanisms of action of thyroid hormones.** *R*, Thyroid receptor; *5'MD*, 5'-monodeiodinase; *TRE*, thyroid-responsive element.

problems are sometimes seen with fibroblasts in the eye (resulting in *exophthalmos*) and the skin of the pretibial region *(pretibial myxedema)*. These problems could be mediated by nonthyroidal TSH receptors.

■ ACTIONS OF THYROID HORMONES (Box 4-5)

Maturational and Differentiational Effects

Thyroid hormones play a crucial role in amphibian metamorphosis. If a tadpole is given excess T_4, it undergoes metamorphosis prematurely and develops into a miniature frog. On the other hand, if thyroid function in the tadpole is blocked with PTU, the tadpole does not undergo metamorphosis. Thyroid hormones actually stimulate synthesis of the enzymes dissolving the tadpole tail.

Thyroid hormones are also important for normal human maturation. Bone maturation is delayed in hypothyroid children (Figure 4-16). These children often show delayed or absent puberty. Thyroid hormones play an important

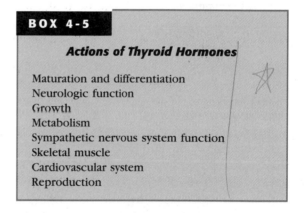

BOX 4-5

Actions of Thyroid Hormones

Maturation and differentiation
Neurologic function
Growth
Metabolism
Sympathetic nervous system function
Skeletal muscle
Cardiovascular system
Reproduction

role in perinatal lung maturation and have been administered in utero to stimulate surfactant formation in high-risk infants.

Neurologic Effects

Thyroid hormones are necessary for normal fetal and neonatal brain development. They regulate neuronal proliferation and differentiation, myelinogenesis, neuronal outgrowth, and synapse formation. There is a critical period of

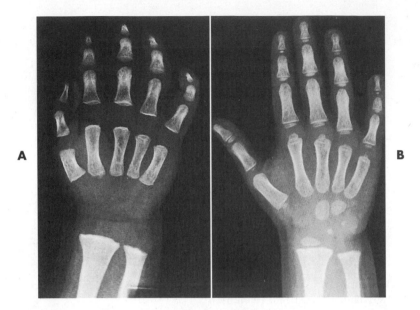

Figure 4-16 ■ **X-ray films of hands of 3-year-old hypothyroid child** (A) **and normal child** (B). **Note marked delay in bone development in hypothyroid child.** (From Besser GM, Thorner MO: *Clinical endocrinology,* London, 1994, Mosby-Wolfe.)

brain development that begins in utero and extends to approximately age 2 years during which a thyroid hormone deficiency results in structural and physiologic impairment. Thyroid hormone replacement subsequent to this period cannot reverse the damage caused by deficiency. Congenital hypothyroidism can result in severe and irreversible brain damage. Because infants with neonatal hypothyroidism (**sporadic congenital hypothyroidism**) who are not treated have severe neurologic impairment, a neonatal thyroid screening program was implemented in the United States. The incidence of sporadic congenital hypothyroidism is approximately 1:4000 to 1:5000 children. The disorder is not always visually apparent at birth. The mental retardation that could result without treatment is severe enough to warrant the cost of routine screening. It is important that the diagnosis be made and treatment initiated within

the first month, and most clinicians attempt to begin replacement therapy as soon as possible within that period. Some people have even attempted hormone replacement in utero.

Thyroid hormones also affect neurologic function subsequent to the critical period, but these changes can be reversed by correcting the thyroid disorder. Hypothyroid adults tend to be dull and lethargic and to have prolonged reflex times. Their thought processes and speech are slow. They often sleep excessively. Hypothyroidism can produce psychological disturbances, leading to **myxedema madness.** Patients who are hyperthyroid tend to be excitable, restless, and distractable; they have insomnia and a decreased reflex time.

Effects on Growth

Adequate thyroid hormone levels are necessary for normal growth. Children with thyroid hormone deficiencies show stunted growth, which can be severe. When thyroid hormone levels are low, growth hormone and IGF secretion decline, which increases growth stunting. However, both thyroid hormones and growth hormone are essential for normal growth.

Metabolic Actions

Thyroid hormones control the **basal metabolic rate (BMR).** They are calorigenic and hence increase oxygen consumption and heat production. This response has a long latent period in vivo. In fact, after serum thyroid hormone levels are increased, it takes approximately 10 days for the BMR to reach a maximal level. Before the advent of RIAs for thyroid hormones, the BMR was used as a clinical test for thyroid disorders. The BMR decreases in hypothyroidism and increases in hyperthyroidism. In hyperthyroidism, mitochondria increase in size and number. The complexity of their cristae increases, as does the concentration of the oxidative phosphorylation enzymes. Some tissues do not respond to T_4 with an increase in oxygen consumption (brain in the adult, spleen, testis); these tissues lack mitochondrial thyroid hormone receptors.

Thyroid hormones increase membrane Na-K adenosine triphosphatase (ATPase) concentration and activity and increase membrane Na^+ and K^+ permeability. As much as 15% to 40% of the basal energy used in the cell is applied to maintaining this electrochemical gradient. Thyroid hormone increases the activity of Na-K ATPase and hence increases energy expenditure in resting cells. Thyroid hormone administration decreases the ratio of intracellular sodium to potassium concentration in liver, skeletal muscle, and heart.

Thyroid hormones increase energy expenditure by increasing futile cycling because they frequently stimulate both anabolic and catabolic enzymes of the same pathways.

In general, thyroid hormones stimulate all metabolic pathways, both anabolic and catabolic (with some exceptions). They stimulate protein synthesis, but they also stimulate protein degradation. The actual effects are dose dependent. Moderate doses of T_4 are protein anabolic in a hypothyroid individual, and these moderate doses decrease nitrogen excretion. However, high doses can lead to net protein catabolism and increased urinary nitrogen excretion. Thyroid hormones stimulate protein turnover. Whether the tissue concentrations of fats, protein, or glycogen change depends on the relative effects on anabolic and catabolic pathways. Thyroid hormones increase cellular uptake of amino acids and incorporation of these amino acids into protein. In hypothyroidism, protein synthesis decreases but so does its degradation. In actuality, the percentage of the body weight that is protein tends to decrease. In hyperthyroidism, both synthesis and degradation increase. Total protein concentration is not necessarily compromised with mild hyperthyroidism, but, if the disturbance is excessive, there may not be adequate substrate available to maintain protein levels. The same can be said about fat and glycogen synthesis and degradation.

Thyroid hormones stimulate lipogenesis. However, they also are lipolytic and can increase hormone-sensitive lipase activity. In general, degradation is affected more than synthesis. Again, fat synthesis and degradation decrease in hypothyroidism. In this case, the percentage of fat in the body increases over time. As expected, hyperthyroidism results in increased lipid synthesis and degradation. Total lipids decrease. Although the liver synthesis of triglycerides increases after thyroid hormone administration, triglyceride clearance from plasma increases because lipoprotein lipase concentration increases. Thyroid hormones can lower serum cholesterol in a euthyroid person, but the effects are transient. Although thyroid hormones increase cholesterol synthesis, they also increase availability of low-density lipoprotein (LDL) receptors, and therefore more cholesterol (predominantly as LDL) is cleared from serum. Serum cholesterol levels increase in hypothyroidism.

Thyroid hormones affect essentially all aspects of carbohydrate metabolism. Blood glucose levels usually are normal in both hypothyroidism and hyperthyroidism. However, a hyperthyroid person often responds abnormally to a glucose tolerance test. After ingestion of the glucose load, blood glucose tends to rise more rapidly than normal. There are several proposals for this abnormality. Thyroid hormones increase the rate the gastrointestinal tract absorbs glucose, and the high hormone levels may increase both insulin resistance and insulin degradation. Glycogen metabolism also is altered in thyroid disorders. In hypothyroidism, liver synthesis and degradation decrease, but glycogen levels increase. With hyperthyroidism, glycogen synthesis and degradation increase, and as substrate availability is compromised, glycogen concentration decreases.

The clinician treating a patient with a thyroid disorder must consider the role of thyroid hormones in turnover within the body. If a patient is hypothyroid, the thyroid disorder may increase the $t_{1/2}$s of medications or hormones. The dosage may have to be decreased. On the other hand, if the patient is hyperthyroid, the dosage may have to be increased.

Actions Mimicking Sympathetic Nervous System Activity

Many actions of excessive thyroid hormone levels resemble those of increased sympathetic nervous system (SNS) activity (increased β-adrenergic receptor stimulation). These actions include increasing the heart rate and producing tremor and excessive sweating. The β-blocker propranolol relieves many of these symptoms without lowering serum T_4 levels. Hyperthyroidism does not increase serum catecholamines, but in some tissues it increases the β-receptor quantity, and in others it increases β-receptor affinity for catecholamines. It might also increase adenylyl cyclase sensitivity to β-adrenergic stimulation.

Actions on Skeletal Muscle

Thyroid hormones have direct actions on muscle. They increase both the content of the plasmalemma electrogenic Na-K pump and increase the resting membrane potential. They also increase the rate and amount of calcium uptake in the sarcoplasmic reticulum, thereby increasing calcium availability on stimulation. They influence the isotype availability of myosin and increase myosin ATPase activity. The maximal shortening velocity can increase after thyroid hormone administration. Myopathies are common in both hypothyroidism and hyperthyroidism. In hypothyroidism, muscle stiffness and discomfort are common, and delayed muscle contraction and relaxation lead to slow movements. Muscle mass may increase, but the mechanism is not understood. Muscle glycogenolysis is impaired, and glycogen accumulates. Hyperthyroidism can also produce myopathy. Muscle weakness, wasting, and fatigability are common. This is seen most often in the proximal muscles of the limbs and can lead to difficulties in climbing stairs. There are probably multiple causes of these myopathies. Thyroid hormone excess can deplete proteins. Furthermore, thyroid hormones can inhibit phosphocreatine kinase and impair the muscle's ability to phosphorylate creatine.

Actions on Cardiovascular System

Thyroid hormones increase the heart rate, myocardial contractility, and consequently the cardiac output. Although these effects can be mediated by potentiating the effects of SNS stimulation as discussed previously, the hormones also have direct actions on the myocardium. They increase actin and myosin concentration, the membrane Na-K ATPase (the electrogenic pump) content, and myosin ATPase activity. In contrast to the effects on skeletal muscle, hyperthyroidism produces myocardial hypertrophy rather than atrophy. Thyroid hormone also acts directly as both a positive inotrope and chronotrope, independent of its action by potentiation of catecholamines. There is an increase in the rate of pressure development (dP/dt) and the maximum velocity of shortening (Vmax). Thyroid hormones also increase the velocity of relaxation by increasing expression of cardiac-specific slow sarcoplasmic reticulum calcium ATPase. Characteristic changes are sometimes seen in the electrocardiogram (ECG) of people with thyroid disorders. The ECG of a hypothyroid person may show inverted T waves (particularly in lead II) and low P, QRS, and T wave amplitudes. The hyperthyroid person may show ECG changes indicative of left ventricular hypertrophy.

In hyperthyroidism, stroke volume, heart rate, and mean systolic ejection velocity increase, accompanied by decreased peripheral resistance. Peripheral resistance is decreased when thyroid hormone levels are high for two reasons: (1) thyroid hormones act directly on vascular smooth muscle to cause vasodilation; (2) in addition, the increased heat and metabolite production results in cutaneous vasodilation. People with hyperthyroidism have warm, moist skin. Because cardiac output increases and peripheral resistance decreases, the pulse pressure increases (Table 4-1).

Heart rate and stroke volume decrease in hypothyroidism, and peripheral resistance is usually increased. Again, the effects on peripheral resistance reflect both the loss of cutaneous vasodilation and the loss of the direct action of thyroid hormones on vascular smooth muscle.

The cutaneous vasoconstriction is responsible for the cold skin of patients with myxedema.

■ PATHOLOGIC CONDITIONS INVOLVING THE THYROID
Hypothyroidism

Children Hypothyroidism in children is different from hypothyroidism in adults because thyroid hormones are important for normal development and maturation. There are multiple causes of hypothyroidism in children. Dietary iodine deficiency beginning in utero impairs the thyroid's ability to synthesize thyroid hormones and results in **endemic cretinism** (Figure 4-17). Although technically the term *cretinism* should be reserved for children with endemic iodine deficiency, the term is often loosely applied to all forms of hypothyroidism beginning at or before birth. For children whose hypothyroidism does not result from iodine deficiency, the term *sporadic congenital hypothyroidism* is more appropriate. There are multiple causes for sporadic congenital hypothyroidism, including thyroid agenesis or dysgenesis and thyroidal defects in hormone biosynthesis, such as organification defects. There are also rare cases of hereditary thyroid hormone resistance. Another cause of neonatal hypothyroidism is the transfer of thyroid-blocking antibodies across the placenta from a mother with autoimmune thyroid disease.

The symptoms of hypothyroidism in newborns can include respiratory distress syndrome, poor feeding, hoarse cry, umbilical hernia, and retarded bone age. Because visible symptoms are not always obvious, routine neonatal thyroid screening is essential to detect the disorder and to begin replacement therapy early enough to prevent mental retardation.

Untreated hypothyroidism in children results in mental retardation and growth stunting. These children may show delayed or absent sexual maturity. However, in a small percentage

TABLE 4-1

Physiologic action of thyroid hormones

	Hypothyroid	Euthyroid	Hyperthyroid
Metabolic rate	Decreased BMR		Increased BMR
Proteins	↓ Synthesis, ↓ degradation, ↓ turnover (% BW as protein will ↓)	Protein anabolic	↑ Synthesis, ↑ degradation, ↑ turnover (catabolic if insufficient dietary protein)
Lipids	↓ Synthesis, ↓ degradation, ↓ turnover (% of BW as lipid increases), ↑ serum cholesterol	↑ Beta oxidation, ↑ lipolysis, ↑ lipogenesis	↑ Synthesis, ↑ degradation, ↑ turnover (% of BW as lipid decreases), ↓ serum cholesterol
Glucose	Normal	Normal	Normal serum glucose; abnormal glucose tolerance test
Glycogen	↓ Synthesis, ↓ degradation, ↓ turnover, glycogen accumulates		↑ Synthesis, ↑ degradation, ↑ turnover, glycogen is depleted
Actions with SNS			Excess mimics effects of ↑ β-adrenergic stimulation; can ↑ number and affinity of β-receptors and ↑ adenylyl cyclase sensitivity
Direct cardiovascular actions	↓ Amplitude of ECG waves	↑ HR, ↑ CO, ↑ contractility, ↑ pulse pressure, ↑ actin and myosin	↑ Amplitude of ECG waves

BMR, Basal metabolic rate; *BW,* body weight; *SNS,* sympathetic nervous system; *HR,* heart rate; *ECG,* electrocardiogram; *CO,* cardiac output.

of cases, precocious puberty may occur. This is possible because the high serum TSH levels in congenital hypothyroidism result in some TSH binding to LH and FSH receptors (remember, all three of these hormones are from the same family of glycoprotein hormones); TSH then mimics the action of these gonadotropins. The developmental and maturational changes discussed previously cannot be entirely reversed by subsequent replacement therapy.

Adults Common symptoms of hypothyroidism in adults are listed in Box 4-6. Hypothyroidism results in a decreased BMR, hypothermia, and cold intolerance. The skin tends to be dry and cool because of decreased sweating, decreased sebaceous gland secretion, and cutaneous vasoconstriction. Sweating decreases in response to lower heat production, and there is insufficient adenosine triphosphate (ATP) for normal sweat formation. These people tend to feel cold in a warm room (Figure 4-18).

There are neurologic symptoms as well. Adults with hypothyroidism tend to become dull and lethargic, their speech rate slows, and

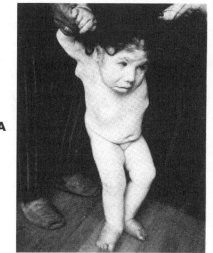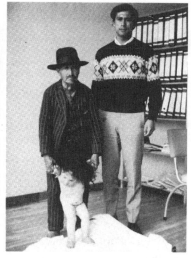

A

B

Figure 4-17 ■ A, **A 28-year-old Ecuadoran woman with endemic cretinism.** B, **She is held by her father and accompanied by a normal-height Ecuadoran man.** (From Fierro-Benitez R, Ramirez I, Garces J, Jaramillo C, Moncayo F, Stanbury JB: *Am J Clin Nutr* 27:531, 1974.)

BOX 4-6

Common Symptoms of Hypothyroidism

Decreased basal metabolic rate	Thick tongue
	Myxedema
Weakness, fatigue, lethargy	Goiter
	Slow speech
Somnolence	Hoarseness
Mental slowness	Amenorrhea
Muscle aches	Psychosis
Cold intolerance	Electrocardiogram changes
Dry cold skin	
Prolonged reflex times	Thin, brittle hair
Decreased sweating	Constipation
Weight gain	

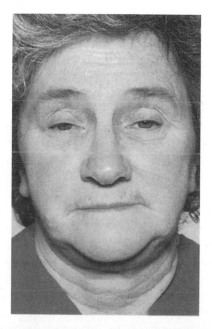

Figure 4-18 ■ **Adult hypothyroidism. Note puffy face, puffy eyes, frowzy hair, and dull, apathetic appearance.** (From Hall R, Evered DC: *Color atlas of endocrinology,* ed 2, London, 1990, Mosby-Wolfe.)

their reflex time is prolonged. They are prone to depression and will frequently sleep excessively. Resultant psychologic problems can reach the level of frank psychosis; the term *myxedema madness* has been used to describe the psychiatric problems that can result.

The patients tend to demonstrate a generalized, nonpitting edema called **myxedema.** This myxedema results from the accumulation of **glycosaminoglycans (GAGs)** (mucopolysaccharides; primarily hyaluronic acid and chondroitin sulfate) in the interstitial spaces, and hence fluid is retained. This swelling leads to the hoarseness frequently described in these people. The skin thickens and coarsens, facial features thicken, the tongue enlarges, and there is noticeable periorbital edema. Although the term *myxedema* is frequently used synonymously with hypothyroidism, its use is not appropriate because myxedema is a descriptive term for a specific type of nonpitting edema; it is also seen in pathologic disorders other than hypothyroidism. In fact, **pretibial myxedema** is a common occurrence in the hyperthyroidism of Graves' disease.

Because thyroid hormones regulate protein metabolism, it is not surprising that changes are seen in hair texture. There are changes in hair follicle function, and the hair becomes thin, coarse, and brittle and lacks luster. The loss of the lateral third of the eyebrows is common. Nail deformities are also noted frequently.

Gastrointestinal disturbances are common in thyroid disorders, and hypothyroid people tend to have problems with constipation. Their appetite and hence food consumption tend to decrease; however, their BMR and therefore their caloric use also decrease. Consequently, these individuals frequently gain weight.

Menstrual irregularities are common in both hypothyroidism and hyperthyroidism. Women with hypothyroidism find it difficult to become pregnant, and when pregnancy occurs, the incidence of spontaneous abortion, stillbirths, and fetal impairment increases.

Cardiovascular signs occurring in hypothyroidism include bradycardia, decreased myocardial contractility, and hence reduced cardiac output. The voltage of the deflections on the ECG is reduced, and there may be pericardial effusion as a result of the interstitial edema. These people may have hypertension because of increased peripheral resistance at rest. Such changes result in decreased pulse pressure. Elevated serum cholesterol and triglyceride levels are common, as is the development of atherosclerosis. At one time, thyroid hormones were used to treat hyperlipemia in euthyroid people, but the effects were transient and the side effects were unacceptable.

Causes of hypothyroidism are listed in Box 4-7. Many of the symptoms of hypothyroidism described for adults are also seen in children. Although most of the symptoms are reversed on correction of the thyroid disorder, developmental disturbances are often not entirely reversible with subsequent treatment.

Hyperthyroidism

Thyrotoxicosis results when tissues are exposed to excessive quantities of thyroid hormones. The most prevalent form of hyperthyroidism is *Graves' disease.* This is an autoimmune disorder in which T lymphocytes become sensitized to antigens within the thyroid gland

---

BOX 4-7

Causes of Adult Hypothyroidism

Destruction of gland
  Surgical
  Irradiation
  Autoimmune (Hashimoto's thyroiditis)
  Cancer
  Thyroiditis
Inhibition of thyroid hormone synthesis
  Dietary iodine deficiency
  Enzyme defects for hormonogenesis
  Antithyroid drugs
Hypothalamic or pituitary disorders
Resistance to thyroid hormone

and subsequently stimulate B lymphocytes to produce antibodies (IgGs) to these antigens. Some of these antibodies can mimic the action of TSH on the thyroidal TSH receptors. They bind to the follicular cell membrane, stimulating cAMP production and hence hormonogenesis and secretion. Like TSH, these antibodies stimulate the growth and vascularity of the thyroid gland. The antibodies are called *thyroid-stimulating immunoglobulins (TSIs)*.

These thyroid-related IgGs are a diverse group of antibodies directed against various different sites within the follicular cell membrane. Some appear to be cytotoxic, some stimulate cAMP, and some block the action of TSH. Individuals with this disorder show an increased frequency of certain haplotypes: HLA-B8 and HLA-DR3 in whites, HLA-BW46 in Chinese, and HLA-BW35 in Japanese. There is strong familial predisposition for the disorder, and women have 7 to 10 times the incidence of men. This antibody production is not related to the circulating levels of pituitary TSH secretion, and hence the feedback loop between the thyroid and the hypothalamus-pituitary is no longer regulating the thyroid. The high circulating T_4

and T_3 levels inhibit pituitary TSH synthesis and secretion.

The symptoms frequently seen in thyrotoxicosis are listed in Box 4-8. Because the antibodies can stimulate thyroid growth, a goiter is usually present. As expected, both the BMR and body heat production increase. Some symptoms of hyperthyroidism result, at least partially, from potentiated catecholamine actions. These include **lid retraction** (resulting in a "wide-eyed" stare), tachycardia, and tremor.

Eye changes (**exophthalmos**) are common in Graves' disease (Figure 4-19). The most common observations are lid lag (upper lid is slow to follow the movement of the gaze downward), upper lid retraction, stare, extraocular muscular weakness, diplopia, periorbital edema, and proptosis. Proptosis may become so severe that the eyelids cannot close and corneal ulceration results. Proptosis occurs because the retroorbital contents increase. Both the retroorbital connective tissue and the muscles are involved. The extraocular muscles can increase to eight times their original volume. Muscle weakness is associated with the muscle enlargement. There is fibroblastic proliferation, and GAGs accumu-

---

BOX 4-8

Symptoms of Hyperthyroidism

Nervousness
Heat intolerance
Palpitations
Muscle weakness
Increased defecation
  frequency
Increased appetite
Moist, warm skin
Bruit over thyroid
Goiter
Tremor

Pretibial myxedema
  (Graves' disease)
Fatigue
Eye problems (Graves'
  disease)
Exophthalmos
Lid retraction
Extraocular muscle
  weakness
Eye irritation

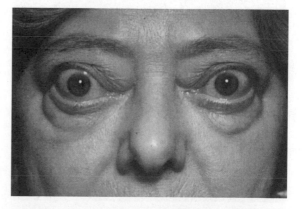

Figure 4-19 ■ **Severe exophthalmos of Graves' disease. Note lid retraction, periorbital edema, and proptosis.** (From Hall R, Evered DC: *Color atlas of endocrinology*, ed 2, London, 1990, Mosby-Wolfe.)

late in the retroorbital tissues (Figure 4-20). The pathogenesis of this ophthalmopathy is not well understood. These ocular abnormalities are immunologically mediated. The ophthalmopathy is not caused by the high levels of serum T_4 and T_3, and correcting the hyperthyroidism does not necessarily prevent progression. The retroorbital fibroblasts and adipocytes are targets of the autoimmune attack. TSH receptors associated with these cells may promote the T lymphocytes activated against the TSH receptor to infiltrate the orbit and skin. These activated cells then release cytokines such as interferon-γ, interleukin-1, and transforming growth factor-β. The cytokines stimulate fibroblasts to produce GAGs that accumulate and produce edema. Edema within the retroorbital muscles and adipose tissue produces proptosis and extraocular muscle dysfunction.

Dermopathy (pretibial myxedema) may be associated with Graves' disease. Between 2% and

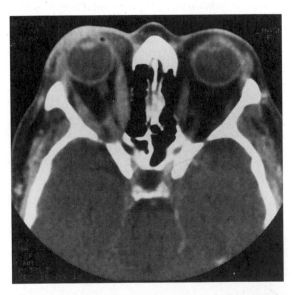

Figure 4-20 ■ CT scan of middle cranial fossa of woman with exophthalmos. Extraocular muscles are enlarged, and eyes protrude beyond rims of orbit. (Courtesy Dr. C. Joe.)

10% of the patients have myxedema in the pretibial area *(pretibial myxedema)* and/or feet. In these regions, the skin thickens and forms "piglike" plaques. The edges of these plaques are well defined, and nodules are sometimes present. As with the myxedema of hypothyroidism, GAGs accumulate in the dermis. These regions itch and are sometimes painful. The pathologic basis of this dermopathy is thought to be an autoimmune disorder. T lymphocytes infiltrate the skin in the pretibial region, where fibroblasts have TSH receptors (type 2); these lymphocytes release cytokines that stimulate GAG production and subsequent edema.

Other forms of thyrotoxicosis include toxic multinodular goiter, toxic adenoma, and sometimes Hashimoto's thyroiditis.

Thyroiditis

Subacute thyroiditis is an acute inflammation of the thyroid that is probably the result of viral infection. The symptoms generally include fever and tenderness of the gland. Symptoms of hyperthyroidism may be present, although the thyroidal status depends on the stage of the inflammation. Although excessive thyroid hormones may be released early in the inflammation, transient hypothyroidism may follow before resolution of the inflammation and restoration of euthyroidism. TSH levels are not generally elevated during the course of the thyroiditis, and elevated radioactive iodide uptake and serum thyroid antibodies are typically not seen. Although approximately 10% of patients have permanent hypothyroidism, more typically the thyroid disorder resolves spontaneously.

Hashimoto's thyroiditis is a common cause of acquired hypothyroidism. It is an autoimmune disorder characterized by the presence of thyroid antibodies. The antibodies are produced by lymphocytes that become sensitized to thyroidal antigens. Common thyroidal antigens are TPO and TG. In Hashimoto's thyroiditis, the gland becomes inflamed and lymphocytes infiltrate the gland. Structural damage of the gland occurs, and TG is released into serum. Hyperthyroidism may be present early in the progression of Hashimoto's thyroiditis, and Hashimoto's thyroiditis and Graves' disease can occur simultaneously. However, as the disease progresses and the gland is destroyed, hypothyroidism develops, serum T_4 and T_3 levels fall, and TSH levels rise. The patient usually has a goiter and most typically is either euthyroid or hypothyroid. Radioactive iodine uptake may be low, normal, or high, depending on the nature of the disorder. However, high antibody titers to TPO or TG are typical. Hashimoto's thyroiditis can sometimes be part of a syndrome involving multiple autoimmune endocrine disorders that can include the adrenals, pancreas, parathyroids, and ovaries (*Schmidt's syndrome*).

Summary

1. The biologically active thyroid hormones are iodothyronines. Whereas T_4 is the predominant hormone secreted by the gland, T_3 is the most potent hormone at the receptor level. Most circulating T_3 is produced peripherally from T_4, and the reaction is catalyzed by 5′-monodeiodinase.

2. Thyroid hormones are major regulators of the body's energy metabolism. They also regulate many aspects of maturation and development as well as growth. They have neurologic, cardiovascular, musculoskeletal, and reproductive functions.

3. Growth of the thyroid is stimulated by TSH; therefore physiologic changes resulting in increased TSH secretion can produce goiters. The size of the gland is not indicative of the level of function of the gland.

4. Congenital hypothyroidism can produce permanent brain damage if it occurs during the "critical period" that begins in utero and extends until age 2.

5. Common symptoms of hypothyroidism include decreased BMR, cold intolerance, prolonged reflex times, myxedema, and constipation. Common symptoms of hyperthyroidism include increased BMR, heat intolerance, shortened reflex times, diarrhea (or frequent bowel movements), and tremor. The most common form of hyperthyroidism is Graves' disease. It is an autoimmune disease associated with the production of antibodies sensitized to the TSH receptor. Exophthalamos is frequently associated with Graves' disease.

■ KEY WORDS AND CONCEPTS

- Bruit
- Follicular cells
- Colloid
- Thyroglobulin (TG)
- Iodothyronines
- Thyroxine (T_4)
- Triiodothyronine (T_3)
- Reverse T_3 (rT_3)
- Iodotyrosines
- Monoiodotyrosine (MIT)
- Diiodotyrosine (DIT)
- Iodide
- Iodide trap
- T/S [I$^-$]
- Thyrotropin, thyroid-stimulating hormone (TSH)
- Thyroid peroxidase (TPO)

- Organification
- Coupling
- Phagosome (endosome)
- Thyroid deiodinase
- Extrathyroidal pools
- Goitrogens
- Thioureas (propylthiouracil [PTU])
- Wolff-Chaikoff effect
- Thyroxine-binding globulin (TBG)
- Transthyretin (TTR), thyroxine-binding prealbumin
- 5'-Monodeiodinase
- 5-Monodeiodinase
- T_2, T_1, T_0
- Triac
- Tetrac
- T_3-amine
- T_4-amine
- Thyrotropin-releasing hormone (TRH)
- Hypothyroid
- Goiter
- Euthyroid
- Hyperthyroid
- Graves' disease
- Thyroid-stimulating antibodies (TSAb), thyroid-stimulating immunoglobulins (TSI)
- Thyroid-responsive element
- Sporadic congenital hypothyroidism
- Myxedema madness
- Basal metabolic rate (BMR)
- Endemic cretinism
- Myxedema
- Glycosaminoglycans (GAGs)
- Pretibial myxedema
- Lid retraction
- Exophthalmos
- Subacute thyroiditis
- Hashimoto's thyroiditis

■ SELF-STUDY PROBLEMS

1. Why is hypercholesterolemia common in hypothyroidism?

2. How does hypothyroidism affect the $t_{1/2}$ of administered drugs?
3. What effect would a decrease in TBG's binding affinity for thyroid hormones have on thyroid function?
4. Why do serum T_4 levels approximately double in pregnancy? Are pregnant women hyperthyroid?
5. What effect does T_4 administration have on the size of the thyroid and the secretion of T_4 and TSH in a euthyroid person?

■ BIBLIOGRAPHY

Bahn RS, Heufelder AE: Retroocular fibroblasts: important effector cells in Graves' ophthalmopathy, *Thyroid* 2:89, 1992.

Chin WW: Current concepts of thyroid hormone action: progress notes for the clinician, *Thyroid Today* 15(3), 1992.

Delange F: The disorders induced by iodine deficiency, *Thyroid* 4:107, 1994.

Heufelder AE, Dutton CM, Sarkar G, Donovan KA, Bahn RS: Detection of TSH receptor RNA in cultured fibroblasts from patients with Graves' ophthalmology and pretibial dermopathy, *Thyroid* 3:297, 1993.

Koenig RJ: Thyroid hormone receptor coactivators and corepressors, *Thyroid* 8:703-713, 1998.

Larsen PR, Davies TF, Hay ID: The thyroid gland. In Wilson JD, Foster DW, Kronenberg HM, Larsen PR, et al, editors: *Williams Textbook of endocrinology,* ed 9, Philadelphia, 1998, WB Saunders.

Lazar MA: Thyroid hormone receptors: multiple forms, multiple possibilities, *Endocr Rev* 14:184, 1993.

Ojamaa K, Klemperer JD, Klein I: Acute effects of thyroid hormone on vascular smooth muscle, *Thyroid* 6:505-512, 1996.

Polikar RA, Burger G, Scherrer U, Nicod P: The thyroid and the heart, *Circulation* 87:1435, 1993.

Porterfield SP, Hendrich CE: The role of thyroid hormones in prenatal and neonatal neurological development—current perspectives, *Endocr Rev* 14:94, 1993.

Weintraub BD: Molecular biology of thyroid disease, *Forum* (Endocrine Fellows Foundation): 13, Pfizer, 1992.

Wiersinga WM: Propranolol and thyroid hormone metabolism, *Thyroid* 1:273, 1991.

Appendix

■ LABORATORY DATA ON THYROID FUNCTION

Hormone Production Rates

1. T_4 production is approximately 90 mg/day.
2. T_3 production is approximately 30 mg/day.
3. Normal serum T_4 levels are 5 to 12 mg/dl.
4. Normal serum T_3 levels are 115 to 190 ng/dl.
5. Serum rT_3 levels are approximately 40 ng/dl.
6. $t_{1/2}$ of T_4: 6 to 8 days.
7. $t_{1/2}$ of T_3: 24 hours.

Tests of Thyroid Function (Table 4-2)

Serum T_4 and T_3 Serum T_4 and T_3 are measured by RIA. These tests measure total serum T_4 or T_3 and do not distinguish bound from free hormone.

T_3 Resin Uptake This test provides an index of TBG levels (or available hormone binding sites). To measure this uptake, a tracer quantity of radioactive T_3 is mixed with serum. The radioactive T_3 should distribute itself between the bound and free forms in accordance with the ratio of bound and free forms for the nonradioactive hormone. A synthetic resin that binds free T_3 is then added. The radioactive T_3 (and cold T_3) that was originally in the free form will now bind to the resin. The resin can be precipitated from the serum and the radioactivity counted. If the levels of free T_3 are high in the original serum, the percentage of resin ^{125}I-T_3 uptake will be high. This could result from low levels of TBG or excessively high levels of free T_3. If serum TBG levels increase and free T_3 is normal, the percentage of free T_3 is low and the relative distribution of the radioactive T_3 between the free and the bound phases decreases. This reduces the free ^{125}I-T_3 available to bind the resin. Hence the percentage of resin uptake will decrease. Because the resin uptake basically provides an index of serum binding capacity (predominantly TBG), either T_3 or T_4 can be used. However, because the percentage of free T_3 is higher than the percentage of T_4, the results of the resin uptake tend to be slightly more accurate if ^{125}I-T_3 is used rather than ^{125}I-T_4.

Free T_4/T_3 Index

$$\text{Free } T_4 \text{ index} = [T_4] \times [T_3 \text{ resin uptake}]$$

$$\text{Free } T_3 \text{ index} = [T_3] \times [T_3 \text{ resin uptake}]$$

TABLE 4-2

Serum tests for thyroid evaluation

	T_4	T_3	Resin T_3 uptake	T_4 index	T_3 index	rT_3	TSH
Hyperthyroidism	↑	↑, N	↑	↑, N	↑	↑	↑, ↓, N
Hypothyroidism	↓	↓, N	↓	↓	↓	↓	↑, ↓, N
↑ TBG	↑	↑	↓	N	N	↑	N
↓ TBG	↓	↓	↑	N	N	↓	N

TSH, Thyroid-stimulating hormone; *N,* normal; *TBG,* thyroxine-binding globulin.

TABLE 4-3
Responses to thyrotropin-releasing hormone challenge

	Basal morning TSH	**Response to TRH**
Normal	0.5-4 μU/ml	6-25 μU/ml; peak at 20-30 min
Hyperthyroid	<0.05 μU/ml	No response
Hypothyroidism		
Primary	>4 μU/ml	Increased response
Secondary	Low to normal	No response
Tertiary	Low to normal	Normal or increased response, often delayed (60 min or later)
Nonthyroidal—illness, starvation	Normal to low	Normal to low
Excess glucocorticoids	Low	Decreased response

TSH, Thyroid-stimulating hormone; *TRH,* thyrotropin-releasing hormone.

These are nondimensional numbers that are an indirect approximation of the true free T_4 or T_3 levels.

Radioactive Iodide Uptake (RAIU) Increased

1. The RAIU increases in hyperthyroidism (especially at 4 hours and it is rarely normal at 24 hours).
2. The RAIU increases in iodine deficiency.

Decreased

1. Hypothyroidism
2. After exogenous T_4, T_3 administration
3. Subacute thyroiditis

Thyroid Antibodies Anti-TPO or anti-TG may be elevated in multiple forms of thyroid disease. Very high titers are common for Hashimoto's thyroiditis.

Serum TG These levels increase in disorders involving destruction of the thyroid, such as thyroid carcinoma and Hashimoto's thyroiditis. Serum TG levels increase when thyroid hormone synthesis and secretion increase.

TRH Challenge to TSH Secretion A bolus injection of TRH is given, and the effects on serum TSH levels are measured. Responses are listed in Table 4-3.

CHAPTER 5

Endocrine Pancreas

Objectives

1. Explain the functional and structural relationship between insulin and proinsulin.

2. Describe the interaction of insulin with the insulin receptor.

3. List the major biologic actions of insulin.

4. Identify the major stimuli and inhibitors of insulin secretion.

5. Explain the relationships between the various forms of glucagon.

6. Identify the major stimuli and inhibitors of glucagon secretion.

7. List the major biologic actions of glucagon.

8. Explain the relationship between somatostatin and insulin and glucagon.

9. Distinguish between non-insulin-dependent diabetes mellitus and insulin-dependent diabetes mellitus.

10. Explain the physiologic basis for the major symptoms of diabetes mellitus.

■ ANATOMY

The pancreas is both an exocrine and an endocrine gland. The exocrine portion is important for the production of both bicarbonate and digestive enzymes.

The islets of Langerhans constitute the endocrine portion of the pancreas (Figure 5-1). Although there are thousands of islets, they are a small fraction of the total pancreatic weight. **Glucagon** is produced by the A (alpha) cells of the islets, **insulin** by the B (beta) cells, and **gastrin** and **somatostatin** by the D (delta)

cells. **Pancreatic polypeptide** is produced by the F cells.

Gap junctions are present between the alpha, beta, and delta cells, and the hormones of these cells probably serve a paracrine role in coordinating the functions of the endocrine pancreas. Blood flow through the islets passes from beta cells, which predominate in the center of the islet, to alpha and delta cells, which predominate in the periphery (see Figure 5-1). Consequently, insulin may have a more important direct paracrine role in the regulation of glucagon and so-

85

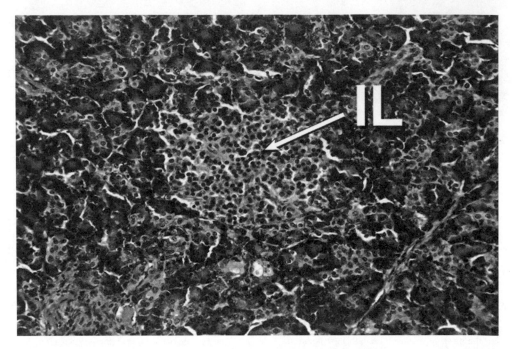

Figure 5-1 ■ Histologic section of rat pancreas. Single islet of Langerhans *(IL)* is surrounded by exocrine pancreas.

matostatin secretion than pancreatic glucagon and somatostatin have on insulin secretion. The F cells are found predominantly in the posterior lobe of the head of the pancreas. This posterior lobe is served by a different vascular supply than the anterior lobe, tail, and body, where most of the alpha, beta, and delta cells are found.

■ INSULIN (Box 5-1)
Structure
Insulin is a protein hormone consisting of two chains, an α chain and a β chain, connected by two disulfide bridges (Figure 5-2). A third disulfide bridge is contained within the α chain. Insulin is synthesized on the polyribosome as pre-proinsulin, and microsomal enzymes cleave the N-signal peptide to produce proinsulin as the peptide enters the endoplasmic reticulum.

> **BOX 5-1**
>
> ### *Overview of Insulin's Actions*
>
> Insulin is an anabolic hormone secreted in times of excess nutrient availability. It allows the body to use carbohydrates as energy sources and store nutrients.

Proinsulin is packaged at the Golgi apparatus into membrane-bound secretory granules. Proinsulin contains the amino acid sequence of insulin plus the 31–amino acid **C (connecting) peptide** and four linking amino acids. The protease that cleaves proinsulin is contained within the secretory granule. On stimulation, the gran-

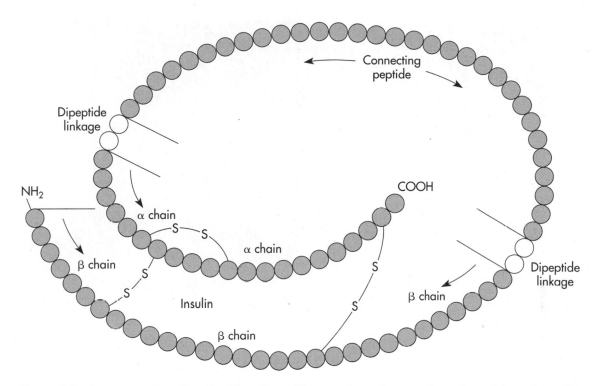

Figure 5-2 ■ Structure of proinsulin. Two dipeptides are cleaved to produce C peptide and insulin. (Modified from Greenspan FS, Strewler GJ, editors: *Basic and clinical endocrinology,* ed 5, Norwalk, Conn, 1997, Appleton & Lange.)

ule's contents are released to the outside of the cell by exocytosis. Release requires a functional microtubular system and is Ca^{2+} dependent. Because the entire contents of the granule are released, equimolar amounts of insulin and C peptide are secreted, as are small amounts of proinsulin. When insulin secretion is rapid, the percentage of proinsulin secreted tends to rise. C peptide has no known biologic activity, and proinsulin has about 7% to 8% the biologic activity of insulin. Measurements of C peptide in the blood are used to quantitate endogenous insulin production in patients receiving exogenous insulin.

Unlike most protein hormones, insulin shows minimal species variability; consequently, bovine and porcine insulin can be used to treat humans. However, antibodies are formed when animal insulins are used for prolonged periods. Recombinant human insulin is now readily available and is generally the treatment of choice.

Insulin has a 5- to 8-minute half-life ($t_{1/2}$) and is cleared rapidly from the circulation. It is degraded by insulinase in the liver, kidney, and other tissues. Because insulin is secreted into the portal vein, it is exposed to liver insulinase before it enters the peripheral circulation; consequently, almost one half of the insulin is degraded before leaving the liver. Thus the peripheral tissues are exposed to only one half the serum concentration as the liver. This produces

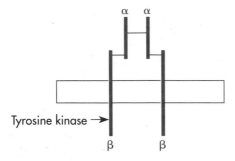

Figure 5-3 ■ **Insulin receptor contains two alpha and two beta subunits.**

problems when diabetic patients are treated with exogenous insulin injected superficially because an adequate dosage for regulating liver metabolism exposes the peripheral tissues to excessive insulin levels.

Receptors

The insulin receptor is a tyrosine kinase–containing receptor. It has two alpha and two beta subunits (Figure 5-3). The alpha subunits are external to the cell membrane and contain the hormone-binding sites. The beta subunits span the membrane and contain tyrosine kinase on the cytosolic surface. Insulin binding to the receptor activates the tyrosine kinase, which then phosphorylates tyrosine residues on the beta subunits. Such autophosphorylation of the beta subunits amplifies and prolongs the signal. Tyrosine kinase also phosphorylates tyrosine residues of cytoplasmic proteins such as the proteins, **insulin receptor substrate 1** and **2 (IRS-1, IRS-2),** which are phosphorylated on tyrosine residues immediately after the cell is stimulated by insulin or IGF-I. These substrates act as intracellular docking proteins for proteins mediating insulin action, such as phosphatidylinositol 3'-kinase. It is not clear whether protein phosphorylation is the primary mechanism for all of insulin's actions. Insulin lowers cyclic

adenosine monophosphate (cAMP) levels in some tissues. Other hormone receptors that regulate tyrosine kinase include the IGF and epidermal growth factor (EGF) receptors.

The insulin-receptor complex can be internalized. This process appears related to insulin degradation rather than to intracellular actions of insulin. Insulin receptors exhibit down regulation when circulating insulin levels are high.

Insulin ultimately stimulates dephosphorylation of many enzymes that play key regulatory roles in intermediary metabolism (Box 5-2).

Control of Secretion

Serum insulin levels normally begin to rise within 10 minutes after food ingestion and reach a peak in 30 to 45 minutes (Figure 5-4). The higher serum insulin level rapidly lowers blood glucose to baseline values.

Fast vs. Slow Insulin Release When insulin secretion is stimulated, insulin is released rapidly (within minutes). If the stimulus is maintained, insulin secretion falls within 10 minutes and then slowly rises over a period of about

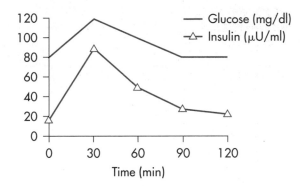

Figure 5-4 ■ Levels of plasma glucose and insulin after meal.

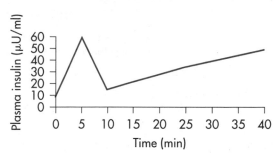

Figure 5-5 ■ Insulin release after perfusion of pancreas with 300 mg/dl glucose.

---

1 hour (Figure 5-5). The latter phase is referred to as the **late phase of insulin release.** The **early phase of insulin release** probably involves release of preformed insulin, whereas the late phase represents the release of newly formed insulin.

Glucose entry into islet cells is facilitated by the GLUT-2 transporter. To stimulate insulin secretion, glucose must be phosphorylated by glucokinase, and insulin secretion is correlated with glucose oxidation. Glucose metabolism increases the intracellular ATP/ADP ratio and closes an ATP-sensitive K^+ channel. The resultant depolarization opens voltage-gated Ca^{2+} channels that activate microtubule-mediated exocytosis of insulin/proinsulin-containing secretory granules.

Regulators of Insulin Secretion Glucose is a major regulator of insulin secretion (Table 5-1). When serum glucose levels rise, insulin secretion is stimulated; when the levels fall, insulin secretion is inhibited. However, there are other stimulators. These include a rise in certain amino acids (arginine and lysine are particularly potent) and serum free fatty acids (FFAs). All of these stimuli are likely to be present immediately after a balanced meal. Other stimuli for insulin secretion include the following gas-

trointestinal hormones: (1) glucagon-like peptide 1, (GLP-1), (2) gastroinhibitory peptide (GIP), (3) gastrin, (4) secretin, and (5) cholecystokinin (CCK). Parasympathetic nervous system stimulation increases insulin secretion, whereas sympathetic nervous system stimulation inhibits it. Somatostatin inhibits both insulin and glucagon secretion.

Actions

Glucose Transport into Cells Glucose transport into cells is in many cases by carrier-mediated facilitated diffusion. Seven glucose transporters have been identified. One of these (**SGLT-1**) is the glucose cotransporter that is involved in the sodium-dependent secondary active transport of glucose by intestinal epithelium and renal tubular cells. The other six are involved in sodium-independent facilitated diffusion of glucose into cells. Several of the major carriers include **GLUT-1** and **GLUT-3,** which seem to be ubiquitous. They mediate basal glucose transport. **GLUT-2** is found in the liver and pancreas and is capable of bidirectional transport, with the direction of transport depending on the relative glucose concentration on each side of the membrane. **GLUT-4** is regulated by insulin. It is present in skeletal muscle, cardiac

TABLE 5-1

Regulators of insulin secretion

Stimulators of insulin secretion	Inhibitors of insulin secretion
↑ Serum glucose	↓ Glucose
↑ Serum amino acids	↓ Amino acids
↑ Serum free fatty acids	↓ Free fatty acids
↑ Serum ketone bodies	
Hormones	Hormones
Gastroinhibitory peptide (GIP)	Somatostatin
Glucagon-like peptide 1 (GLP-1)	Epinephrine (α-receptor)
Gastrin	Leptin
Cholecystokinin (CCK)	
Secretin	
Vasoactive intestinal peptide (VIP)	
Epinephrine (β-receptor)	
Parasympathetic nervous system	Sympathetic nervous system stimulation

muscle, and adipose tissue and may be present in other cell types as well.

A pool of GLUT-4 is available in the cytoplasm of cells that have insulin-sensitive transport systems. Insulin stimulates the transporters to migrate from the cytosol to the cell surface, making them more readily available. It also regulates the synthesis of new transporter. These tissues are said to have **insulin-sensitive transport systems.** Glucose can enter these tissues even without insulin because transporters such as GLUT-1 are present, but the transport rate is inadequate to maintain normal metabolism in the absence of insulin. When insulin is not present, these tissues show changes in intermediary metabolism typical of starvation. Those tissues with insulin-sensitive glucose transport systems are normally responsible for approximately 40% of the body's total glucose metabolism. Skeletal muscle accounts for 80% of insulin-mediated glucose uptake. Glucose transport is the rate-limiting step in glucose use in most tissues.

Insulin does not directly regulate glucose transport into liver cells. The liver has a GLUT-2 transport system that is bidirectional and insulin independent. However, insulin indirectly alters glucose transport because it influences the fate of glucose once it enters the cell; insulin activates glucokinase, the enzyme regulating glucose phosphorylation.

Insulin does not regulate glucose transport into important tissues like the brain—except for the pituitary and regions of the hypothalamus (amygdala, ventrolateral nucleus, ventromedial nucleus)—red blood cells, lens of the eye, mucosa of the small intestine, and renal tubular brush border.

Action on Carbohydrate Metabolism Insulin lowers blood glucose levels because it stimulates glucose transport into tissues with insulin-sensitive transport systems and increases glucose use as an energy source. Insulin is the only major hormone producing hypoglycemia **(hypoglycemic hormone).** Although the IGFs can lower blood glucose, they are not considered physiologic regulators of blood glucose. Many hormones elevate blood glucose **(hyperglycemic hormones).** These include glucagon

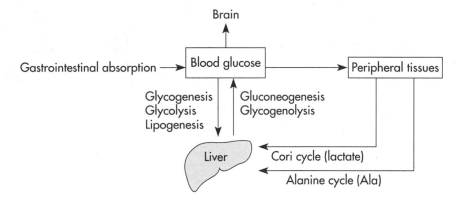

Figure 5-6 ■ Control of blood glucose. The blood glucose level is a function of glucose entering the serum from gastrointestinal absorption and tissue production and of glucose leaving serum because of tissue uptake and metabolism.

and catecholamines (the most important hyperglycemic hormones) as well as cortisol and growth hormone (GH). These hormones are counterregulatory to insulin.

Liver Insulin increases the liver uptake of glucose (unless hypoglycemia is present) by increasing glucokinase activity and thereby increasing glucose phosphorylation. Insulin increases glycolysis as well as the incorporation of glucose into glycogen and synthesis of fatty acids (Box 5-3).

The liver plays an important role in "buffering" blood glucose (Figure 5-6). When blood glucose levels are high, the liver takes up glucose and uses it or stores it as glycogen. When levels are low, the liver releases glucose into serum. This glucose can come from glycogen, from gluconeogenesis, or both. Because insulin increases liver glycolysis and glycogenesis and decreases liver gluconeogenesis and glycogenolysis, it influences the glucoregulatory functions of the liver.

Actions of insulin on the liver's metabolism are shown in Figure 5-7.

Muscle and Adipose Tissue Insulin directly stimulates glucose transport into muscle (Boxes

---

BOX 5-3

Actions of Insulin on Liver

↑ Glucose uptake (if blood glucose level is high)
↑ Glucose use
  ↑ Glycogenesis, ↓ glycogenolysis
  ↑ Glycolysis, ↓ gluconeogenesis
↑ Fatty acid synthesis and very-low-density lipoprotein formation, ↓ ketogenesis
↓ Urea cycle activity

5-4 and 5-5). Most of this glucose is either oxidized or stored as glycogen. Muscle and adipose tissue can be readily converted to fat catabolism for an energy source when blood glucose levels fall. However, the brain requires glucose for energy metabolism and consequently is sensitive to large decreases in blood glucose.

Acute hypoglycemia produces symptoms such as restlessness, irritability, motor incoordination, confusion, tingling sensation, headache, sweating, and even loss of consciousness, coma, and death. When the fall in blood glucose is

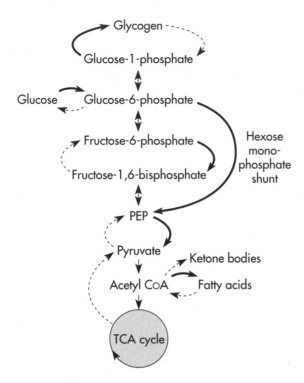

Figure 5-7 ■ **Actions of insulin on liver glucose metabolism.** *Heavy arrows,* Pathways stimulated by insulin. *PEP,* phosphoenolpyruvate; *TCA,* tricarboxylic acid; *Acetyl CoA,* acetyl coenzyme A.

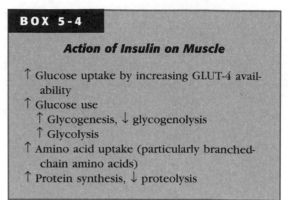

BOX 5-4

Action of Insulin on Muscle

↑ Glucose uptake by increasing GLUT-4 availability
↑ Glucose use
  ↑ Glycogenesis, ↓ glycogenolysis
  ↑ Glycolysis
↑ Amino acid uptake (particularly branched-chain amino acids)
↑ Protein synthesis, ↓ proteolysis

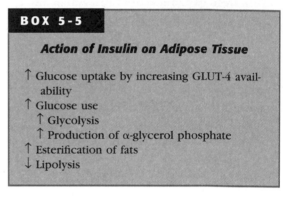

BOX 5-5

Action of Insulin on Adipose Tissue

↑ Glucose uptake by increasing GLUT-4 availability
↑ Glucose use
  ↑ Glycolysis
  ↑ Production of α-glycerol phosphate
↑ Esterification of fats
↓ Lipolysis

gradual, the brain can adapt by using ketone bodies for energy, but this process requires several weeks. Fortunately, tissue response to insulin is such that this hormone (or lack thereof) provides an effective mechanism for channeling glucose away from muscle and adipose tissue, which can readily use fats, to the brain, which has an absolute requirement for glucose. When blood glucose falls and hence insulin secretion falls, the glucose transport via GLUT-4 transporters into muscle and adipose tissue decreases. These tissues have less intracellular glucose, resulting in decreased glycolysis, increased gluconeogenesis, and increased fat mobilization and use for energy. The brain, however, has a transport system that is not insulin dependent. Consequently, as serum insulin levels drop, glucose transport to the brain continues. Thus glucose is preferentially channeled into the brain and away from adipose tissue and muscle.

Because muscle accounts for the largest single portion of the body's metabolism, insulin's action on this tissue has a significant impact on whole-body metabolism. As discussed earlier, if insulin is deficient, plasmalemma GLUT-4 levels drop appreciably because GLUT-4 is internalized. This does not block all glucose transport, but it decreases intracellular levels to the point at which insufficient glucose is available for normal metabolism, and the resulting metabolic changes—decreased glycolysis and increased gluconeogenesis and glycogenolysis—

are characteristic of starvation. Fats, rather than glucose, now provide a greater proportion of the acetyl coenzyme A (acetyl CoA) used for energy production in the tricarboxylic acid (TCA) cycle. When blood glucose levels rise, glucose uptake by muscle rises despite low insulin levels because there is a high glucose gradient for GLUT-1 transport. This transport remains inadequate for normal cellular metabolism.

Exercise increases glucose transport into muscle, even in the absence of insulin. It appears that the decreased tissue oxygen levels directly stimulate GLUT-4 migration to the cell membrane. The effect of exercise on glucose transport is an important consideration for diabetic patients; when they anticipate strenuous exercise, they must lower the insulin dose or consume additional carbohydrates to prevent hypoglycemia.

Actions on Protein Metabolism Insulin stimulates cells to take up amino acids and incorporate them into protein. When amino acids are absorbed in the small intestine, gluconeogenic amino acids such as alanine, glutamine, and glutamate are taken up primarily by the liver, whereas the **branched-chain amino acids** (leucine, isoleucine, valine) are taken up primarily by muscle. Insulin stimulates muscle uptake of these branched-chain amino acids, thereby lowering serum levels. These amino acids are then incorporated into proteins. When insulin levels are low, muscle proteolysis increases. At this time muscle releases the gluconeogenic acids alanine, glutamine, and glutamate in concentrations higher than those found in muscle protein. Obviously, there is considerable muscle protein transamination. Ninety-seven percent of the muscle alanine output has been shown to come from pyruvate and lactate. Glutamine shuttles amine groups to the kidney, and glutamine serves as a substrate for ammonium production. Alanine and glutamate transport amines to the liver for the urea

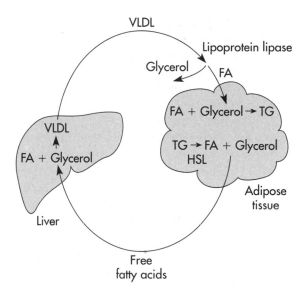

Figure 5-8 ■ **Production and transport of very-low-density lipoprotein** *(VLDL)* **and fatty acid** *(FA)* **between liver and adipose tissue.** *TG*, Triglyceride; *HSL*, **hormone-sensitive lipase.**

cycle and provide important substrates for gluconeogenesis.

Actions on Fat Metabolism In humans, most fatty acid synthesis occurs in the liver. *Lipogenesis is favored when insulin levels are high* because insulin activates pyruvate kinase, pyruvate dehydrogenase, acetyl-CoA carboxylase, and glycerol phosphate acyltransferase. When excess nutrients are available, insulin decreases acetyl CoA entry into the TCA cycle while directing it toward fat synthesis. There is increased substrate flux through the hexosemonophosphate shunt, thereby producing NADPH for lipogenesis. The fatty acids must then be transported to the storage depots (predominantly adipose tissue). These fatty acids are esterified with α-glycerol phosphate in the liver to produce triglycerides and transported, predominantly in the very-low-density lipoprotein (VLDL) fraction, to the adipocyte (Figure 5-8). Insulin increases the level of the enzyme **lipopro-**

tein lipase that is found in the capillary endo-thelium of adipose tissue and many other tissues. This enzyme hydrolyzes triglycerides in VLDLs to monoglycerides and fatty acids. An isomerase allows this reaction to proceed to fatty acids and glycerol. Glycerol does not readily enter the adipocyte, but the membrane-permeable fatty acids do. However, because insulin increases glucose transport into adipose tissue by GLUT-4 transporters, and subsequently increases glycolysis, it increases the production of the α-glycerophosphate needed for fat esterification. Once in the adipocyte (or other cell), the fatty acid is re-esterified with α-glycerophosphate to produce neutral fats (triglycerides). Fats are stored as triglycerides.

Insulin acts on adipocytes to inhibit lipolysis and fat mobilization by inhibiting the enzyme **hormone-sensitive lipase (HSL)** that hydrolyzes neutral fats to fatty acids and glycerol. This enzyme is activated in catabolic states when fat mobilization becomes important.

When insulin is deficient, serum very-low-density lipoprotein (VLDL) levels rise because VLDLs are no longer effectively cleared from serum. Rising serum levels of free fatty acids reflect increased adipocyte lipolysis. Consequently, patients with diabetes mellitus have hyperlipemia. Serum cholesterol (carried predominantly in the low-density lipoprotein [LDL] fraction) is cleared by cellular uptake; this uptake required functional cell surface LDL receptors. In diabetes, LDL receptors decrease, which increases serum LDL levels.

Actions on Potassium Shifts Insulin increases the net movement of potassium into liver and muscle cells, even in the absence of glucose movement or pH changes. This is thought to be a direct action of insulin. Insulin increases Na-K adenosine triphosphatase activity and therefore increases the cell's transmembrane potential. The clinician must remember

---

this action of insulin because, when insulin levels drop in diabetes, there is a net shift of potassium out of the cells and into the extracellular compartment, where it is lost via the kidneys.

■ GLUCAGON (Box 5-6)
Structure

Proglucagon-derived peptides can be found in the brain, pancreas, and gastrointestinal tract (Figure 5-9). Posttranslational processing of proglucagon yields many compounds. The predominant form secreted by the pancreas is a 29–amino acid polypeptide referred to as glucagon. Surprisingly, this hormone has the same structure in all mammals studied except the guinea pig. Other compounds produced from proglucagon include **glicentin, glucagon-related polypeptide (GRPP),** and **glucagon-like peptides 1** and **2 (GLP-1, GLP-2).**

Only about 30% to 40% of the immunoreactive glucagon measured in serum comes from the pancreas; the remainder is from the gastrointestinal tract. Glicentin is the predominant glucagon secreted from the intestine; for this reason it is sometimes referred to as enteroglucagon. This compound is larger and contains within its structure the amino acid sequences of glucagon and glucagon-related polypeptide. Some of the proglucagon-derived peptides stimulate insulin secretion, suppress glucagon secretion, and inhibit gastric secretion.

Preproglucagon

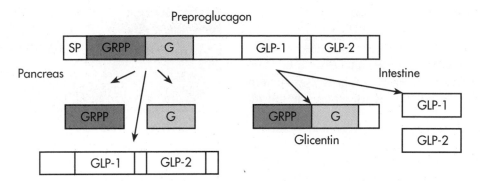

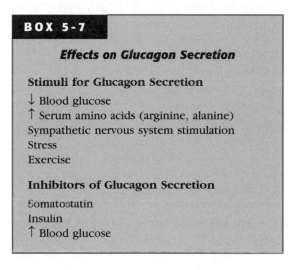

Figure 5-9 ■ **Compounds derived from preproglucagon.** *GLP-1,* Glucagon-like peptide-1; *GLP-2,* glucagon-like peptide-2; *G,* glucagon; *GRPP,* glucagon-related polypeptide; *SP,* signal peptide.

Control of Secretion

The predominant site of glucagon degradation is the liver, which degrades as much as 80% of the circulating glucagon in one pass. Because glucagon (either from the pancreas or the gut) enters the hepatic portal vein and is carried to the liver before reaching the systemic circulation, a large portion of the hormone never reaches the systemic circulation. The liver is the primary target organ of the hormone, and its direct peripheral effects are small. Like insulin, glucagon is carried unbound in serum and has a short t½ (about 6 minutes).

The major stimuli for glucagon secretion are (1) drop in blood glucose, (2) rise in serum amino acids (particularly arginine and alanine), and (3) sympathetic nervous system stimulation. An increase in blood glucose concentration inhibits glucagon secretion, as do somatostatin and insulin (Box 5-7).

Receptors

Glucagon binds to extracellular receptors that have G_s proteins. Consequently, glucagon increases intracellular cAMP levels. The increase in cAMP initiates the cascade of metabolic changes associated with enzyme phosphorylation.

BOX 5-7

Effects on Glucagon Secretion

Stimuli for Glucagon Secretion

↓ Blood glucose
↑ Serum amino acids (arginine, alanine)
Sympathetic nervous system stimulation
Stress
Exercise

Inhibitors of Glucagon Secretion

Somatostatin
Insulin
↑ Blood glucose

Actions

The primary target organ for glucagon is the liver. Glucagon's actions on the liver are antagonistic to those of insulin. Glucagon increases cAMP production and the phosphorylation, and hence activation, of many catabolic enzymes.

Actions on Carbohydrate Metabolism

Liver Glucagon increases liver glucose output. The glucose comes from both glycogenolysis and gluconeogenesis. Liver glycolysis decreases.

Muscle Glucagon does not directly affect skeletal muscle glucose uptake or use. However, glucagon increases serum FFAs, which inhibits glucose uptake and use by muscle and adipose tissue.

Actions on Fat Metabolism

Liver Glucagon increases beta oxidation of fats. When beta oxidation is high, reduced nicotinamide adenine dinucleotide levels (NADH) increase and nicotinamide adenine dinucleotide (NAD) levels drop. The decrease in NAD reduces the ability of acetyl CoA to be oxidized via the TCA cycle. As a result, acetyl CoA levels rise, and ketone body formation increases. This rise in acetyl CoA also suppresses glycolysis. The ketone bodies can serve as a metabolic alternative to glucose in some tissues, including the brain (if sufficient time is allowed). However, if too many ketone bodies are formed, they accumulate and produce ketoacidosis.

Adipose Tissue Glucagon increases adipocyte cAMP, which stimulates HSL and promotes lipolysis and release of fatty acids.

Actions on Protein Metabolism Glucagon increases liver uptake of gluconeogenic precursors such as alanine, glutamate, pyruvate, and lactate. Greater quantities of these gluconeogenic precursors are converted to glucose. Liver urea cycle activity increases, urinary nitrogen excretion increases, and a negative nitrogen balance is produced.

■ SOMATOSTATIN (Box 5-8)

Somatostatin is a 14–amino acid polypeptide (there is also a larger 28–amino acid prohormone) that is produced in the delta cells of the pancreas and in many other locations, including the gastrointestinal tract and the hypothalamus (somatostatin is growth hormone–inhibiting hormone). It serves as part of a complex control

---

> **BOX 5-8**
>
> ### *Overview of Somatostatin's Actions*
>
> Somatostatin has many actions, all of them inhibitory.

---

system for nutrient flux that involves the alpha, beta, and delta cells and gastrointestinal hormones. Somatostatin has a short circulating $t_{1/2}$ (about 2 minutes), and its predominant actions are paracrine in nature.

Control of Secretion

The stimuli for somatostatin release from the gut or pancreas are the same as those for insulin. An increase in serum glucose, serum amino acids, or serum fatty acids is an effective stimulus. In addition, many gastrointestinal hormones such as secretin and CCK stimulate somatostatin release from pancreas and gut.

Actions

Somatostatin acts broadly; its known actions are all inhibitory. Somatostatin decreases gut motility and secretion. It inhibits the release of the hormones gastrin, secretin, CCK, and GIP. It decreases gastric acid and pancreatic exocrine secretion. It decreases gastric emptying, gallbladder contraction, and intestinal absorption of glucose, amino acids, fats, and other nutrients. It decreases splanchnic blood flow. It inhibits pancreatic insulin and glucagon secretion. It may provide a mechanism for regulating gastrointestinal absorption of nutrients to match the efflux of these nutrients to tissues. The exact role of somatostatin in the regulation of islet cell function is not well understood.

Somatostatin analogs have been used pharmacologically for many purposes, including suppressing glucagon secretion in insulin-dependent diabetes mellitus and insulin secre-

TABLE 5-2

Effects of hormones on regulation of islet cell secretion and tissue metabolism

Hormone	Glucagon secretion	Insulin secretion	Muscle glucose uptake	Liver glucose production	Lipolysis
Glucagon		↑	Not directly	↑	↑
Insulin	↓	↓	↑	↓	↓
Catecholamines	↑	↓	↓	↑	↑
Cortisol	↑	Indirectly ↑	↓	↑	↑ (Weak)
Growth hormone		↑	↓	↑	↑

tion from insulinomas, treating acromegaly, reducing gastrointestinal secretion in diarrhea, and reducing blood flow in gastrointestinal bleeding.

The effects of stress hormones on the regulation of islet cell secretion and tissue metabolism are listed in Table 5-2.

■ PANCREATIC POLYPEPTIDE

Pancreatic polypeptide (PP) is a 36–amino acid peptide found in the F cells of the pancreas. Several conditions stimulate secretion of PP: (1) ingestion of a protein-rich meal, (2) hypoglycemia, and (3) strenuous exercise. Some of these effects might be mediated via the vagus nerve. PP inhibits gallbladder contraction and pancreatic exocrine secretion.

■ GASTRIN

A functional role for pancreatic gastrin has not been established, but a pathologic disorder called **Zollinger-Ellison syndrome** is caused by a functional gastrin-secreting tumor, which is typically a pancreatic tumor.

■ SIGNIFICANCE OF INSULIN/GLUCAGON RATIO

The ratio of insulin to glucagon (I/G ratio) may be more important than the levels of the individual hormones. A high I/G ratio produces an anabolic state with more nutrient incorporation into peripheral tissues. A high ratio is associated with low levels of cAMP and a respiratory quotient close to 1 (indicating that carbohydrates are the predominant energy source). When the I/G ratio is low, a catabolic state is produced in which nutrients are mobilized and cAMP levels are high. The normal I/G ratio on a balanced diet is about 2.3, but it can drop to as low as 0.4 within 3 days during starvation. After a high-carbohydrate, low-protein meal, it can rise to as high as 400.

Normally, insulin and glucagon are inversely regulated. However, there is one exception. A diet that is low in carbohydrate but high in protein will simultaneously stimulate the release of both hormones. After this meal, serum amino acid levels rise, but glucose levels do not. If only insulin were secreted, serum glucose would fall excessively. The presence of glucagon prevents the blood glucose from falling excessively, whereas the presence of insulin allows the cells to take up amino acids and synthesize proteins.

■ DIABETES MELLITUS

Diabetes mellitus is a pathologic disorder characterized by an absolute or a relative deficiency of insulin. It is accompanied by an absolute or a relative excess of glucagon. The disorder is a heterogeneous disease with many different forms and probably many causes. The major types are characterized as **insulin-dependent diabetes mellitus (IDDM)** and as **non–insulin-dependent diabetes mellitus (NIDDM).**

Insulin-Dependent Diabetes Mellitus

The characteristics of this disorder are as follows:

1. People with IDDM need exogenous insulin to maintain life and prevent ketosis; there is virtually no pancreatic insulin production.
2. There is histologic damage to the pancreatic beta cells; insulinitis with pancreatic mononuclear cell infiltration is a characteristic feature at the onset of the disorder. Cytokines may be involved in the early destruction of the pancreas.
3. People with IDDM are prone to ketosis.
4. Ninety percent of the cases begin in childhood, mostly between 10 and 14 years of age. This common observation led to application of the term *juvenile diabetes* to the disorder. This term is no longer used because IDDM can present at any time of life, although juvenile onset is the typical pattern.
5. Islet cell autoantibodies are frequently present around the time of onset. People demonstrating autoantibodies only transiently may have virally induced diabetes. Occasionally, antibodies will persist long term, particularly if they are associated with other autoimmune disorders. The persistence of autoantibodies suggests an autoimmune disorder.

Most people with IDDM are classified as having type I diabetes, and many use the two terms synonymously. Type I diabetes is related to problems with the major histocompatibility complex on chromosome 6. *It is correlated with increased frequencies of certain human leukocyte antigen (HLA) alleles.* The HLA types DR3 and DR4 are most commonly associated with diabetes mellitus.

Non–Insulin-Dependent Diabetes Mellitus

This form of the disease is sometimes called type II diabetes. There are many forms of NIDDM, and the distinction between NIDDM and IDDM is not always very clear. The characteristics of this disorder are as follows:

1. Individuals with NIDDM do not need exogenous insulin to maintain life (although insulin may facilitate management for some). The serum insulin levels can be low, normal, or even high. Often there is a decreased sensitivity to insulin.
2. People with NIDDM are not ketosis prone.
3. This disorder is not linked to HLA markers or associated with islet cell antibodies.
4. Of those with NIDDM, 85% are obese, and, as they lose weight, management of the diabetes improves, and the diabetes may even be ameliorated.

There are probably many causes of this form of diabetes. Some people have problems with the control of insulin secretion. Beta cells may respond to hyperglycemia slowly or inappropriately. The early phase of insulin secretion is often seriously impaired. Certain oral medications used to treat this disorder act by stimulating beta cell insulin secretion. Some people with NIDDM are hyperinsulinemic; they commonly show insulin resistance. Obesity can decrease insulin sensitivity.

Diabetes can result from excessive amounts of hormones antagonistic to insulin. These antagonistic hormones include *cortisol, GH, epinephrine, glucagon, oral contraceptives, progesterone, and human placental lactogen (hPL).* A diabetic patient requires more insulin during periods of stress because the **stress hormones** *(cortisol, GH, epinephrine, glucagon)* are elevated. *The diabetogenicity of pregnancy*

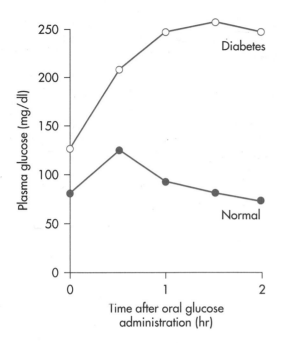

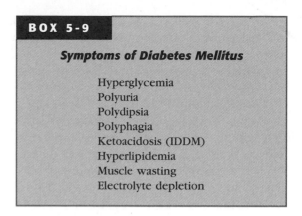

Figure 5-10 ■ Oral glucose tolerance test. Fasting glucose should be less than 115 mg/dl; when measured at 2 hours, level should be less than 140 mg/dl and not greater than 200 mg/dl. If 2-hour measurement plus level at one other measurement exceeds 200 mg/dl, preliminary diagnosis of diabetes is made. (Redrawn from Ganong WF: *Review of medical physiology*, ed 18, Norwalk, Conn, 1997, Appleton & Lange.)

is thought to result from high levels of hPL, estrogen, and progesterone.

In some instances, abnormal forms of insulin are secreted by the beta cells; in other cases, receptor function is compromised. Diabetes can also be caused by a postreceptor defect that decreases insulin response.

Glucose Tolerance Test

The glucose tolerance test is used in the initial screening for diabetes. Ideally, the individual is maintained on a balanced diet for 3 days (this step is often omitted) and must fast overnight before being administered the test. The patient is given a bolus amount of glucose (usually 75 g) orally, and blood glucose levels are measured over time (typically 2 to 4 hours) (Figure 5-10). The glucose is administered orally rather than intravenously (IV) because the insulin response to an oral glucose load is faster and greater than the response to an IV load. When glucose is absorbed in the gut, gastrointestinal hormones that are potent stimulators of insulin secretion are released. These hormones include GIP, GLP-1, glicentin, secretin, CCK, and other gastrointestinal hormones. If the glucose is administered IV, the release of these gastrointestinal hormones is not stimulated. The oral glucose tolerance test result is normal if the fasting glucose level is less than 115 mg/dl, the 2-hour level is below 140 mg/dl, and none of the values exceeds 200 mg/dl. The National Institutes of Health criteria (1979) for the diagnosis of diabetes are (1) fasting (overnight) glucose levels greater than 126 mg/dl on at least two separate occasions and (2) at least two blood glucose measurements equal to or greater than 200 mg/dl, including the 2-hour sample.

Symptoms of Diabetes Mellitus

Box 5-9 lists the symptoms of diabetes mellitus.

Hyperglycemia Hyperglycemia, or high blood glucose concentration, occurs because when the I/G ratio is low, glucose uptake and utilization are decreased, as is liver glucose production.

Diabetes mellitus is characterized by hyperglycemia and the "three polys"—**polyuria, polydipsia,** and **polyphagia.**

Polyuria Polyuria refers to excessive urine production. As serum glucose levels rise, glucose is presented to the renal tubules (filtered load) at a rate that exceeds the glucose tubular maximum (Tm). As the renal threshold is exceeded, glucose begins to appear in the urine (glucosuria) and acts as an osmotic diuretic. Glucosuria generally becomes evident at blood sugar levels between 150 and 200 mg/dl. As dehydration progresses, polyuria eventually leads to hemoconcentration and circulatory failure because of decreased circulating blood volume. Oliguria, or scant urination, results from reduced glomerular filtration because of decreased glomerular hydrostatic pressure.

Polydipsia Polydipsia, or increased thirst, is a result of the dehydration that results from the osmotic diuresis.

Polyphagia Polyphagia, or excessive eating, occurs because the areas of the hypothalamus that regulate appetite (ventrolateral and ventromedial nuclei) have insulin-sensitive transport systems. Consequently, intracellular glucose levels remain low although serum glucose levels are high; intracellular glucose availability is a regulator of appetite and satiety.

Ketoacidosis Many diabetic symptoms resemble those associated with starvation; these symptoms result from the inability of many cells to take up and use glucose appropriately. Ketoacidosis is acidosis caused by excessive ketone body production. It is a symptom of IDDM that results from both low serum insulin levels and high (relative to blood glucose) glucagon levels. These endocrine changes *increase HSL activity,* which mobilizes lipids, and produce an *elevated level of serum FFA.* Liver FFA uptake and beta oxidation increase. The low I/G ratio inhibits glycolysis and hence the production of malonyl CoA, which is the first committed intermediate in fatty acid synthesis. Malonyl CoA is a competitive inhibitor of carnitine palmitoyltransferase I. When malonyl CoA levels drop, carnitine palmitoyltransferase I activity increases. This enzyme transesterifies fatty acyl CoA to fatty acylcarnitine. In this form, it can traverse the inner mitochondrial membrane, thereby becoming accessible to the enzymes for beta oxidation and ketogenesis. The elevated acetyl CoA production accompanied by a decreased TCA cycle activity (the result of NAD depletion) increases ketone body production. Because production exceeds the peripheral use, ketosis, or abnormally high ketone body levels, results. Ketosis is not thought to be a problem in patients with NIDDM because these patients have some insulin. The insulin present is adequate to prevent ketosis but not to maintain normal carbohydrate metabolism.

The high serum ketone body level reduces serum pH (acidosis) because ketone bodies are acidic. In addition, as hypovolemia (low blood volume) leads to circulatory collapse, tissue perfusion decreases. This results in hypoxia (low tissue oxygenation) and subsequent increased lactic acid production. The majority of the metabolic acidosis and the increased anion gap result from high ketone body levels.

Hyperlipemia Hyperlipemia (abnormally high serum lipid levels) is typical of IDDM. VLDL levels rise because of decreased clearance resulting from lower lipoprotein lipase activity. High serum FFA levels reflect the increase in HSL activity and resultant fat mobilization. Insulin deficiency decreases LDL receptor availability, which decreases serum cholesterol clearance. This decreased clearance produces hypercholesterolemia, or high blood cholesterol.

Protein Wasting Net protein loss occurs because insulin is needed for normal amino acid uptake into cells and protein synthesis. Furthermore, because cellular glucose uptake is impaired, proteins are mobilized as an energy source. Serum branched-chain amino acids (leucine, isoleucine, valine) increase because their use in muscle protein synthesis decreases.

Electrolyte Depletion When insulin is deficient, there is a net shift of potassium from the intracellular compartment to the extracellular compartment. This potassium is lost in the urine, so serum potassium levels may appear normal but total body potassium is low. The glucosuria and ketonuria produce diuresis, which results in obligatory loss of many electrolytes. Additional sodium is lost as a result of renal acid secretion and cellular dehydration. Additional phosphate is lost in association with acid excretion and because acidosis lowers the phosphate tubular maximum. Bicarbonate is lost because of acidosis. A physician must be careful when beginning to treat a patient with poorly controlled diabetes. Insulin administered too rapidly and not supplemented with potassium can produce hypokalemia as potassium shifts intracellularly.

Complications of Diabetes Mellitus

Diabetic Ketoacidosis Diabetic ketoacidosis is a serious consequence of poorly controlled IDDM. It is characterized by elevated blood glucose level, ketonemia, increased serum osmolarity (because of the high serum glucose concentration), and elevated stress hormone levels (the counterregulatory hormones to insulin—cortisol, GH, glucagon, epinephrine). These elevated hormones aggravate the metabolic disorder. The patients have acidosis and decreased vascular volume. The neurologic symptoms can include an altered cog-

nitive state, but the patients may not lose consciousness.

Nonketotic Hyperosmolar Coma A nonketotic hyperosmolar coma can occur with either IDDM or NIDDM. People with nonketotic hyperosmolar coma have extremely high serum hyperosmolarity and glucose. When they become dehydrated to the point of oliguria, the last significant route for disposing of excess glucose is lost, so serum glucose levels rise more rapidly. The hyperosmolarity causes cellular dehydration. By definition, ketoacidosis is not present. This type of coma is characterized by extreme dehydration. When ketoacidosis occurs, the patient frequently becomes nauseated, vomits, and exhibits obvious signs of acidosis, such as increased ventilation. Consequently, patients with ketosis frequently receive medical attention sooner than patients without. However, people in nonketotic hyperosmolar coma are likely to have more severe cellular dehydration by the time they receive medical care.

Insulin Shock Administering excessive amounts of insulin can lead to hypoglycemia, which can cause confusion, convulsions, loss of consciousness, and even death.

Long-Term Sequelae of Diabetes Mellitus

Long-term problems associated with diabetes mellitus include neuropathies, nephropathies, microangiopathies, macroangiopathies, and retinopathies.

Neuropathies Peripheral nerve damage (neuropathy) can occur as a result of metabolic or osmotic damage to neurons or Schwann cells. Schwann cells are among those shown to accumulate sorbitol as a result of hyperglycemia. Diabetic patients can exhibit sensory loss, paresthesias, and even pain as a result of the neurologic damage. Neuronal transmission is slowed. The sensory loss is more apparent in the extremities, particularly the lower portions of the legs and feet. This poses particular problems because, as diabetic patients lose cutaneous sensation in the feet, they become unaware of poorly fitting shoes and are more prone to injuries. Poor peripheral circulation aggravates this problem. Because diabetic patients have impaired wound healing, foot ulcerations can become a serious threat.

Nephropathies Diabetes is a common cause of renal failure (nephropathy). The glomerular capillary basement membrane thickens, which is thought to produce glomerulosclerosis and subsequent renal insufficiency.

Microangiopathies Microscopic changes occur in the microcirculation (microangiopathies). Particularly prominent are thickened capillary basement membranes.

Macroangiopathies Atherosclerosis develops in diabetic patients at an accelerated rate (macroangiopathies). Diabetic patients are more likely to have coronary artery disease and myocardial infarction than are nondiabetic individuals.

Retinopathies Retinal abnormalities (retinopathies) develop in diabetic patients and are a major cause of blindness in the United States. The retinal changes are characterized by microaneurysms, increased capillary permeability, small retinal hemorrhages, and excessive microvascular proliferation. Proliferative retinopathy is caused by impaired blood flow to the retina and subsequent tissue hypoxia. Subsequent vascular degeneration can produce vitreal hemorrhage and retinal detachment.

Nonretinal Visual Problems As blood glucose and therefore blood osmolarity rise, the volume of the lens changes, distorting vision. Diabetic patients commonly have cataracts, and sorbitol and glycosylated protein accumulation have been proposed as mechanisms for inducing cataract formation.

• • •

The current thinking is that long-term sequelae develop more slowly with improved diabetes management. However, careful diabetes control does not entirely prevent the development of these secondary problems. There are multiple proposals to explain the tissue damage that occurs in diabetes. One is that tissue damage is due to **nonenzymatic glycosylation of proteins.** When blood glucose becomes high, abnormal protein glycosylations are seen, such as the glycosylation of hemoglobin A to produce **hemoglobin A_{1c} (HbA$_{1c}$),** which is a useful marker for long-term glucose regulation. A red blood cell has a 120-day life span; once glycosylation occurs, the hemoglobin remains glycosylated for the remainder of the red blood cell's life span. The proportion of HbA$_{1c}$ present in a nondiabetic person is low. However, a diabetic patient who has had prolonged periods of hyperglycemia over the last 8 to 12 weeks will have elevated levels. HbA$_{1c}$ measurements are clinically useful for checking treatment compliance. Another check is to measure blood fructosamines. Glucose combines with albumin and other serum proteins to produce **fructosamines.** These levels indicate blood glucose maintenance over a 2- to 3-week period. It has been proposed that tissue damage occurs as a result of protein glycosylation in tissues such as capillary basement membranes. Glycosylation of lens proteins may be involved in diabetic cataract development.

When blood glucose levels rise in diabetes, some tissues produce more **sorbitol.** In these tissues, the enzyme **aldose reductase** converts glucose to sorbitol. Sorbitol is not readily removed from cells. When intracellular glucose, and hence sorbitol, levels rise, intracellular osmolarity also rises. This can lead to tissue swelling, hypoxia, and subsequent tissue damage. Neurons, the kidneys, blood vessels, and the

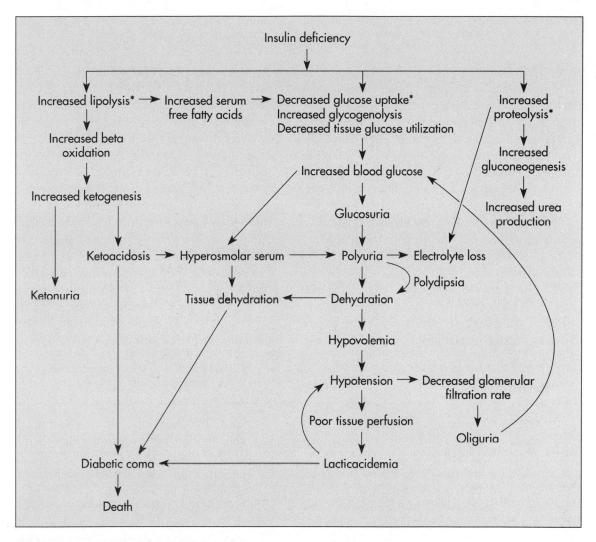

Figure 5-11 ■ **Summary of biologic effects of insulin deficiency.** *Asterisk,* **Point at which elevated stress hormone levels will aggravate problem.**

lenses of the eyes have aldose reductase, and hyperglycemia is thought to produce tissue damage in these tissues as a result of sorbitol accumulation.

The effects of insulin deficiency are summarized in Figure 5-11.

■ ORAL HYPOGLYCEMICS

Because insulin is a protein hormone, it can be given only by injection. No forms of insulin can be given orally because the protein would be hydrolyzed and absorbed as amino acids. The oral medications used to treat diabetes can be used only in patients who have some insulin present.

Sulfonylureas

The sulfonylureas are oral hypoglycemic agents that work by increasing pancreatic insulin secretion. It has also been proposed that they might potentiate the peripheral effects of insulin at the receptor or postreceptor level, but this action has not been conclusively shown in humans in vivo. These drugs include tolbutamide (Orinase), tolazamide (Tolinase), acetohexamide (Dymelor), glyburide (Micronase), glipizide (Glucotrol), and chlorpropamide (Diabinese).

Biguanides

The biguanides do not act on the pancreatic beta cells but rather act to lower blood glucose by decreasing gastrointestinal absorption of glucose and acting on the liver to decrease glucose

output. This group of drugs includes phenformin, buformin, and metformin.

■ PROBLEMS ASSOCIATED WITH DIABETES MANAGEMENT

Sometimes a diabetic patient will awaken in the morning with hyperglycemia, even before eating. One cause of this preprandial hyperglycemia is the *Somogyi effect,* which results from nocturnal hypoglycemia that stimulates secretion of the stress or counterregulatory hormones (glucagon, cortisol, GH, and epinephrine) that act to elevate blood glucose. People with this problem generally need a lower nighttime insulin dose. The *dawn phenomenon* is thought to be a result of sleep-induced GH secretion that antagonizes insulin's effect, thereby producing hyperglycemia. This problem can sometimes be prevented by administering the evening insulin dose at bedtime rather than at dinnertime.

Summary

1. The endocrine pancreas produces the hormones insulin, glucagon, somatostatin, gastrin, and pancreatic polypeptide.
2. Insulin is an anabolic hormone that is secreted in times of excess nutrient availability. It allows the body to use carbohydrates as energy sources and store nutrients.
3. Major stimuli for insulin secretion include increased serum glucose, amino acids, and fatty acids. The GI tract releases many hormones that stimulate pancreatic insulin secretion. Gastroinhibitory peptide (GIP) is a particularly potent stimulator of insulin secretion.
4. Insulin increases liver glucose uptake (unless blood glucose levels are low) and increases glycogenesis, glycolysis, and fatty acid synthesis. It increases muscle glucose uptake, glycogenesis, and glycoly-

sis. It increases muscle amino acid uptake and protein synthesis. Insulin also increases adipocyte glucose uptake and glycolysis, adipocyte fatty acid esterification, lipoprotein lipase activity, and decreases hormone-sensitive lipase (HSL) activity.
5. Glucagon is a catabolic hormone. Its secretion increases during periods of food deprivation, and it acts to mobilize nutrient reserves. It also mobilizes glycogen, fat, and even protein.
6. Glucagon is released in response to decreased serum glucose and increased serum amino acid levels.
7. The primary target organ for glucagon is the liver. Glucagon increases liver glucose output by increasing glycogenolysis and gluconeogenesis. It increases beta oxidation of fatty acids and ketogenesis.

8. Diabetes mellitus is classified as insulin-dependent diabetes mellitus (IDDM) and non–insulin-dependent diabetes mellitus (NIDDM), according to whether the pancreas can or cannot produce insulin.

9. Major symptoms of diabetes mellitus include hyperglycemia, polyuria, polydipsia, polyphagia, muscle wasting, electrolyte depletion, and ketoacidosis (in IDDM).

■ KEY WORDS AND CONCEPTS

- Glucagon
- Insulin
- Gastrin
- Somatostatin
- Pancreatic polypeptide
- Proinsulin
- C (connecting) peptide
- Insulin receptor substrate (IRS-1, IRS-2)
- Late phase of insulin release
- Early phase of insulin release
- SGLT-1
- GLUT-1
- GLUT-3
- GLUT-2
- GLUT-4
- Insulin-sensitive transport systems
- Hypoglycemic hormone
- Hyperglycemic hormones
- Branched-chain amino acids
- Lipoprotein lipase
- Hormone-sensitive lipase (HSL)
- LDL receptors
- Glicentin
- Glucagon-related polypeptide
- Glucagon-like peptide 1 (GLP-1)
- Glucagon-like peptide 2 (GLP-2)
- Zollinger-Ellison syndrome
- Insulin/glucagon (I/G) ratio
- Insulin-dependent diabetes mellitus (IDDM)
- Non–insulin-dependent diabetes mellitus (NIDDM)
- Stress hormones
- Glucose tolerance test
- Polyuria
- Polydipsia
- Polyphagia
- Ketoacidosis
- Hyperlipemia
- Diabetic ketoacidosis
- Nonketotic hyperosmolar coma
- Insulin shock
- Neuropathies
- Nephropathies
- Microangiopathies
- Macroangiopathies
- Retinopathies
- Nonenzymatic glycosylation of proteins
- Hemoglobin A_{1c} (HbA_{1c})
- Fructosamines
- Sorbitol
- Aldose reductase

■ SELF-STUDY PROBLEMS

1. What is the difference between insulin released in the early phase of secretion and that released in the late phase?
2. What is meant by the term *hypoglycemic hormone?*
3. Why do serum concentrations of branched-chain amino acids increase in patients with poorly managed diabetes mellitus?
4. Why do serum lipid concentrations rise in patients with poorly managed diabetes mellitus?
5. What is the basis for ketoacidosis in patients with poorly managed diabetes mellitus?
6. Why is the response to an oral glucose tolerance test more rapid and greater in magnitude than the response to an IV glucose challenge?
7. What happens to serum glucagon levels during a glucose tolerance test?

■ BIBLIOGRAPHY

Abello J, Ye F, Bosshard A, Bernard C, Cuber J, Chayvialle J: Stimulation of glucagon-like peptide-1 secretion by muscarinic agonist in a murine intestinal endocrine cell line, *Endocrinology* 134:2011, 1994.

Baskin DG, Schwartz MW, Sipols AJ, D'Alessio DA, Goldstein BJ, White MF: Insulin receptor substrate-1 (IRS-1) expression in rat brain, *Endocrinology* 134:1952, 1994.

Fehmann H, Goke R, Goke B: Cell and molecular biology of the incretin hormones glucagon-like peptide-I and glucose-dependent insulin releasing polypeptide, *Endocr Rev* 16:390, 1995.

Hofmann CA, Edwards CW III, Hillman RM, Colca JR: Treatment of insulin-resistant mice with the oral antidiabetic agent pioglitazone: evaluation of liver GLUT-2 and phosphoenolpyruvate carboxykinase expression, *Endocrinology* 130:735, 1992.

Howard BV, Howard WJ:Dyslipidemia in non–insulin-dependent diabetes mellitus, *Endocr Rev* 15:263, 1994.

Kono S, Kuzuya H, Yamada K, Yoshimasa Y, Okamoto M, Inoue G, Hayashi T, Suga J, Imura H, Nakao K: A novel substrate for insulin-sensitive serine/threonine kinase in intact cells, *Endocrinology* 135:1529, 1994.

Mitanchez D, Doiron B, Chen R, Kahn: Glucose-stimulated genes and prospects of gene therapy for type I diabetes, *Endocr Rev* 18:520, 1997.

CHAPTER 6

Endocrine Regulation of Calcium and Phosphate Metabolism

Objectives

1. Explain how serum calcium is regulated.

2. Explain how serum phosphate is regulated.

3. Describe the role of osteoblasts, osteocytes, and osteoclasts in bone metabolism.

4. Describe the control of parathyroid hormone secretion.

5. List the major actions of parathyroid hormone on bone, kidney, and gut.

6. Describe the control of calcitonin secretion.

7. List the major actions of calcitonin on bone and kidney.

8. Describe the control of 1,25-dihydroxycholecalciferol (calcitriol) production.

9. List the major actions of calcitriol on bone and gut.

10. Describe the physiologic bases for the pathologic symptoms produced by hyperparathyroidism, hypoparathyroidism, and vitamin D deficiency.

11. Explain the physiologic basis for bone loss in renal failure.

■ CONTROL OF CALCIUM HOMEOSTASIS

Role of Calcium in the Body

Serum calcium levels are tightly regulated. This is important because calcium is critical for many physiologic processes. The following processes depend on calcium:

1. **Neuromuscular excitability.** Normal neuromuscular excitability (membrane stability) depends on appropriate extracellular calcium levels. When extracellular calcium levels fall, membrane permeability increases nonselectively. The increased permeability increases neuromuscular excitability. If serum calcium levels drop too low, spontaneous skeletal muscle contractions (tetany) result.

2. **Secretion.** Calcium is essential for the secretion of many hormones and neurotransmitters. When serum calcium levels drop, both hormone and neurotransmitter secretion is impaired.

3. **Other actions of calcium.** Calcium is essential for **blood clotting** and **excitation-contraction coupling.** It serves as a **second messenger** for the action of many hormones. Excessive levels of calcium cause calcification of soft tissues.

Overview

Serum or extracellular fluid (ECF) calcium levels are a function of the calcium entering serum from gastrointestinal (GI) absorption and the skeleton and the calcium leaving serum to enter bone or be excreted in the urine. Therefore the regulation of serum calcium levels occurs primarily through the GI tract, skeleton, and kidney. Changes in the inflow or outflow from serum that result in changes in serum calcium levels will stimulate changes in the secretion of the regulatory hormones: parathyroid hormone (PTH), calcitonin, and 1,25-dihydroxycholecalciferol (calcitriol).

Serum Calcium Levels (Box 6-1)

Serum calcium levels normally average about 9.5 mg/dl (about 2.5×10^{-3} mol/L). This level normally changes less than 10%. Extracellular fluid (ECF) calcium levels are much higher than intracellular fluid (ICF) levels. The ICF calcium concentration is 10^{-8} to 10^{-7} mol/L. These low intracellular levels are essential for many aspects of cell signalling, including calcium-regulated excitation-contraction coupling and excitation-secretion coupling. Calcium concentrations in intracellular fluid can change rapidly through transmembrane flux and/or release from calcium stores.

Serum calcium is present in both a free and a bound form. Approximately 50% of serum calcium is free, whereas 40% is bound to protein. The remaining 10% is complexed with substances such as citrate. Free calcium is the physiologically active form for the processes listed previously. Changes in serum pH alter the ratio between free and bound calcium. When serum pH rises, calcium binding to protein increases, thereby lowering free serum calcium levels. Consequently, alkalosis increases manifestations of symptoms of neuromuscular hyperexcitability, such as tingling in the extremities or tetany. Pain can stimulate hyperventilation and thereby cause muscle cramping or even tetany.

Serum Calcium Balance

Serum calcium levels depend on the rate of gastrointestinal (GI) calcium absorption, bone demineralization, renal calcium clearance, and bone mineral formation (Figure 6-1).

Input to Serum Calcium The active vitamin D_3 metabolite, **1,25-dihydroxycholecalciferol (calcitriol),** increases GI calcium absorption. In addition, dietary factors decreasing calcium solubility in chyme, such as high dietary phosphate, fat, or oxylate levels, will decrease calcium absorption. Corticosteroids also inhibit GI calcium absorption. *Most calcium absorption occurs in the proximal small intestine,* and absorption efficiency decreases in the more distal portions of the small intestine. Calcium is absorbed by both diffusion and carrier-mediated (calbindin) energy-dependent transport. In normal adults, less than 50% of dietary calcium is absorbed. GI calcium secretion results from secretion of calcium-containing digestive juices. Because this calcium secretion is relatively constant, it is not included in the balance diagram (see Figure 6-1). Calcium is continually exchanged between serum and bone.

Output from Serum Calcium When serum calcium levels are high, calcium tends to leave serum and enter bone. Low serum calcium levels increase calcium flux out of bone. The hormones parathormone (PTH), calcitonin, and calcitriol regulate this flux. The kidney readily filters free, but not protein-bound, serum calcium. Approximately 98% of filtered calcium is normally reabsorbed. *Calcium reabsorption occurs predominantly in the proximal tubule* (about 60%) *and in the loop of Henle* (about 25%). Fine regulation of calcium reabsorption occurs in the distal nephron.

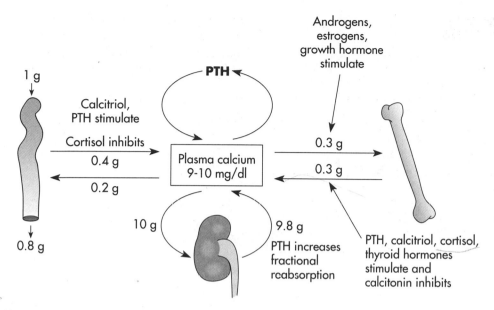

Figure 6-1 ■ Hormonal regulation of calcium balance. Parathormone *(PTH)*, calcitonin, and other hormones regulate plasma calcium levels by controlling GI absorption, renal excretion, and bone calcium flux.

■ CONTROL OF PHOSPHATE (PHOSPHORUS) HOMEOSTASIS

Role of Phosphate (Phosphorus) in the Body

Phosphate is important in all biologic systems. It is a constituent of glycolytic intermediates such as glucose-6-phosphate. Many of the high-energy compounds are phosphorylated. Phosphorylated compounds are important components of all cells. As with calcium, large amounts of phosphate are present in the skeleton, and the skeleton acts as a phosphate reservoir. Phosphate is a major intracellular ion, and intracellular levels are much greater than extracellular levels. Consequently, soft tissues, as well as bone, serve as phosphate reservoirs.

Serum Phosphate (Phosphorus) Levels

Although only 50% of serum calcium is in the free, ionized form and hence biologically active, almost 85% of plasma phosphorus is in the free form. Most serum phosphorus is present as phosphate.* Normal serum inorganic phosphate levels are about 3 to 4 mg/dl. Unlike the tightly regulated serum calcium levels, serum phosphate levels vary widely during the day.

Serum Phosphate Balance

Phosphate enters serum from GI absorption, bone, and soft tissue. It leaves serum from renal excretion, entry into bone, and entry into soft tissue (Figure 6-2).

Input to Serum Phosphate Unlike GI calcium absorption, GI phosphate absorption is relatively efficient. At low levels of GI phosphate, 80% to 90% is absorbed. Consequently,

---

* At physiologic pH, phosphate exists primarily as HPO_4^- and $H_2PO_4^-$. For simplicity, these ions are referred to collectively as phosphate.

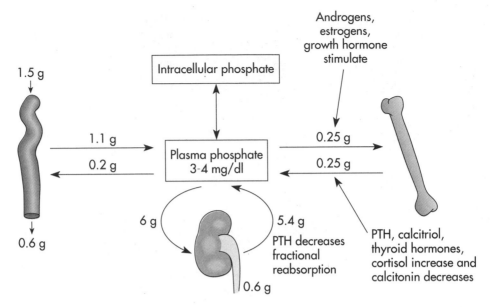

Figure 6-2 ■ Hormonal regulation of phosphate balance. Parathormone *(PTH),* calcitonin, and other hormones regulate plasma phosphate levels by acting on GI phosphate absorption, renal phosphate excretion, and bone mineral flux.

decreased GI phosphate absorption is not typically a cause of hypophosphatemia. Bone and soft tissues also serve as sources for serum phosphate, and phosphate from these tissues is readily exchanged with phosphate in serum.

Output from Serum Phosphate Inorganic phosphate is freely filtered by the kidney, and approximately 90% is reabsorbed. The bulk of reabsorption is in the proximal tubule. It is tubular maximum (Tm) regulated and the Tm value is close to that of the filtered load. Consequently, the urinary phosphate excretion can be regulated by changing the Tm or changing the filtered load. PTH decreases the Tm in the proximal tubule and therefore increases phosphate excretion in the urine. Factors increasing the filtered load will also increase renal phosphate excretion. For example, in soft tissue damage, intracellular phosphate is released into serum, which increases serum phosphate levels. This

increases the filtered load and thereby increases renal phosphate excretion.

Consequences of Severe Hypophosphatemia

When serum phosphate levels are low, nerve conductance decreases and bone mineralization is defective. In addition, hemolytic anemia can occur because red blood cell adenosine triphosphate decreases.

■ BONE

Bone is composed of an organic matrix (**osteoid**) impregnated with mineral salts (Figure 6-3). The predominant component of the organic matrix is collagen. It is a highly vascular tissue that receives approximately 10% of the cardiac output. Bone is a dynamic structure that is remodeled throughout life. Changes in total bone mass depend on the relative balance be-

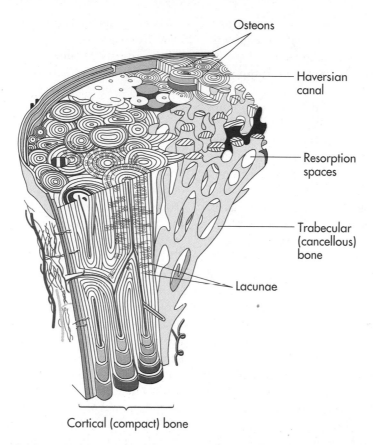

Osteons

Haversian
canal

Resorption
spaces

Trabecular
(cancellous)
bone

Lacunae

Cortical (compact) bone

Figure 6-3 ■ Some of primary features of microstructure of mature bone, shown in both transverse section *(top)* and longitudinal section. Areas of cortical (compact) and trabecular (cancellous) bone are indicated. Note general construction of osteons, distribution of osteocyte lacunae, Haversian canals, resorption spaces, and different views of structural basis of bone lamellation. (Redrawn from Warwick R, Williams PL: *Gray's anatomy,* ed 35 [British edition], Philadelphia, 1973, WB Saunders.)

tween bone formation (accretion) and breakdown (resorption). Bone resorption results from bone matrix degradation and dissolution of bone minerals. Bone accretion entails the synthesis of the organic matrix and the subsequent deposition of minerals in this matrix. Until early in the second decade of life, bone accretion exceeds resorption and bone mass increases. After the bone mass remains relatively stable for a decade, at about age 30 years, resorption begins to

exceed accretion, and bone mass progressively decreases thereafter. Bone loss accelerates in women after menopause. The structural function of bone is obvious; however, bone also plays a major role in the regulation of ECF calcium, phosphate, and magnesium homeostasis. Large quantities of these minerals are stored in bone. Other minerals, such as fluoride and lead, are also stored in bone, as are some drugs such as tetracycline. In addition, bone matrix is a source of numerous growth factors that are synthesized in the bone cells. Many of these growth regulators are hormonally regulated and are involved in the control of bone resorption and accretion.

Bone osteoid is produced by bone-forming cells called **osteoblasts.** These cells are derived from mesenchymal stem cells called **osteoprogenitor cells.** Osteoblasts synthesize the organic matrix. They are characterized by having receptors for the hormones PTH and calcitriol and by having the ability to synthesize matrix proteins such as **collagen** and **osteocalcin.** Once the matrix is synthesized by the osteoblast, it is calcified. The osteoblast creates an environment conducive to mineralization. The osteoblast produces **alkaline phosphatase,** which hydrolyzes phosphate esters and hence locally raises phosphate levels. As local phosphate concentrations increase, the tendency of calcium-phosphate salts to precipitate increases. Serum alkaline phosphatase and osteocalcin are used as markers for osteoblastic activity.

Bone mineral is composed predominantly of **hydroxyapatite** $(Ca_{10}[PO_4]_6[OH]_2)$. Other minerals, particularly magnesium, contaminate the hydroxyapatite. The minerals in bone are continually exchanged with minerals in ECFs, and a dynamic equilibrium exists between bone and ECF calcium and phosphate. Although this exchange can occur in the absence of PTH, vitamin D, and calcitonin, these hormones influence this flux.

Osteoblasts that become entrapped in the bone matrix become **osteocytes.** These osteocytes are found within **lacunae** and are interconnected with one another through processes that extend through the interconnecting channels, called **canaliculi,** that run between lacunae. There are gap junctions between these cells. These cells play a major role in regulating the flux of minerals in and out of the adjacent bone matrix.

Osteoclasts are large, multinucleate cells derived from hematopoietic stem cells similar to monocytes. They are located external to the bone-lining layer of surface osteoblasts.

Bone resorption takes place as osteoclasts penetrate the bone lining and attach to bone matrix. When these cells are stimulated, they develop characteristic changes in a portion of the cell membrane referred to as the ruffled border. Bone is resorbed under the ruffled border, forming scalloped-appearing surfaces called **Howship's lacunae.** Osteoclasts phagocytose the matrix and, as a result both of a proton pump and the presence of carbonic anhydrase at the ruffled border, produce an acid environment in the Howship's lacunae. This lower pH increases hydroxyapatite solubility and hence promotes bone mineral dissolution. Mature osteoclasts lack receptors for PTH and calcitriol but have calcitonin receptors. PTH is thought to stimulate osteoclastic bone resorption by acting on osteoblasts to promote the formation of osteoclast-activating factors such as the cytokines interleukin-1 (IL-1), tumor necrosis factor (TNF-α and TNF-β), and interferon-γ.

Bone remodeling continues throughout life. It has been estimated that as much as 18% of the adult skeleton may turn over in a year. Actively forming bone surfaces are covered with osteoblasts, whereas resorption areas contain numerous osteoclasts. Bone resorption is closely linked with bone accretion, so that as bone is resorbed, new bone formation, and hence remodeling, is stimulated. These processes are thought to be linked through local production of osteoclast-activating factors.

Bone Fluid

Bone fluid is found in the lacunae and canaliculi. Its ionic composition differs from that of ECF. Bone fluid is separated from ECF by a layer of bone-lining cells (surface osteoblasts) (Figure 6-4). This layer of bone cells plays an active role

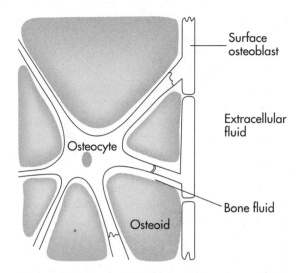

Figure 6-4 ■ Bone fluid. Surface osteoblasts regulate calcium flux between bone fluid and extracellular fluid (*ECF*). Calcium passively enters bone fluid by diffusing from ECF or from osteoid exchange. Calcium from bone fluid is taken up by osteocytes and transported through processes to surface osteoblasts, where it can be actively transported to ECF.

in determining the level of calcium flux between bone fluid and ECF. These cells have processes that connect with osteocytes. Calcium levels in bone fluid are approximately one third those in ECF. Therefore there is a concentration gradient for calcium to enter bone. Surface osteoblasts control bone fluid calcium levels by actively pumping calcium out of the cell and into the ECF.

The mineral exchange is between bone salts and bone fluid. The large aggregate surface area of the lacunae and canaliculi provides a sizable surface for mineral exchange. Osteocytes influence the equilibrium between bone minerals and bone fluid minerals by two mechanisms. First, they produce acids and therefore decrease the pH of the surrounding bone fluid. This pH drop at the bone–bone fluid interface increases bone salt solubility, thereby promoting dissolu-

tion of bone mineral. Second, on PTH stimulation, calcium influx increases, which serves to locally lower bone fluid calcium concentrations.

■ MAJOR GROWTH FACTORS IN BONE
Fibroblast Growth Factors

Fibroblast growth factors (FGFs) are polypeptide mitogens that are synthesized in many tissues, including bone. They stimulate bone-cell proliferation and collagen synthesis.

Insulin-like Growth Factors

Insulin-like growth factors (IGFs) are mitogenic polypeptides that resemble insulin in structure and function. These compounds are present in bone matrix. They stimulate bone and cartilage growth and increase osteoblast proliferation, collagen deposition, and bone mineralization. Although their synthesis can be regulated by growth hormone, there are other factors, including insulin, that control their production. Many hormones, such as estrogens and PTH, known to act on bone have been shown to increase synthesis of bone IGFs. IGFs were once called sulfation factors because they increased incorporation of sulfate into collagen in vitro.

Transforming Growth Factors

Transforming growth factors (TGFs) are polypeptides found in both normal and neoplastic tissues. TGF-α is a relatively small growth factor that shares homology with epidermal growth factor (EGF). TGF-βs are larger compounds and resemble platelet-derived growth factor (PDGF). Both groups of compounds stimulate bone resorption. They may be important in linking bone formation with resorption.

Cytokines

Cytokines are compounds synthesized from mononuclear or lymphocytic cells, although these are not the only sites of synthesis. The cytokines IL-1, TNF-α, TNF-β, colony-stimulating factor, and interferon-γ are known to have effects on bone remodeling.

■ PARATHYROID HORMONE

Structure

The primary parathyroid hormone **(PTH, parathormone)** secreted is an 84–amino acid protein. It is secreted by the chief cells of the gland. It is originally synthesized as **preproparathyroid hormone,** which is cleaved to **proparathyroid hormone** on entry into the endoplasmic reticulum. Typical of protein hormones, there is considerable species variation. Consequently, PTH obtained from species such as cattle is not suitable for long-term use in humans because of antibody formation. Ninety percent of circulating PTH is degraded in the liver and kidney, and the circulating half-life (t½) is short.

Control of Secretion

A drop in serum calcium concentration stimulates the secretion of PTH (Figure 6-5), and this effect is mediated through calcium-sensing receptors. Although a rise in serum calcium decreases PTH secretion, secretion is not abolished at high calcium levels, thereby producing a sigmoidal relationship between serum calcium

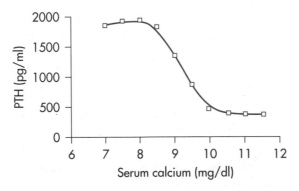

Figure 6-5 ■ Relationship between serum calcium and parathormone *(PTH).* (Redrawn from Felsenfeld AJ, Llach F: *Kidney Int* 43:771, 1993).

and serum PTH levels (see Figure 6-5). An increase in serum phosphate indirectly stimulates PTH secretion by decreasing serum calcium. Magnesium has the same action on PTH secretion but it is one half as potent. Paradoxically, magnesium is necessary for parathyroid function, and consequently severe hypomagnesemia impairs PTH secretion.

Actions

Actions on Bone [PTH directly increases bone resorption and calcium mobilization from bone. Its administration indirectly increases the number and activity of osteoclasts and increases osteoclastic bone dissolution. In addition, it increases bone remodeling. When bone resorption increases, bone formation secondarily increases because these two processes are normally closely coupled. Although PTH receptors have been demonstrated on osteoblasts, most investigators have not been able to show their presence on mature osteoclasts. [However, the hormone alters osteoclastic function both by increasing the quantity of osteoclasts indirectly by stimulating differentiation of osteoclast precursors into osteoclasts and by stimulating the release of cytokines from osteoblasts that act to increase osteoclastic activity.]

[PTH increases osteoblast and osteocyte calcium permeability, resulting in increased calcium flux from bone fluid into the cells. Calcium may be transported across gap junctions from osteocytes to surface osteoblasts. PTH stimulates active calcium transport out of surface osteoblasts and into ECFs. These processes decrease bone fluid calcium concentration and increase ECF calcium concentration. As the calcium concentration in the fluid immediately bathing bone minerals (bone fluid) decreases, the equilibrium between calcium in bone mineral and calcium in bone fluid shifts so that it favors bone demineralization.] Although passive exchange of calcium between bone minerals and bone fluid occurs continually, PTH, by stimulating calcium pumping from bone fluid into ECF, shifts this equilibrium toward bone demineralization. This process, termed **osteocytic osteolysis,** decreases bone mineral but does not destroy osteoid (Figure 6-6).

In the absence of PTH, serum calcium drops to approximately 7 mg/dl, a level that is below the threshold for tetany in humans. However, a new equilibrium is established between bone and serum calcium. PTH increases the set-point

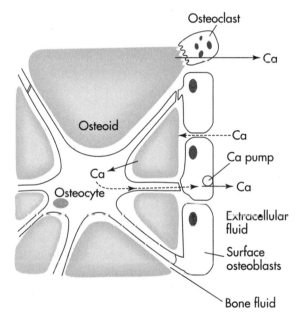

Figure 6-6 ■ Osteocytic osteolysis. PTH opens calcium channels in osteocytes and surface osteoblasts so that calcium *(Ca)* flux from bone fluid into these bone cells increases. This lowers concentration of calcium in bone fluid, thereby favoring demineralization of bone. Calcium entering osteocytes is transferred to osteoblasts through long cytoplasmic processes extending through lacunae that form gap junctions with surface osteoblasts. As calcium is pumped out of surface osteoblasts into ECF, the gradient for calcium flux into bone cells is maintained.

for this equilibrium so that serum calcium is higher and bone calcium is lower.

Actions on Kidney PTH increases calcium reabsorption in the thick ascending loop of Henle. The bulk of calcium reabsorption occurs in the proximal tubule; this is not regulated by PTH. However, because the kidneys filter and reabsorb a sizable amount of calcium in a day, regulation of even a relatively small percentage can have major effects. PTH regulates approximately 10% of calcium reabsorption. However, because PTH increases serum calcium, the filtered load for calcium increases. Although this hormone increases fractional reabsorption of calcium, urinary calcium typically increases because of the greater filtered load. Although PTH acts through multiple mechanisms, the renal action of PTH is predominantly mediated through cyclic adenosine monophosphate (cAMP), and an increase in urinary cAMP is evident after PTH administration.

Renal Actions on Phosphate Reabsorption PTH lowers the Tm for phosphate reabsorption in the proximal tubule (Figure 6-7). The Tm decrease lowers the fractional reabsorption of phosphate and therefore produces phosphaturia. This action is so potent that when PTH is given, which increases the flux of phosphate from bone to serum and increases GI absorption of phosphate, serum phosphate usually drops because of the increased renal phosphate excretion.

Renal Actions on Bicarbonate Reabsorption PTH decreases renal bicarbonate reabsorption. Because renal bicarbonate reabsorption and chloride reabsorption tend to be inversely related, PTH increases serum chloride concentrations. Consequently, excess PTH produces hyperchloremic acidosis. The acidosis aids in bone demineralization.

Gastrointestinal Absorption PTH stimulates renal 1α-hydroxylase and therefore increases vitamin D_3 activation to calcitriol. Calcit-

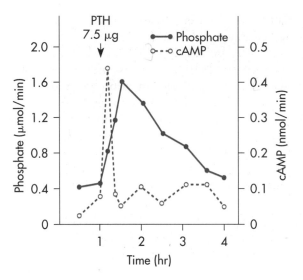

Figure 6-7 ▪ Effect of parathormone *(PTH)* on excretion of phosphate and cyclic adenosine monophosphate *(cAMP)* in a parathyroidecto-mized rat. PTH was given at time indicated by *arrow*. Note that cAMP excretion preceded phosphate excretion and how quickly both substances appeared in urine. Note also that phosphate excretion is given in units of micromoles (10^{-6} mol), whereas cAMP is in nanomoles (10^{-9} mol). (Redrawn from Chase LR, Auerbach GD: *Proc Natl Acad Sci USA* 58:518, 1967.)

riol increases GI calcium and phosphate absorption.

▪ CALCITONIN

Structure

Calcitonin is a 32–amino acid polypeptide produced by the thyroid parafollicular cells (Figure 6-8). Because there is minimal species variation, calcitonin from other species is biologically active in humans. In fact, salmon calcitonin is about 20 times more potent in humans than human calcitonin and can therefore be used to decrease bone turnover in high-turnover bone disorders such as **Paget's disease.** Normal serum calcitonin levels are about 10 to 50 pg/ml, and

its $t_{1/2}$ in circulation is less than 1 hour. Because the primary site of inactivation is the kidney, serum calcitonin levels are often elevated in renal failure. Alternative splicing of the calcitonin gene in other tissues can produce calcitonin gene-related peptide (CGRP), which is a potent vasodilator and positive cardiac inotrope.

Actions

The primary actions of calcitonin are on bone and kidney. Calcitonin lowers serum calcium and phosphate levels, primarily by inhibiting bone resorption, in many species of animals. However, although it can lower serum calcium and phosphate levels in humans, it takes high doses to show this effect. There are no definitive complications from calcitonin deficiency or excess in humans. For this reason, some have questioned the physiologic role for calcitonin in humans. Medical interest in calcitonin is primarily because potent forms of calcitonin can be used therapeutically in the treatment of high-turnover bone disorders.

Actions on Bone Calcitonin inhibits osteoclastic bone resorption. The hormone decreases osteoclastic differentiation from precursor cells and decreases the activity of existing osteoclasts. Osteoclasts have calcitonin receptors, and the action of calcitonin on these cells is mediated by cAMP. Calcitonin does not have direct actions on bone formation.

Actions on Kidney Calcitonin increases renal clearance of both calcium and phosphate. These actions on the kidney are transient and probably are not physiologically significant.

Control of Secretion

An increase in serum calcium concentration stimulates calcitonin secretion. Many GI hormones such as gastrin, glicentin, secretin, and cholecystokinin-pancreozymin also stimulate its release. This has led to the suggestion that the primary role of calcitonin in humans is to

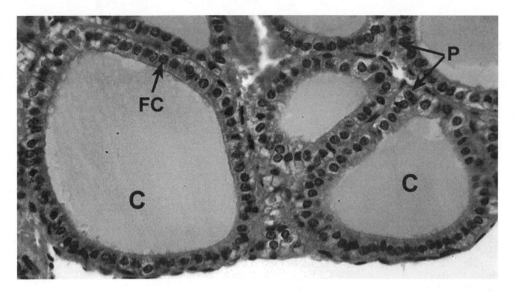

Figure 6-8 ■ Histologic view of thyroid gland of rat. Parafollicular *(P)* cells are indicated in the walls of follicles. *FC,* follicular cell. *C,* colloid.

increase calcium deposition in bone when serum calcium levels rise postprandially. Calcitonin is degraded primarily in the kidneys; its t½ is less than 10 minutes.

■ VITAMIN D

Structure, Synthesis, and Control of Secretion

Vitamin D_3 (cholecalciferol) can be obtained through both diet and synthesis in the skin in the presence of sunlight from the cholesterol derivative **7-dehydrocholesterol** (Figure 6-9). Vitamin D_3 is a **secosteroid,** which means it is a steroid in which one of the rings has been opened. Vitamin D_3 is not the active form. It must be 25-hydroxylated in the liver to 25-hydroxycholecalciferol and then 1α-hydroxylated by the proximal tubules of the kidney to the most active form, 1,25-dihydroxycholecalciferol (calcitriol). Both serum PTH and serum phosphate directly regulate **1α-hydroxylase** activity. PTH stimulates synthesis of the enzyme in

the kidney and thereby regulates calcitriol production. A decrease in serum phosphate stimulates enzymatic activation. A decrease in serum calcium can indirectly stimulate 1α-hydroxylase activity because hypocalcemia increases PTH secretion. Although the kidney also has a 24α-hydroxylase that converts 25-hydroxycholecalciferol ($25\text{-}[OH]_2D_3$) to 24,25-dihydroxycholecalciferol ($24,25\text{-}[OH]_2D_3$) or 1,25-dihydroxycholecalciferol ($1,25\text{-}[OH]_2D_3$) to 1,24,25-trihydroxycholecalciferol ($1,24,25\text{-}[OH]_3D_3$), these compounds are less potent and their specific physiologic functions remain to be defined. Other factors that enhance $1,25\text{-}(OH)_2D_3$ production include estrogen, growth hormone, and prolactin.

Calcitriol is only sparingly soluble in blood and hence is transported bound (>99% bound) to the plasma protein **transcalciferin.** Because of the protein binding, the hormone has a long circulating t½. Its t½ has been variously reported to be between 5 and 24 hours.

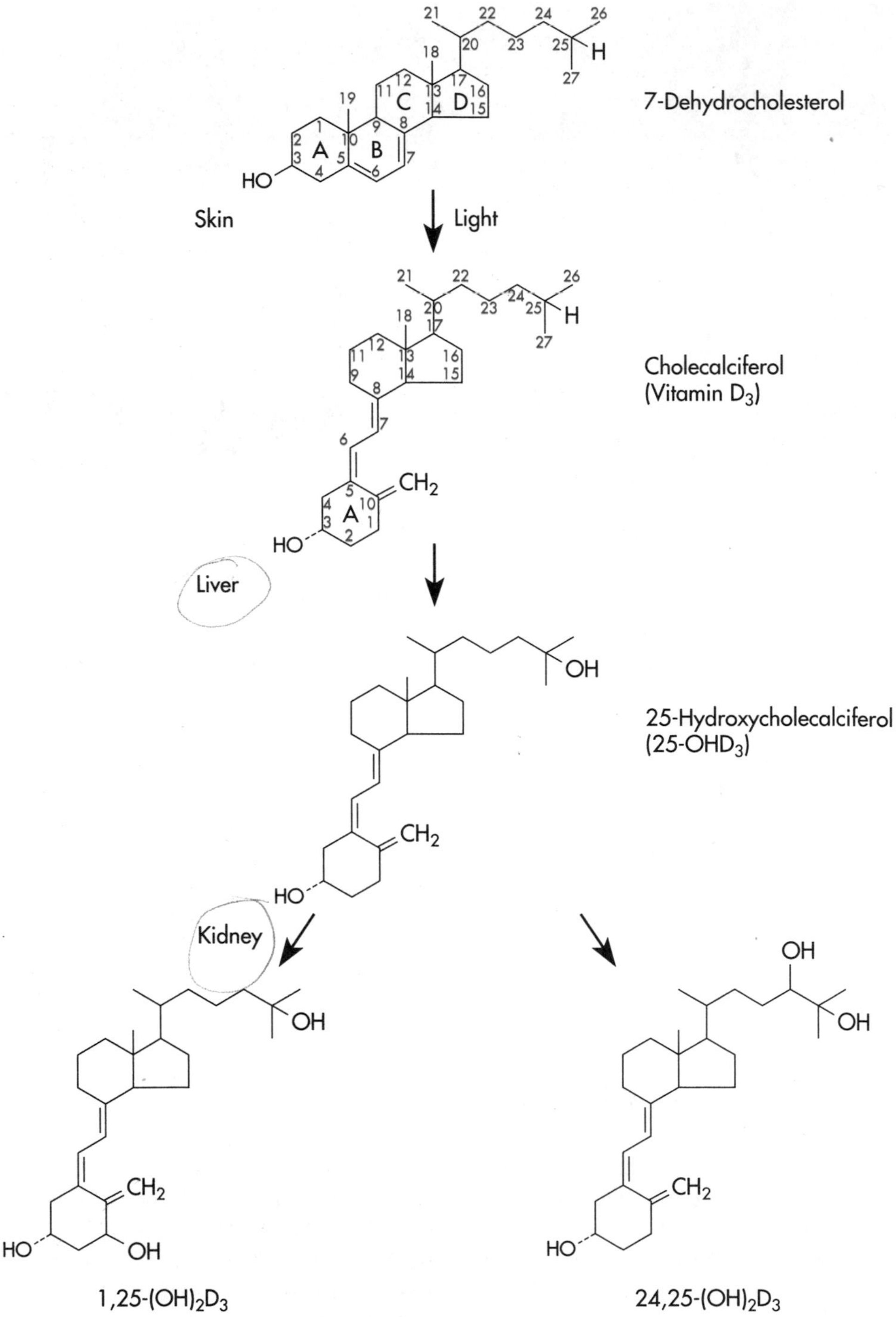

7-Dehydrocholesterol

Skin   Light

Cholecalciferol
(Vitamin D$_3$)

Liver

25-Hydroxycholecalciferol
(25-OHD$_3$)

Kidney

1,25-(OH)$_2$D$_3$ 24,25-(OH)$_2$D$_3$

Figure 6-9 ■ Biosynthesis of 1,25-dihydroxycholecalciferol.

Actions

The primary role of calcitriol is to increase serum calcium (and phosphate) levels and hence make conditions favorable for bone mineralization. Calcitriol accomplishes this primarily through its potent actions to increase GI calcium (and phosphate) absorption. The primary target organs for vitamin D in the regulation of calcium-phosphate balance are the gut and bone. The actions on the kidney are minimal. Vitamin D receptors have been found in tissues other than bone, gut, and kidney, which suggests that it may have actions on other tissues.

Calcitriol may play a role in muscle function, hematopoietic-lymphoreticular function, and tumor development or suppression. Many tumor cell lines have calcitriol receptors. Calcitriol inhibits cellular proliferation in some tumors and in psoriasis.

Serum calcitriol levels increase in pregnancy, leading to a concomitant increase in the efficiency of GI calcium absorption.

Figure 6-10 shows the response of the PTH-calciferol axis to mithramycin-induced hypocalcemia. Table 6-1 summarizes the actions of the calcium regulatory hormones.

Actions on Gastrointestinal System Calcitriol increases the fractional absorption of calcium and, to a lesser extent, phosphate and magnesium. The intestinal mucosal epithelium contains a calcium-binding protein called **calbindin** that facilitates calcium, magnesium, and phosphate transport from the mucosal surface to the serosal surface. Synthesis of this transport protein is regulated by calcitriol. If vitamin D (calcitriol) is deficient, GI calcium and phosphate absorption are impaired, which prevents normal bone mineralization.

Actions on Bone Calcitriol synergizes with PTH on bone and therefore increases osteoclastic activity and bone turnover. PTH has little effect on bone in the absence of vitamin D. Although calcitriol stimulates bone turnover, it is

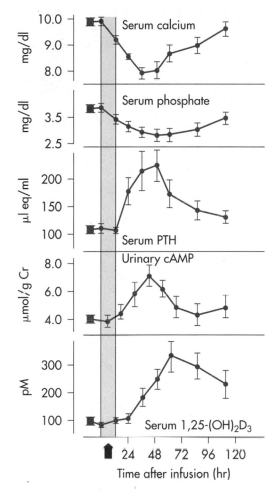

Figure 6-10 ■ Response of parathormone-calciferol axis to hypocalcemia. **Eight patients with Paget's disease received mithramycin (25 μg/kg) by infusion *(shaded band)*. Note that response of serum 1,25-(OH)$_2$D$_3$ lags 12 to 24 hours behind changes in serum parathormone *(PTH)* and urinary cyclic adenosine monophosphate *(cAMP)*.** (Redrawn from Bilezikian JP, et al: *N Engl J Med* 299:437, 1978.)

essential for normal bone mineralization because it provides for adequate GI absorption of calcium and phosphate and therefore ultimately provides the high bone fluid calcium and phosphate concentrations necessary for bone mineralization.

TABLE 6-1			
Actions of calcium regulatory hormones			
	Bone	**Kidney**	**GI tract**
PTH	Increases bone resorption and osteocytic osteolysis	Increases renal calcium reabsorption; lowers Tm for phosphate reabsorption; increases renal conversion of 25-(OH)D$_3$ to 1,25-(OH)$_2$D$_3$	No direct action; stimulates activation of vitamin D$_3$, which stimulates calcium and phosphate absorption
Calcitonin	Decreases bone resorption	Decreases calcium and phosphate reabsorption	No direct action
Vitamin D	Synergizes with PTH on bone; stimulates calcium pump on ECF interface of surface osteoblasts	Minimal renal actions; renal actions appear to increase calcium reabsorption	Increases GI calcium and phosphate absorption

GI, Gastrointestinal; *PTH,* parathormone; *Tm,* tubular maximum; *ECF,* extracellular fluid.

Vitamin D deficiency states result in impaired bone mineralization. In children this is seen as **rickets** and in adults it is seen as **osteomalacia.**

Actions on Renal System As it does in the gut, active vitamin D stimulates renal calcium-binding protein (calbindin) synthesis, which facilitates renal calcium reabsorption.

■ ACTIONS OF OTHER HORMONES ON BONE

Estrogens

There are estrogen receptors on osteoblasts, and estrogens may have direct stimulatory effects on osteoblastic function. Shortly after the onset of menopause, estrogen administration decreases urinary hydroxyproline levels and decreases the deficit between bone formation and bone loss. At this time, the hormone is not thought to be capable of stimulating net bone formation; rather it acts to decrease the rate of bone loss. Androgens can have the same effect as estrogens on bone.

Glucocorticoids

Glucocorticoids directly decrease the active component of GI calcium absorption. In addition, glucocorticoid administration in humans increases urinary calcium excretion. Glucocorticoids act on the kidney to decrease fractional reabsorption of calcium. Both of these actions of cortisol lower blood calcium, which produces mild secondary hyperparathyroidism. In addition, glucocorticoids act through glucocorticoid receptors on osteoblasts to depress osteoblastic bone formation. This is reflected in a decrease in synthesis of collagen and the bone protein osteocalcin. Glucocorticoid excess can produce osteoporosis.

Thyroid Hormones

Excessive levels of thyroid hormones can produce osteoporosis; this effect is thought to be mediated by a direct action stimulating bone turnover. Mildly elevated serum calcium levels are common in hyperthyroid patients because of this high bone turnover. Bone resorption tends to exceed accretion.

■ PATHOLOGIC DISORDERS OF CALCIUM AND PHOSPHATE BALANCE

Hyperparathyroidism (Primary)

Patients with primary hyperparathyroidism have high serum calcium levels and, in most cases, low serum phosphate levels. Hypercalcemia is a result of bone demineralization, increased GI calcium absorption (mediated by calcitriol), and increased renal calcium reabsorption. The major symptoms of the disorder are directly related to increased bone resorption, hypercalcemia, and hypercalciuria (Figure 6-11). High serum calcium levels decrease neuromuscular excitability. People with hyperparathyroidism often show psychologic disorders, particularly depression, that may be associated with increased serum calcium levels (Box 6-2). Other neurologic symptoms include fatigue, mental confusion, and, at very high levels (greater than 15 mg/dl), coma. Hypercalcemia can cause cardiac arrest. Kidney stones (nephrolithiasis) are common because hypercalcemia eventually leads to hypercalciuria and increased phosphate clearance leads to phosphaturia. The high urinary calcium and phosphate concentrations increase the tendency for precipitation of calcium-phosphate salts in the soft tissues of the kidney.

Hypercalcemia can result in peptic ulcer formation because calcium increases gastrin secretion. When serum calcium levels exceed about 13 mg/dl with a normal phosphate level, the calcium-phosphate **solubility product** is exceeded. At this level, insoluble calcium-phosphate salts form, which results in calcification of soft tissues such as blood vessels, skin, lungs, and joints. People with hyperparathyroidism have evidence of increased bone turnover, such as elevated levels of serum alkaline phosphatase and osteocalcin, which indicate high osteoblastic activity, and increased urinary hy-

---

BOX 6-2

Symptoms of Hyperparathyroidism

Kidney stones
Osteoporosis
Gastrointestinal disturbances, peptic ulcers, nausea, constipation
Muscle weakness, decreased muscle tone
Depression, lethargy, fatigue, mental confusion
Polyuria
High serum calcium concentration, low serum phosphate concentration

---

droxyproline levels, which indicates high bone resorptive activity. Hydroxyproline is an amino acid characteristically found in type I collagen. When the collagen is degraded, urinary hydroxyproline excretion increases. Although hyperthyroidism will eventually cause **osteoporosis** (bone loss involving both osteoid and mineral), it is not necessarily the presenting symptom. However, bone demineralization is apparent. These individuals frequently exhibit **hyperchloremic acidosis.** They also show high urinary cAMP levels. Some people with hyperparathyroidism have the bone disorder **osteitis fibrosa cystica,** which is characterized by bone pain, multiple bone cysts, a tendency for pathologic fractures of long bones, and histologic abnormalities of the bone.

Hypercalcemia of Malignancy

Many malignant tumors produce hypercalcemia as a result of tumor production of bone-mobilizing substances that can act like PTH. Some tumors produce substances that are structurally and functionally similar to PTH. These compounds, termed **PTH-related protein (PTHrP),** cross-react with the PTH receptors. They stimulate local production of bone-mobilizing substances such as prostaglandins and osteoclastic-activating factors such as IL-1,

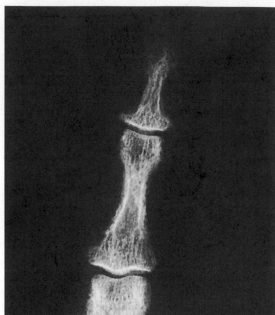

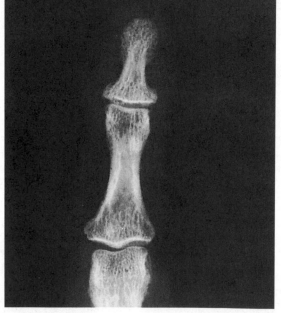

Figure 6-11 ■ **Primary hyperparathyroidism.**
X-ray films of middle and distal phalanges of
index finger show subperiosteal bone resorp-
tion of shafts and tip of distal phalanx (A). Second x-ray film was taken after bone had healed
after treatment by removal of parathyroid he-
matoma (B). (From Besser GM, Thorner MO: *Clinical*
endocrinology, London, 1994, Mosby-Wolfe.)

as well as increase calcitriol production. In general, serum PTH levels are suppressed in these individuals because of the high serum calcium levels. The antibiotic mithramycin (plicamycin) is sometimes used in the treatment of hypercalcemia of malignancy because it inhibits bone resorption. PTHrP can also be produced in normal tissue and may play a role in calcium balance in the fetus and infant.

Pseudohypoparathyroidism

Pseudohypoparathyroidism is a rare familial disorder characterized by tissue resistance to PTH. In many instances, the problem is thought to originate with the PTH receptor. Often there is a decrease in levels of the guanine nucleotide-binding protein, Gs. Individuals with pseudohypoparathyroidism demonstrate increased PTH secretion and low serum calcium levels, sometimes associated with congenital defects of the skeleton including shortened metacarpal and metatarsal bones.

Hypoparathyroidism

Hypoparathyroidism is associated with low serum calcium levels and high serum phosphate levels. The hypocalcemia results from both a PTH and a calcitriol deficiency. Consequently, there is a decrease in bone calcium mobilization by both osteoclastic resorption and osteocytic osteolysis. Because calcitriol is deficient, GI absorption of calcium is impaired. The PTH deficiency decreases renal calcium reabsorption, thereby decreasing fractional calcium reabsorption. Although fractional calcium reabsorption decreases, the urinary calcium level is generally low. Urinary cAMP concentration also decreases (Figure 6-12). Alkalosis occurs because bicarbonate excretion decreases; this further lowers the free calcium level in serum. Although the serum calcium level is low, bone demineralization is usually not a problem because of the high serum phosphate level. Hypocalcemia increases

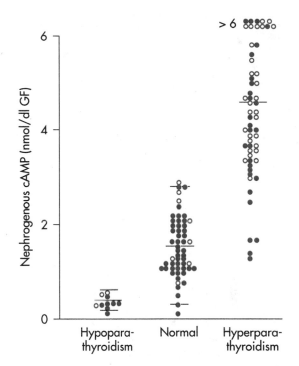

Figure 6-12 ■ Nephrogenous cyclic adenosine monophosphate *(cAMP),* **expressed as function of glomerular filtration rate in control subjects and patients with primary hypoparathyroidism and hyperparathyroidism.** *Open circles,* **Patients with renal impairment;** *closed circles,* **subjects with normal renal function;** *long horizontal bars,* **mean values;** *short bars,* **±2 SD;** *GF,* **glomerular filtrate.** (Redrawn from Broadus AD, et al: *J Clin Invest* 60:77, 1977.)

neuromuscular excitability, increasing the possibility of tetany and even convulsions. Hypocalcemia alters cardiac function. It can produce a first-degree heart block. The low serum calcium level decreases myocardial contractility.

The most prominent symptom of hypoparathyroidism is increased neuromuscular excitability (Box 6-3). Low serum calcium concentrations decrease the neuromuscular threshold. This can be manifested as repetitive responses to a single stimulus and as spontaneous neuromuscular discharge. The increased neuromuscular excitability can result in tingling in the fingers or toes (paresthesia), muscle cramps, or even tetany. Laryngeal spasms can be fatal. Sometimes the serum calcium level is not low enough to produce overt tetany, but a latent tetany can be demonstrated by inflating a blood pressure cuff on the arm to a pressure greater than systolic pressure for 2 minutes. The resultant oxygen deficiency precipitates overt tetany as demonstrated by **carpal-pedal spasms.** This is called **Trousseau's sign** (Figure 6-13, *A*). Another test is to tap the facial nerve, which evokes facial muscle spasms **(Chvostek's sign).**

Treatment of hypoparathyroidism is difficult because of the lack of readily available effective human PTH. The disorder is frequently treated with a high-calcium diet, vitamin D (calcitriol), and occasionally thiazide diuretics to decrease renal calcium clearance. Thiazide diuretics increase calcium reabsorption in the thick ascending limb of the loop of Henle. Acute hypocalcemia can be treated with intravascular calcium gluconate infusion.

Hypomagnesemia resulting from either severe malabsorption or chronic alcoholism can cause hypoparathyroidism. Hypomagnesemia impairs the secretion of PTH and decreases the biologic response to PTH.

Vitamin D Deficiency

Vitamin D deficiency produces hypocalcemia and hypomagnesemia and decreases GI absorption of calcium and phosphate. The drop in the serum calcium level stimulates PTH secretion, which stimulates renal phosphate clearance, thereby aggravating the serum phosphate loss. Because the level of the calcium-phosphate product in serum, and hence in body fluids, is low, bone mineralization is impaired and demineralization is increased. This leads to osteomalacia in adults or rickets in children. The secondary elevation in PTH can produce osteoporosis. Rickets and osteomalacia are disorders in which bone mineralization is defective. Osteoid is formed, but it does not mineralize adequately. If the calcium-phosphate product level or the pH in bone fluid bathing the osteoid is low, demineralization rather than mineralization is favored. *Rickets* is caused by a calcium (calcitriol) deficiency before skeletal maturation; it involves problems in not only the bone but also the cartilage of the growth plate (Figure 6-13, *B* and *C*). *Osteomalacia* is the term used when inadequate bone mineralization occurs after skeletal growth is complete and the epiphyses have closed.

Paget's Disease

Paget's disease results in bone deformities. It is characterized by an increase in bone resorption followed by an increase in bone formation. The new bone is generally abnormal and often irregular. Serum alkaline phosphatase and osteocalcin levels are increased, as are those of urinary hydroxyproline. Pain, bone deformation, and bone weakness can occur (Figure 6-13, *D*).

Bone Problems of Renal Failure (Renal Osteodystrophy)

Approximately 0.9 g, or more than 50% of dietary phosphate, is normally lost in the urine in a day. Consequently, the kidney serves as the

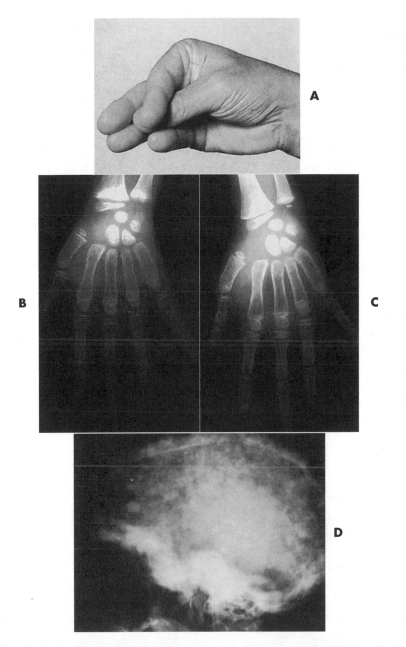

Figure 6-13 ■ A, Position of hand in hypocalcemic tetany. B, X-ray film of left hand of 9-year-old boy with rickets caused by malnutrition. He would eat only potato chips. All of bony structures are osteopenic. Note widening of space between provisional zone of calcification and epiphysis of left radius. C, After 2 months of force feedings, rickets has subsided. Note decreased width of space between provisional zone of calcification and epiphysis of radius and increased bone calcification. D, X-ray film of skull of patient with Paget's disease. Thickness of skull is increased and sclerotic changes are seen scattered throughout skull, consistent with healing phase of Paget's disease. (A from Hall R, Evered DC: *Color atlas of endocrinology,* ed 2, London, 1990, Mosby-Wolfe. **B** to **D** courtesy Dr. C. Joe.)

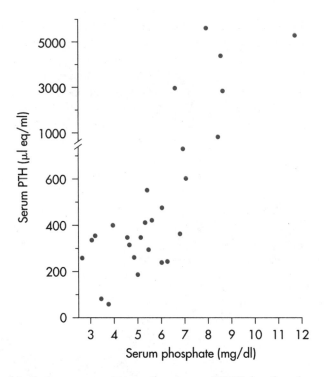

Figure 6-14 ■ Relationship between serum parathormone *(PTH)* level and serum phosphate level in patients with renal failure. (Redrawn from Bordier PF, Marie PF, Arnaud CD: *Kidney Int* 7[suppl 2]:102, 1975.)

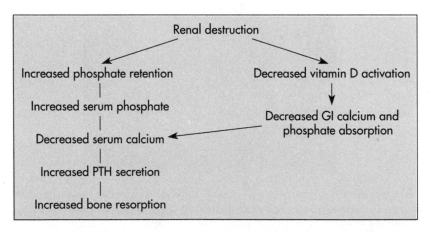

Figure 6-15 ■ The physiologic basis of bone loss in renal failure. *PTH,* Parathormone; *GI,* gastrointestinal.

major excretory route for phosphate. As renal function, and hence phosphate clearance, decreases, the serum phosphate concentration rises (Figure 6-14). The increase in serum phosphate concentration will lower serum calcium levels by exceeding the solubility product and hence increasing calcium-phosphate precipitation. A drop in the serum calcium level is an effective stimulus for PTH, and serum PTH levels rise. In addition, vitamin D activation by 1α-hydroxylase occurs in the renal proximal tubules. In kidney failure, vitamin D activation is impaired, which decreases GI absorption of calcium and phosphate. This results in a further drop in the serum calcium level and aggravates the preexisting problem with excess PTH secretion. The result is to stimulate bone resorption and demineralization. As bone demineralization occurs, it will aggravate the hyperphosphatemia because the renal mechanisms of counteracting the hyper-phosphatemia are now defective.

Figure 6-15 shows the effect of renal impairment on phosphate, calcium, vitamin D, and PTH.

Pregnancy

The placenta plays a major role in regulating calcium flux to the fetus. PTHrP is produced and released from the placental trophoblast in response to a decrease in extracellular calcium concentration, and this may regulate fetal calcium availability.

Summary

1. Serum calcium levels are a function of the rate calcium enters from GI absorption and bone demineralization and leaves through bone mineralization, GI secretion, and renal excretion. PTH, calcitonin, and calcitriol regulate the flux of calcium into and out of serum. Serum calcium levels are normally maintained within a narrow range.

2. Serum phosphate levels are determined by the rate phosphate enters from GI absorption, soft tissue efflux, and bone demineralization and leaves through GI secretion, soft tissue influx, bone mineralization, and renal excretion. Serum phosphate levels normally fluctuate over a relatively wide range.

3. The major hormones regulating serum calcium and phosphate levels are PTH, calcitonin, and calcitriol.

4. Osteoblasts are bone-forming cells that are of mesenchymal origin. They synthesize bone matrix and produce an environment that promotes bone mineralization. Osteocytes are osteoblasts that have become entrapped in bone. Osteoclasts are large, multinucleate cells derived from hematopoietic stem cells. They resorb bone.

5. PTH acts to raise serum calcium levels and lower phosphate levels. It stimulates bone calcium and phosphate loss by osteoclastic resorption and osteocytic osteolysis. It increases the fractional reabsorption of calcium in the kidney. However, because the filtered load of calcium increases, renal excretion of calcium typically increases after PTH administration. PTH decreases renal bicarbonate reabsorption and increases renal 1α-hydroxylase activity.

6. The major action of calcitonin is to decrease osteoclastic bone resorption.

7. Vitamin D can be synthesized from 7-dehydrocholesterol in skin in the presence of ultraviolet light. It is hydroxylated to 25-hydroxycholecalciferol in the liver and activated by renal 1α-hydroxylase to 1,25-dihydroxycholecalciferol (calcitriol).

8. Calcitriol increases GI absorption of calcium

and phosphate by increasing production of calbindin. It synergizes with PTH on bone.

9. Patients with hyperparathyroidism typically have hypercalcemia, hypophosphatemia, hyperchloremia, and acidosis. They are prone to kidney stones because of hypercalciuria and hyperphosphaturia.

10. Patients with hypoparathyroidism typically have hypocalcemia, hyperphosphatemia, hypochloremia, and alkalosis. They may show symptoms of increased neuromuscular excitability such as paresthesias, muscle cramps, and tetany.

11. Children with a vitamin D deficiency are prone to develop rickets, whereas adults with a vitamin D deficiency develop osteomalacia. The vitamin D deficiency results in decreased GI absorption of calcium, phosphate, and magnesium.

■ KEY WORDS AND CONCEPTS

- 1,25-dihydroxycholecalciferol (calcitriol)
- Osteoid
- Osteoblasts
- Collagen
- Osteocalcin
- Alkaline phosphatase
- Hydroxyapatite
- Osteocytes
- Lacunae
- Canaliculi
- Osteoclasts
- Howship's lacunae
- Bone fluid
- Parathormone (PTH)
- Preproparathyroid hormone
- Proparathyroid hormone
- Osteocytic osteolysis
- Calcitonin
- Paget's disease
- 7-Dehydrocholesterol
- Secosteroid
- 1α-Hydroxylase
- Transcalciferin
- Calbindin
- Rickets
- Osteomalacia
- Solubility product
- Osteoporosis
- Hyperchloremic acidosis
- Osteitis fibrosa cystica
- PTH-related protein
- Hyperparathyroidism
- Pseudohypoparathyroidism
- Hypoparathyroidism
- Carpal-pedal spasms
- Trousseau's sign
- Chvostek's sign
- Renal osteodystrophy

■ SELF-STUDY PROBLEMS

1. Although PTH increases renal calcium reabsorption, excess PTH typically increases urinary calcium excretion. Why does this occur?

2. Why would long-acting forms of calcitonin be useful in the treatment of Paget's disease?

3. What is the physiologic basis for cardiac arrest in hyperparathyroidism?

4. What is the physiologic basis for polyuria and nocturia in hyperparathyroidism?

5. Why would hyperchloremic acidosis develop in people with hyperparathyroidism?

6. Why would urinary cAMP increase after PTH administration?

7. Why are the urinary calcium level and fractional reabsorption of calcium typically low in hypoparathyroidism?

8. Why would the alkalosis produced by hypoparathyroidism decrease serum free calcium levels?

9. Why does the low serum calcium level produced by hypoparathyroidism decrease myocardial contractility?

10. What is indicated when serum alkaline phosphatase, hydroxyproline, and osteocalcin levels increase?

■ BIBLIOGRAPHY

Arnaud CD, Kolb FO: The calciotropic hormones and metabolic bone disease. In Greenspan FS, editor: *Basic and clinical endocrinology,* ed 3, Norwalk, Conn, 1991, Appleton & Lange, pp 247-322.

Aurbach GD, Marx SJ, Spiegel AM: Metabolic bone disease. In Wilson JD, Foster DW, editors: *Williams' textbook of endocrinology,* ed 8, Philadelphia, 1992, WB Saunders, pp 1477-1518.

Aurbach GD, Marx SJ, Spiegel AM: Parathyroid hormone, calcitonin and the calciferols. In Wilson JD, Foster DW, editors: *Williams' textbook of endocrinology,* ed 8, Philadelphia, 1992, WB Saunders, pp 1397-1476.

Bikle DD, Pillai S: Vitamin D, calcium, and epidermal differentiation, *Endocr Rev* 14:3, 1993.

Felsenfeld AJ, Llach F: Parathyroid gland function in chronic renal failure, *Kidney Int* 43:771, 1993.

Guise TA, Mundy GR: Cancer and bone, *Endocr Rev* 19:18-54, 1998.

Hodgson SF: Corticosteroid-induced osteoporosis, *Endocrinol Metab Clin North Am* 19:95, 1990.

Holick MF, Krane SM, Potts JT: Calcium, phosphorus, and bone metabolism: calcium-regulating hormones. In Wilson JD et al, editors: *Harrison's principles of internal medicine,* ed 12, New York, 1991, McGraw-Hill, pp 1888-1901.

Ohlsson C, Bengtsson B, Isaksson OGP, Andreassen TT, Slootweg MC: Growth hormone and bone, *Endocr Rev* 19:55-79, 1998.

Suda T, Takahashi N, Martin TJ: Modulation of osteoclast differentiation, *Endocr Rev* 13:66, 1992.

Tetradis S, Pilbeam CC, Liu Y, Herschman HR, Kream BE: Parathyroid hormone increases prostaglandin G/H synthase-2 transcription by a cyclic adenosine 3′,5′-monophosphate-mediated pathway in murine osteoblastic MC3T3-E1 cells, *Endocrinology* 138:3594-3600, 1997.

Adrenal Gland

Objectives

1. Describe the anatomic and functional relationship between the adrenal medulla and the adrenal cortex.
2. Explain the role of tyrosine hydroxylase and phenylethanolamine *N*-methyltransferase in adrenal catecholamine synthesis.
3. List the major hormones produced in the adrenal and the site of their production.
4. List the major actions of the adrenal hormones.
5. Diagram the major pathways for steroid hormone synthesis in the zona glomerulosa, zona fasciculata, and zona reticularis.

6. Explain the regulatory mechanisms controlling synthesis and secretion of adrenal hormones.
7. List and explain the physiologic basis for the abnormalities seen in pheochromocytoma, Addison's disease, Cushing's syndrome, Conn's syndrome, and congenital adrenal hyperplasia.
8. List pathologic and physiologic conditions that can result in adrenal hyperplasia.

THE ADRENAL GLAND IS BILATERALLY located immediately above the kidneys (*ad*, near; *renal*, kidney). It is a unique gland because, like the pituitary, it is essentially two endocrine tissues within one organ. The inner portion, the adrenal medulla (Figure 7-1), is neurologic tissue, whereas the adrenal cortex is glandular tissue. The two regions of the gland serve different functions and produce structurally different types of hormones. The medulla is the site of production of the **catecholamines epinephrine, norepinephrine,** and **dopamine,** and the adrenal cortex is the site of pro-

duction of steroid hormones that include the **mineralocorticoids,** the **glucocorticoids,** and some **sex hormones.**

■ ADRENAL MEDULLA (Box 7-1)
Anatomy

The adrenal medulla represents approximately 20% of the adrenal gland by weight, but this proportion is variable among individuals. It is derived from neuroectodermal cells of the neural crest. These cells are **chromaffin cells (pheochromocytes)** (Figure 7-2). The adrenal medulla is a component of the sympathetic

131

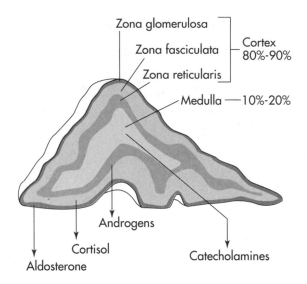

Figure 7-1 ▪ Adrenal gland. Medulla is neuroectoderm tissue and produces catecholamines. Cortex is mesoderm and produces steroids.

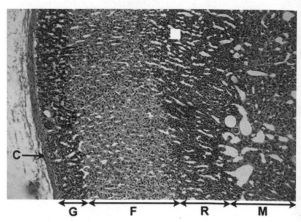

Figure 7-2 ▪ Histologic section of adrenal gland. Adrenal capsule (C), zona glomerulosa (G), zona fasciculata (F), and zona reticularis (R) are visible, as is portion of adrenal medulla (M).

BOX 7-1

Overview

The adrenal gland is a hybrid gland consisting of a cortex and a medulla. The hormones of the adrenal are important regulators of metabolism, and they serve an important role in adaptation to stress. The hormone aldosterone is critical for normal salt balance and hence water balance. Because of the wide range of actions of adrenal corticosteroids, synthetic analogs are widely used in the treatment of disorders ranging from skin rashes to arthritis.

nervous system (SNS), and pheochromocytes are not unique to the medulla. They are seen throughout the SNS. Stimuli for the SNS also stimulate secretion of adrenal medullary hormones.

The adrenal medulla is homologous to a large sympathetic ganglion without postganglionic processes. Instead of being secreted into a synapse, as is done in postganglionic terminals, the catecholamines are secreted into the blood and hence are hormones rather than neurotransmitters. The adrenal medulla is innervated by typical sympathetic preganglionic fibers that release acetylcholine. The chromaffin cells, like postganglionic cells, release norepinephrine on stimulation; however, they also release epinephrine. Although dopamine is present in the adrenal and serves as a precursor for norepinephrine and epinephrine, minimal dopamine secretion occurs and the role of adrenal dopamine is not known. Dopamine is, however, an important neurotransmitter in the central nervous system (CNS). The primary secretory product of the human adrenal medulla is epinephrine, although the ratio of epinephrine to norepinephrine se-

BOX 7-2

Key Enzymes in Catecholamine Synthesis

Tyrosine hydroxylase
Phenylethanolamine *N*-methyltransferase (PNMT)

cretion can vary. These cells are called chromaffin cells because they contain granules that stain readily with chromium stains. These **chromaffin granules** are membrane-bound granules that contain the catecholamine hormones, adenosine triphosphate (ATP), and the protein **chromagranin.** On stimulation, these granules are transported to the cell surface via the microtubular system (a calcium-dependent process), and the contents of the vesicles are released by exocytosis.

Although circulating epinephrine is derived entirely from the adrenal medulla, only about 30% of the circulating norepinephrine comes from the medulla. The remaining 70% is released from nerve terminals and diffused into the vascular system. Because the adrenal medulla is not the sole source of catecholamine production, this tissue is not essential for life.

Metabolism of Catecholamines

Synthesis of Catecholamines The steps of catecholamine synthesis are shown in Figure 7-3. Catecholamines are synthesized from the amino acid tyrosine. The rate-limiting step for catecholamine synthesis is the conversion of tyrosine to **dihydroxyphenylalanine (DOPA),** a reaction that is catalyzed by **tyrosine hydroxylase** (Box 7-2). SNS preganglionic stimulation of the adrenal increases activity of tyrosine hydroxylase and increases release of the contents of the chromaffin granules to the cell surface. Catecholamine synthesis begins in the cytoplasm because tyrosine hydroxylase is located in the cytosol. However, the intermediate DOPA is then ac-

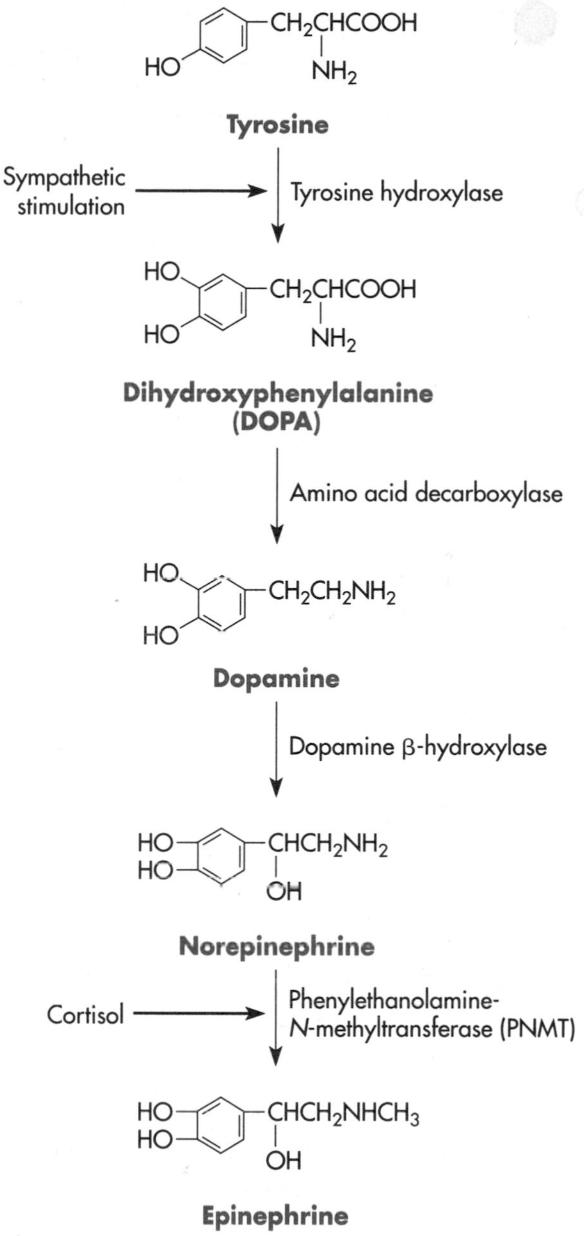

Figure 7-3 ■ Steps in synthesis of catecholamines.

tively transported into the granule, where the next enzymatic reaction occurs. The final step in the epinephrine synthesis is the conversion of norepinephrine to epinephrine, a reaction that is catalyzed by the enzyme **phenylethanolamine N-methyltransferase (PNMT).** Because this is also a cytosolic enzyme, the norepinephrine must diffuse out of the granule to be methylated by PNMT in the cytosol. The product, epinephrine, is then actively transported into the granule again where it is stored complexed with ATP and chromagranin (as is the norepinephrine that remains in the granule). The ratio of catecholamines to ATP is generally 4:1 in the granules. Some granules contain only norepinephrine, whereas others contain both norepinephrine and epinephrine. Release of the two types of granules can be controlled independently so that the ratio of epinephrine to norepinephrine secreted by the adrenal can vary. The enzyme PNMT is induced by the hormone cortisol. Blood flowing to the adrenal medulla has already passed through the adrenal cortex and therefore is high in adrenocortical hormones. In the absence of adrenal cortisol production, the medullary norepinephrine/epinephrine ratio increases. The adrenal medulla and a few regions of the brain are the only locations in the body where the enzyme PNMT is found.

Degradation of Catecholamines There are two primary enzymes involved with degradation of catecholamines: **monoamine oxidase (MAO)** and **catechol-O-methyltransferase (COMT).** Although MAO is the predominant enzyme in neuronal mitochondria, both enzymes are found in many nonneuronal tissues, including liver and kidney. The neurotransmitter norepinephrine is degraded by MAO and COMT after uptake of the compound into the presynaptic terminal. This mechanism is also involved in the catabolism of circulating adrenal catecholamines. However, the predominant fate of adrenal catecholamines is methylation by COMT in nonneuronal tissues such as the liver and kid-

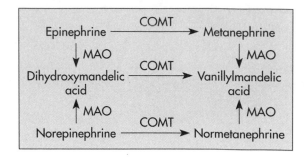

Figure 7-4 ■ Degradative metabolism of catecholamines. Monoamine oxidase *(MAO)* stimulates deamination; catechol-O-methyltransferase *(COMT)* stimulates methylation.

ney. The metabolism of catecholamines is shown in Figure 7-4. Urinary **vanillylmandelic acid (VMA)** and **metanephrine** are sometimes used clinically to assess the level of catecholamine production in a patient. Much of the urinary VMA and metanephrine is derived from neuronal, rather than adrenal, catecholamines.

Actions of Catecholamines

Catecholamines act via α and β receptors (Table 7-1). There are α_1, α_2, β_1, and β_2 receptors (the less prevalent β_3 receptors are not discussed). These receptors are characterized according to the relative potency of various agonists. Epinephrine has a greater effect on β_2 receptors than norepinephrine does, but both hormones have similar effects on β_1, α_1, and α_2 receptors. Because different actions are mediated through different types of receptors, the actions of the two major catecholamines differ. The mechanism of action of the hormone depends on the receptor involved. The α_1 receptors have G_q-associated receptors, which function by stimulating the turnover of phosphatidylinositols; α_2 receptors have G_i-associated receptors, which act by suppressing cyclic adenosine monophosphate (cAMP) production; β_1 and β_2 receptors have G_s-associated receptors, which act by stimulating cAMP production.

	TABLE 7-1		

Catecholamine receptors

Receptor type	Primary mechanism of action	Examples of tissue distribution	Agonist potency
α_1	↑ IP_3, DAG	Adrenergic postsynaptic nerve terminals	Epinephrine ≈ norepinephrine
α_2	↓ cAMP	Adrenergic presynaptic terminals (↓ norepinephrine release)	Epinephrine ≈ norepinephrine
β_1	↑ cAMP	Heart	Epinephrine = norepinephrine
β_2	↑ cAMP	Liver	Epinephrine >> norepinephrine

IP_3, Inositol triphosphate; *DAG*, diacylglycerol; *cAMP*, cyclic adenosine monophosphate.

	TABLE 7-2	

Actions of catecholamines

β_2 Effects	α Effects
Epinephrine >> norepinephrine	Epinephrine ≈ norepinephrine
Metabolic	Metabolic
Glycogenolysis	Gluconeogenesis
Lipolysis	
Calorigenesis	
Increases insulin secretion	Decreases insulin secretion
Vasodilator in skeletal muscle	Vasoconstrictor in most tissues including skeletal muscle
No change in mean arterial pressure	Increases mean arterial pressure
Bronchodilation	Dilation of pupils
	Sweating
	Sphincter contraction

Metabolic Actions Epinephrine is the predominant circulating catecholamine regulating metabolism because circulating norepinephrine rarely reaches levels at which it has significant metabolic actions via the β_2 receptors. Norepinephrine plays a major role in metabolic regulation as an SNS neurotransmitter (Table 7-2).

Catecholamines are major regulators of blood glucose. They increase serum glucose levels by stimulating glycogenolysis and by increasing gluconeogenesis. They also decrease insulin-mediated transport of glucose into muscle and adipose tissue, thereby preferentially channeling glucose to the brain. They stimulate muscle Cori cycle activity whereby muscle glycogenolysis increases and lactate production rises. The lactate becomes a gluconeogenic substrate for the liver.

Catecholamines activate the enzyme **hormone-sensitive lipase (HSL)** in adipose tissue. This is a cAMP-regulated enzyme (β_2) that catalyzes the hydrolysis of the stored triglycerides in the adipocyte to fatty acids and glycerol. The fatty acids are released into the circulation, increasing serum levels of free fatty acids. These fatty acids are taken up by the liver and oxidized by beta oxidation. Acetyl coenzyme A (acetyl CoA) is produced faster than it can enter the tricarboxylic acid (TCA) cycle, so its levels rise; consequently, there is an increase in conversion of acetyl CoA into the ketone bodies **acetoacetic acid, β-hydroxybutyric acid, and acetone.** Therefore catecholamines are ketogenic hormones.

Catecholamines can increase the basal metabolic rate (calorigenic effect), but thyroid hormones and cortisol must be present for the calorigenic effect of catecholamines.

Cardiovascular Effects The α-receptor stimulation of the vasculature produces vasoconstriction. However, β_2 receptors are found in blood vessels in skeletal muscle and liver, and β_2 stimulation causes vasodilation. For this reason, although norepinephrine is a potent vasoconstrictor, the effects of epinephrine are variable and dose dependent. Epinephrine acts through α receptors to cause vasoconstriction but acts through β receptors in skeletal muscle and liver to cause vasodilation. Consequently, epinephrine, unlike norepinephrine, often decreases peripheral resistance.

The adrenergic receptors of the myocardium are β_1 receptors, and both epinephrine and norepinephrine have comparable effects on β_1 receptors. The effect of β-receptor stimulation of the heart is to increase heart rate (chronotropic effect) and myocardial contractility (inotropic effect). However, the actions of the catecholamines on cardiac function in vivo can be complicated by the baroreceptor reflex. Because norepinephrine is a more potent vasoconstrictor than epinephrine, norepinephrine administration increases systolic pressure, diastolic pres-

sure, and mean arterial pressure. The rise in arterial pressure can precipitate a baroreceptor-mediated drop in heart rate (rather than the rise that norepinephrine would produce in a denervated heart). Epinephrine does not produce the intense vasopressive effect of norepinephrine, so epinephrine administration does not necessarily induce a baroreceptor response. Therefore epinephrine often increases heart rate and myocardial contractility. This relationship is shown in Figure 7-5.

Nervous System Effects The adrenal catecholamines cannot cross the blood-brain barrier and therefore do not have direct actions on the CNS. They do have indirect CNS actions, which are probably mediated through changes in cardiovascular function and in levels of blood-borne nutrients or electrolytes that cross the blood-brain barrier. The behavioral effects in-

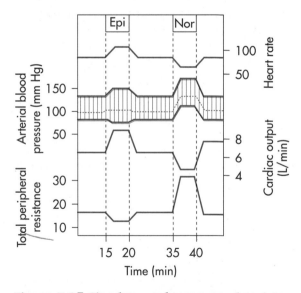

Figure 7-5 ■ **Circulatory changes produced in humans by slow intravenous infusion of epinephrine *(Epi)* and norepinephrine *(Nor).*** (Adapted from Barcroft H, Swan HJC: *Sympathetic control of human blood vessels,* 1953, Arnold; in Ganong WF: *Review of medical physiology,* ed 18, Norwalk, Conn, 1997, Appleton & Lange.)

duced by epinephrine administration are greater than those induced by norepinephrine. Although both catecholamines increase arousal, the sensation associated with epinephrine administration is often described as anxiety or a feeling of impending doom.

Pathologic Conditions Involving the Adrenal Medulla

A **pheochromocytoma** is a tumor of the chromaffin tissue that produces excessive quantities of catecholamines. These commonly are adrenal medullary tumors, but they can occur in other chromaffin cells of the autonomic nervous system. Although pheochromocytomas are not common tumors, they are the most common source of hyperadrenal medullary function and are often used as an example to demonstrate the functions of the adrenal medulla. The catecholamine most frequently elevated in pheochromocytoma is norepinephrine. For unknown reasons, the symptoms of excessive catecholamine secretion (Box 7-3) are often sporadic rather than continuous. The symptoms include hypertension, headaches (from hypertension), sweating, anxiety, palpitations, and chest pain. In addition, patients with this disorder may show orthostatic hypotension (despite the tendency for hypertension). This occurs because hypersecretion of catecholamines can decrease the postsynaptic response to norepinephrine as a result of down regulation of the

BOX 7-3
Common Symptoms Associated with Pheochromocytoma

Hypertension	Palpitations
Headaches	Chest pain
Sweating	Orthostatic hypotension
Anxiety	

receptors. Consequently, the baroreceptor response to the blood shifts occurring on standing is blunted.

■ ADRENAL CORTEX
Anatomy

The adrenal cortex (see Figure 7-1) comprises the bulk of the adrenal gland and is the site of synthesis of many types of steroid hormones. The fetal adrenal plays a critical role in certain definitive steps in the synthesis of the placental steroids. Consequently, the gland forms relatively early in development and is actively involved in steroidogenesis by 8 weeks of gestation. At this stage, the **fetal zone** comprises the bulk of the adrenal cortex. The other region of the adrenal cortex is called the **definitive zone.** At birth, the adrenal is large, and as the fetal zone is gradually lost after birth, the size of the adrenal decreases. The definitive zone differentiates into the three layers associated with the nonfetal adrenal cortex. The outermost layer of the cortex is the **zona glomerulosa;** it is the only one of the three layers that has the enzymes necessary to convert corticosterone to the mineralocorticoid hormone aldosterone. This region lacks the enzyme 17α-hydroxylase/17,20-lyase (CYP17) and therefore cannot produce cortisol or the sex steroids. This region of the adrenal cortex is regulated primarily by angiotensin II. Angiotensin II stimulates both the growth of the zona glomerulosa and the synthesis of aldosterone. The middle layer is the **zona fasciculata,** and the innermost layer is the **zona reticularis.** Although the zona fasciculata is often associated primarily with glucocorticoid production and the zona reticularis with androgen production, the functional distinction between the two layers is blurred and they appear to function as a unit. These inner two layers cannot produce aldosterone, but they do have the enzyme 17α-hydroxylase/17,20 lyase (CYP17) that is necessary for the production of glucocorticoids and sex hormones. The inner two layers are regulated by the anterior pituitary hormone adrenocorticotropic hormone (ACTH), which stimulates both growth of the inner two layers and the synthesis of steroids.

The adrenal cortex is essential for life. If the adrenal cortex is removed or destroyed, perpetual administration of mineralocorticoids and glucocorticoids is imperative. Three groups of steroids are produced in the adrenal cortex; these compounds are classified according to their major actions. These groups are the **mineralocorticoids, glucocorticoids,** and **sex hormones.**

The primary action of the mineralocorticoids is to regulate mineral metabolism. The prototype for this group is **aldosterone.** Aldosterone stimulates renal retention of sodium and promotes secretion of hydrogen and potassium. The increased retention of sodium chloride is accompanied by water reabsorption. **Deoxycorticosterone (DOC)** is the next most potent natural mineralocorticoid. The mineralocorticoids are 21-carbon steroids, as are the glucocorticoids.

The glucocorticoids are important regulators of blood glucose (in actuality, they have many diverse actions). The most potent natural glucocorticoid is the hormone **cortisol.** There is overlap in function between the two groups; cortisol has some mineralocorticoid activity, and aldosterone has some (minimal) glucocorticoid activity.

The predominant sex steroids produced in the adrenal cortex are the weak androgens **dehydroepiandrosterone (DHEA)** and **androstenedione.** These compounds can be converted to more potent androgens, including testosterone, and to estrogens in peripheral tissues. The adrenal cortex is capable of producing testosterone and even estrogens, but there is minimal production of these hormones in the normal adrenal. Naturally occurring androgens have 19 carbons, and estrogens have 18 carbons. The hormone progesterone (21 carbons) is found in all layers of the adrenal cortex and can serve as a precursor of the other biologically active cortical hormones. Although the adrenal androgens are not adequate to replace testicular androgens, they are the major source of androgens in women and are responsible for pubic and axillary hair growth in women. The levels of these adrenal androgens can become clinically significant in some adrenal disorders.

Mineralocorticoids and glucocorticoids can interact with each other's receptors; therefore there is overlap in biologic activity. Table 7-3

TABLE 7-3

Relative potencies of corticosteroids compared with cortisol

	Glucocorticoid activity	Mineralocorticoid activity
Cortisol	1.0	1.0
Corticosterone	0.3	15
Aldosterone	0.3	3000
Deoxycorticosterone	0.2	100
Cortisone	0.7	1.0
Prednisolone	4	0.8
Dexamethasone	25	About 0

compares the relative potencies of some natural and synthetic corticosteroids with respect to their glucocorticoid and mineralocorticoid activity.

Synthesis of Adrenal Corticosteroids

Cholesterol is the precursor for the steroids of the adrenal cortex. The rate-limiting enzyme for the formation of steroids is the **side-chain cleavage (SCC) enzyme** (CYP11A1), which catalyzes the removal of six carbons from cholesterol to produce the 21-carbon steroid pregnenolone. SCC enzyme is induced by ACTH in the zona fasciculata and zona reticularis and by angiotensin II in the zona glomerulosa. An overview of the general pathways for steroid hormone synthesis is shown in Figure 7-6. Note that many biologically active steroids, such as progesterone, serve as precursors for other biologically active steroids. If there is an enzyme blockage and the precursors formed before the blockage accumulate, the nature of the hormones secreted by the endocrine organ can change markedly. This is what happens in **adrenogenital syndrome.** Adrenogenital syndrome occurs when the ability to produce cortisol is impaired, thereby resulting in excessive adrenal androgen production and subsequent masculinization. Women may show symptoms of excessive androgen production such as abnormal sexual hair development **(hirsutism),** male pattern baldness, and clitoral enlargement.

Aldosterone

The hormone aldosterone is the strongest naturally occurring mineralocorticoid in humans. There is some overlap in biologic activity between aldosterone and the glucocorticoids, which is typical of the corticosteroids.

Regulation of Secretion Because steroid hormones cross cell membranes freely, they are not stored in the endocrine gland. Hence regulation of synthesis results in regulation of secretion (Box 7-4). **Angiotensin II** is a potent stimulus for aldosterone production. There are volume receptors in the renal afferent arteriole in the region of the juxtaglomerular apparatus. A decrease in vascular volume (detected as a decrease in stretch of the vessel wall) in this region results in the release of the enzyme **renin,** which is produced and stored in the juxtaglomerular cells. Renin acts on the plasma 14–amino acid peptide **angiotensinogen** (angiotensin substrate) to convert it to angiotensin I (10 amino acids). **Angiotensin I** is converted to angiotensin II (eight amino acids) by **angiotensin-converting enzyme (ACE)** in the lungs.

Angiotensin II has multiple actions (Box 7-5). As the name suggests, it is a potent vasoconstrictor and plays a direct role in compensation for

---

BOX 7-4

Stimuli for Aldosterone Secretion

Angiotensin II is produced in response to the following stimuli:

- Decrease in vascular volume
- Sympathetic nervous system stimulation of renin secretion
- Rise in serum potassium concentration

BOX 7-5

Actions of Angiotensin II

Vasoconstrictor
Increased growth and vascularity of zona glomerulosa
Increased side-chain cleavage enzyme activity
Increased aldosterone synthesis

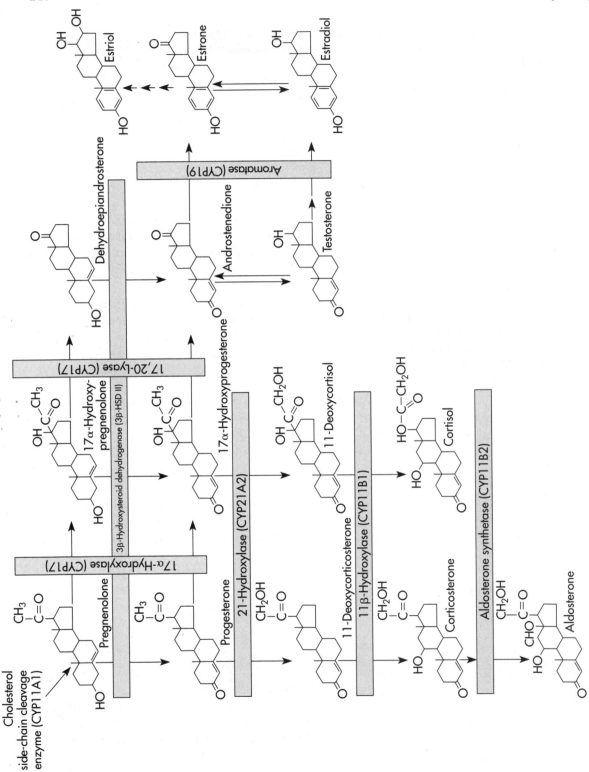

Figure 7-6 ■ Steroid synthesis. Not all intermediates are included, and only enzymes of clinical significance are listed.

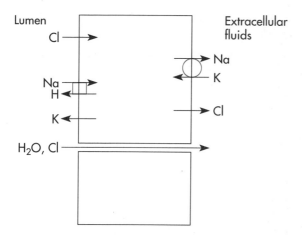

Lumen ... Extracellular fluids

Figure 7-7 ■ **Action of aldosterone on distal nephron. Aldosterone increases active sodium-potassium pump on basilar surface. It increases luminal permeability to sodium *(Na)* and potassium *(K)*. As sodium reabsorption is stimulated, there is increase in reabsorption of sodium chloride and water *(H₂O)* and increase in secretion of hydrogen *(H)* and potassium. *Cl,* Chloride.**

BOX 7-6

Actions of Aldosterone

Renal sodium retention
Water retention resulting from sodium retention
Potassium and hydrogen secretion in kidney

vascular volume depletion. Angiotensin II also acts on the zona glomerulosa to stimulate growth and vascularity of the region and to increase the activity of SSC enzyme and thereby increase the synthesis of aldosterone (Figure 7-7). These actions of angiotensin II on the zona glomerulosa are mediated by stimulating phosphatidylinositol turnover and hence activating protein kinase C. SNS stimulation can also release renin from the juxtaglomerular apparatus both directly and indirectly (by stimulating constriction of the afferent arteriole). In addition to the action of angiotensin II on aldosterone secretion, aldosterone synthesis is stimulated by a rise in serum potassium levels. Rising serum potassium levels depolarize the glomerulosa cell membrane, thereby stimulating voltage-sensitive calcium channels to open. The resultant calcium influx stimulates aldosterone production.

Transport in Blood Aldosterone binds with low affinity to plasma albumin, transcortin, and a specific aldosterone-binding globulin. The affinity for these proteins is low, and therefore only about 50% to 70% of the circulating aldosterone is bound. Consequently, the circulating half-life (t½) of aldosterone, approximately 20 minutes, is relatively low for a steroid. Aldosterone, as is typical of steroids, is metabolized and conjugated primarily in the liver and excreted in the urine.

Actions The primary action of aldosterone is to maintain extracellular volume by promoting sodium retention (Box 7-6). Aldosterone acts on the distal nephron (the latter portion of the distal convoluted tubule and the cortical collecting duct) to increase sodium reabsorption (see Figure 7-7). It increases the number of sodium-permeable channels in the luminal membrane, which increases the sodium permeability of the luminal membrane, thereby increasing intracellular sodium levels. It also increases basilar sodium-potassium adenosine triphosphatase activity (the sodium pump). As it stimulates sodium reabsorption, it also stimulates potassium and hydrogen secretion so that hyperaldosteronism leads to **hypokalemic alkalosis** (Figure 7-8). Aldosterone decreases the sodium in sweat, saliva, and gastric juices and stimulates the sodium-potassium pump in muscle. Although the bulk of sodium reabsorption occurs before the distal nephron (the site of action of

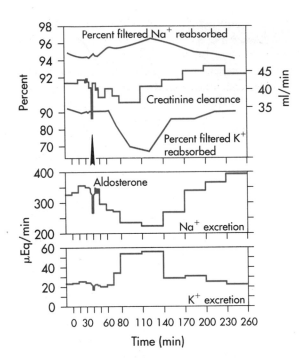

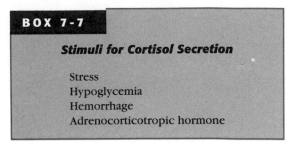

BOX 7-7

Stimuli for Cortisol Secretion

Stress
Hypoglycemia
Hemorrhage
Adrenocorticotropic hormone

Figure 7-8 ▪ **Effect of single dose of aldosterone on electrolyte excretion in adrenalectomized dog.** *Na,* Sodium; *K,* potassium. (Redrawn from Ganong WF: *Medical physiology,* ed 16, Norwalk, Conn, 1993, Appleton & Lange.)

aldosterone), aldosterone plays a critical role in the regulation of sodium balance.

Continuous aldosterone administration will result in **aldosterone escape** in 2 to 3 days. Initially there will be sodium retention and volume expansion, but the volume expansion will not continue indefinitely. As extracellular volume and therefore vascular volume increases, the glomerular filtration rate increases. This increases the rate of sodium delivery to the nephron and therefore the rate of renal sodium excretion, which limits the ability of aldosterone to continue expanding extracellular volume. Furthermore, the increase in vascular volume will stimulate the release of **atrial natriuretic peptide (ANP),** which promotes renal excretion. However, "escape" from the ef-

fects of aldosterone on potassium and hydrogen ion secretion does not occur, and potassium depletion and metabolic alkalosis can persist.

Cortisol and Glucocorticoids

Cortisol is produced in the zona fasciculata and zona reticularis. The zona glomerulosa cannot produce cortisol because it lacks the enzyme 17α-hydroxylase, which is necessary for the hydroxylation of pregnenolone or progesterone. The zona glomerulosa does, however, produce the compounds DOC and **corticosterone.** Although DOC and corticosterone have significant mineralocorticoid activity, they also have some glucocorticoid activity. Steroidogenesis in the zona fasciculata and zona reticularis are regulated by ACTH. ACTH stimulates growth and vascularity of these regions of the adrenal cortex. After hypophysectomy, the loss of ACTH results in atrophy of the zona fasciculata and zona reticularis. Cortisol exerts a negative feedback on ACTH and corticotropin-releasing hormone (CRH) secretion.

Regulation of Cortisol Secretion Cortisol is one of the "stress hormones," and its release is a critical component of the stress response (Box 7-7). The response to stress is mediated through the CNS. Stress increases the secretion of CRH, and CRH stimulates the reticular activating system and the pituitary secretion of ACTH. Stress also stimulates hypothalamic production of antidiuretic hormone (ADH), which can potentiate the effect of CRH on ACTH secretion, thereby amplifying the signal. The response to some

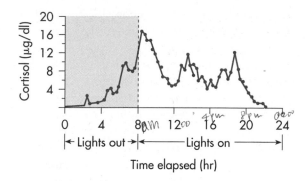

Figure 7-9 ■ Pattern of cortisol secretion over 24-hour period in normal subject. (Redrawn from Weitzman ED, et al: *J Clin Endocrinol Metab* 33:14, 1971.)

forms of intense stress is so potent that ACTH is stimulated even in the presence of high cortisol levels. Other stimuli for cortisol secretion include hypoglycemia and hemorrhage.

ACTH secretion and therefore cortisol secretion show marked diurnal variation. This variation is a function of the diurnal secretion of CRH. ACTH secretion rises progressively at night, with a peak generally occurring just before rising in the early morning. ACTH levels then fall progressively during the day to a low in the evening (Figure 7-9). Unlike the case with growth hormone secretion, the rise in ACTH that occurs at night is not a direct response to sleep, and the rise will occur even if sleep is withheld for several days. This rhythm appears to be a true diurnal rhythm that is entrained to 24 hours by the influences of multiple factors including light-dark patterns, sleep-wake patterns, and eating. After a person changes time zones, it takes approximately 2 weeks for the rhythm to become entrained to the new time schedule.

Mechanism of Action of Adrenocorticotropic Hormone ACTH acts on membrane receptors in the zona fasciculata and zona reticularis to increase cAMP levels. This is in contrast to the mechanism of action of angiotensin II on the zona glomerulosa, which acts through G_q-associated receptors that stimulate phosphatidylinositol turnover.

Mechanism of Action of Corticosteroids The adrenal steroids, like other steroid hormones, diffuse into the target cells and interact with intracellular receptors (see Figure 1-10). Glucocorticoids bind with high affinity to specific glucocorticoid receptors. This receptor is bound to other proteins, including a heat shock protein (HSP). The hormone binds to the receptor-HSP complex, which then dissociates and releases the HSP. The activated hormone-receptor complex now has a high affinity for the steroid-responsive element of the DNA. The exposed zinc fingers of the receptor bind to the steroid-responsive element in the promoter of the DNA. Once bound to DNA, the hormone-receptor complex acts as a transcription factor to regulate gene expression and hence formation of specific messenger RNAs.

Transport and Inactivation of Cortisol Cortisol is transported in blood predominantly bound to proteins. The binding protein **transcortin** (also called **corticosteroid-binding globulin [CBG]**) binds about 75% of the circulating cortisol. Albumin binds approximately 15% of the circulating hormone. The liver is the predominant site of steroid inactivation. It not only inactivates the hormones but also conjugates them with glucuronide or sulfate so they can be excreted more readily by the kidney. The circulating $t_{1/2}$ of cortisol is about 70 minutes.

Actions of Cortisol

Metabolic Actions Cortisol is a potent proteolytic and gluconeogenic hormone (Box 7-8). Like growth hormone, epinephrine, and glucagon, it raises blood glucose. It accomplishes this by two mechanisms: (1) it antagonizes the action of insulin on muscle and adipose tissue glucose uptake and use, thereby sparing glucose for the brain (the rapid initial rise in serum glucose following cortisol administration results

---

BOX 7-8

Biologic Actions of Cortisol

Metabolic
  Hyperglycemic
  Glycogenic
  Gluconeogenic
  Lipolytic
  Protein catabolic
  Insulin antagonist in muscle and adipose
    tissue
Inhibits bone formation, stimulates bone
  resorption
Necessary for vascular response to cate-
  cholamines
Antiinflammatory
Suppresses immune system
Inhibits antidiuretic hormone secretion and
  action
Stimulates gastric acid secretion
  Necessary for integrity and function of
    gastrointestinal tract
Stimulates red blood cell production
Alters mood and behavior
Permissive for catecholamines' calorigenic,
  lipolytic effects

---

from decreased lymphocyte glucose uptake), and (2) it increases liver output of glucose. The liver-generated glucose does not come from glycogenolysis; in fact, as the blood glucose level rises, glycogenesis increases. Instead, it is produced from gluconeogenesis, with amino acids as the predominant carbon source.

Cortisol is permissive for the lipolytic action of catecholamines. Catecholamines activate the lipolytic enzyme, HSL. The lipolytic effect of cortisol is so minor that if high insulin levels are present, lipogenesis rather than lipolysis may predominate. When excess cortisol is present, total body fat increases. This increase in body fat results from two factors: (1) cortisol stimulates appetite (a CNS effect), so the obesity is a result of increased caloric consumption; and (2) corti-

sol increases the blood glucose level, which increases insulin secretion. Insulin is a strong lipogenic hormone, whereas cortisol is a weak lipolytic hormone. Insulin probably plays an important role in the increased adipose tissue mass typically seen with hypercortisolism. For reasons not currently understood, hypercortisolism is associated with a peculiar pattern of fat deposition, which is called **centripetal fat distribution** because the fat is concentrated in the trunk but wasting is seen in the arms and legs. Fat tends to accumulate in the abdomen and subclavicular fat pads. The latter produces the **buffalo hump** characteristic of hypercortisolism (Table 7-4).

Because there are many hyperglycemic hormones, a cortisol deficiency is not likely to produce hypoglycemia unless food is withheld or the person is stressed. However, cortisol is essential for proper mobilization of proteins for glucose production. Changes in the serum after cortisol administration include increased blood urea nitrogen; decreased serum alanine (because it is used in gluconeogenesis); an increase in the branched-chain amino acids leucine, isoleucine, and valine; and sometimes an increase in serum fatty acid levels. The change in branched-chain amino acid levels is indicative of decreased muscle protein synthesis and increased proteolysis, whereas the increase in fatty acids reflects adipose tissue lipolysis.

Actions on Bone Glucocorticoids increase bone resorption. They have multiple actions that alter bone metabolism. Glucocorticoids decrease intestinal calcium absorption and decrease renal calcium reabsorption. Both mechanisms serve to lower serum calcium concentrations. As the serum calcium level drops, the secretion of parathyroid hormone (PTH) increases, and PTH mobilizes calcium from bone both by stimulating resorption of bone and by increasing demineralization of bone (osteocytic osteolysis). In addition to this action, glucocorticoids are thought to act directly on osteoblasts where they inhibit bone formation and suppress

TABLE 7-4	
Clinical manifestations of hypercortisolism	
Symptom	**Metabolic results**
Weight gain	Centripetal fat distribution, increased appetite
Protein wasting	Thin skin, abdominal striae
	Capillary fragility (ecchymoses)
	Muscle wasting, muscle weakness
	Osteoporosis
	Poor wound healing
	Growth retardation
Carbohydrate intolerance	Impaired glucose use, hyperglycemia
	Insulin resistance
Mineralocorticoid effects of cortisol	Hypertension, hypokalemia
Immunologic suppression	Increased susceptibility to infections
Other manifestations	Hirsutism, oligomenorrhea, polycythemia, personality changes

collagen formation. Although glucocorticoids are useful for treating the inflammation associated with arthritis, excessive use will result in bone loss (osteoporosis).

Cardiovascular Actions Cortisol is permissive for the vasoconstrictive actions of catecholamines. In the absence of cortisol, peripheral resistance drops. Orthostatic hypotension (inability to maintain normal mean arterial pressure when going from lying to standing position) occurs because of decreased baroreceptor-mediated vasoconstriction. Cortisol stimulates **erythropoietin** synthesis and hence increases red blood cell production. Anemia occurs when cortisol is deficient, and **polycythemia** occurs when cortisol levels are excessive.

Actions on Connective Tissue Cortisol inhibits fibroblast proliferation and collagen formation. In the presence of excessive amounts of cortisol, the skin thins and is more readily damaged. The connective tissue support of capillaries is impaired, and capillary injury, or bruising, is increased.

Actions on Kidney Cortisol inhibits ADH secretion and action, so it is an ADH antagonist. In the absence of cortisol, the action of ADH is potentiated, making it difficult to increase the free water clearance in response to a water load and increasing the likelihood of water intoxication. Cortisol also has weak mineralocorticoid activity and can stimulate sodium and water reabsorption. Cortisol increases the glomerular filtration rate by both increasing cardiac output and acting directly on the kidney.

Actions on Muscle Cortisol actions on muscle are complex. When cortisol levels are excessive, muscle weakness is typical. The weakness has multiple origins. In part it is a result of the excessive proteolysis that cortisol produces. High cortisol levels can result in hypokalemia (via the mineralocorticoid actions), which can produce muscle weakness because it hyperpolarizes and stabilizes the muscle cell membrane, making stimulation more difficult.

Gastrointestinal Actions Cortisol exerts a trophic effect on the gastrointestinal (GI) mucosa. In the absence of cortisol, GI motility decreases, GI mucosa degenerates, and GI acid and enzyme production decrease. Because cortisol stimulates appetite, hypercortisolism is frequently associated with weight gain. The cortisol-mediated stimulation of gastric acid and pepsin secretion increases the risk of ulcer development.

Antiinflammatory and Immunosuppressive Actions Analogs of glucocorticoid are frequently used pharmacologically because of their **antiinflammatory properties.** The inflammatory response to injury consists of local dilation of capillaries and increased capillary permeability with a resultant local edema and accumulation of white blood cells. These steps are mediated by prostaglandins, thromboxanes, and leukotrienes. Cortisol inhibits phospholipase A_2, a key enzyme in prostaglandin, leukotriene, and thromboxane synthesis. Cortisol also stabilizes lysosomal membranes, thereby decreasing the release of the proteolytic enzymes that augment local swelling. In response to injury, leukocytes normally migrate to the site of injury and leave the vascular system. These changes are inhibited by cortisol, as is the phagocytic activity of the neutrophils, although bone marrow release of neutrophils is stimulated. Cortisol decreases the number of circulating eosinophils. The fibroblastic proliferation involved in inflammation is also inhibited. This latter response is important in the formation of barriers to the spread of certain infectious agents. When cortisol levels are high, many of the body's defense mechanisms against infection are inhibited. For this reason, glucocorticoid therapy is contraindicated as the sole medication for the treatment of infections.

Cortisol inhibits the immune response, and for this reason glucocorticoid analogs have been used as immunosuppressants in organ transplants. High cortisol levels decrease the number of circulating T lymphocytes (particularly helper T lymphocytes) and decrease their ability to migrate to the site of antigenic stimulation. Although corticosteroids inhibit cellularly mediated immunity, antibody production by B lymphocytes does not appear to be impaired.

Psychologic Actions Glucocorticoids can alter mood and behavior. Psychiatric disturbances are associated with either excessive or deficient levels of corticosteroids. Excessive corticosteroids can initially produce a feeling of well-being, but continued excessive exposure eventually leads to emotional lability and depression. Frank psychosis can occur with either excess or deficient hormone. Cortisol has been shown to increase the tendency for insomnia and decrease rapid-eye-movement (REM) sleep. People who are deficient in corticosteroids tend to be depressed, apathetic, and irritable.

Adrenal Androgens

The primary site of adrenal sex hormone production is the zona reticularis. DHEA and androstenedione are the predominant androgens produced by the adrenal. Although these are weak androgens, they can be converted to stronger androgens like testosterone or even to estrogens in peripheral tissues. The adrenal cortex produces very small quantities of testosterone and estrogens, and these quantities are not sufficient to replace testicular androgens in men. The adrenal is the major source of androgens in women; these androgens stimulate pubic and axillary hair development in pubertal females. In certain adrenal pathologic conditions, adrenal androgen production can increase to the level at which the androgens produce masculinization of females or premature puberty in males.

Pathologic Conditions Involving the Adrenal Cortex

When the pituitary-adrenal system is suppressed by exogenous administration of corticosteroids, both the corticotropes and the adrenal cortex (zona fasciculata and zona reticularis) atrophy. If steroid administration is withheld, acute adrenal insufficiency will result, which can be unpleasant and even life threatening. It takes months to restore normal function of the corticotropes after long-term glucocorticoid treatment (Figure 7-10).

***Adrenocortical Insufficiency* Addison's disease** is primary adrenal insufficiency; typically both mineralocorticoids and glucocorticoids are deficient. The most prevalent cause of Addison's disease is autoimmune destruction of the adrenal cortex, and tuberculosis is the second most common cause of the disorder. Because of the cortisol deficiency, ACTH secretion increases. ACTH can cause skin darkening, so an increase is seen in skin pigmentation (Figure 7-11), particularly in skin creases, scars, and gums. The loss of the mineralocorticoids results in contraction of extracellular volume, producing circulatory hypovolemia and therefore a drop in blood pressure. Because the loss of cortisol decreases the vasopressive response to catecholamines, peripheral resistance drops, thereby adding to the tendency toward hypotension. Hypotension predisposes people to circulatory shock. These people are also prone to have hypoglycemia when stressed or fasting. The hyperglycemic actions of other hormones, such as glucagon, epinephrine, and growth hormone, generally will prevent hypoglycemia at other times. Although volume depletion occurs because of the loss of mineralocorticoids, water intoxication can develop if a water load is given. The loss of cortisol impairs the ability to increase free water clearance in response to a water load and hence rid the body of the excess water. Patients with this condition will exhibit **hyperkalemic acidosis.** Because cortisol is important for muscle function, muscle weakness occurs in cortisol deficiency. The loss of cortisol results in anemia, decreased GI motility and secretion, and decreased iron and vitamin B_{12} absorption. The appetite will decrease because of the cortisol deficiency, and this decreased appetite coupled with the GI dysfunction will predispose these persons to weight loss. These patients often show disturbances in mood and behavior and are more susceptible to depression (Box 7-9).

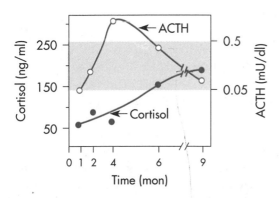

Figure 7-10 ■ Recovery of hypothalamic-pituitary-adrenal axis after long-term glucocorticoid treatment. *ACTH,* **Adrenocorticotropic hormone.** (Data from Graber AL, et al: *J Clin Endocrinol Metab* 25:11, 1965.)

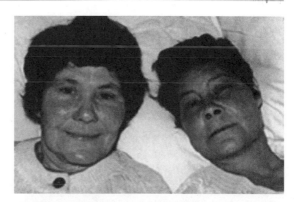

Figure 7-11 ■ Woman on right has Addison's disease. Note increased pigmentation relative to her healthy twin sister on left. (From Hall R, Evered DC: *Color atlas of endocrinology,* ed 2, London, 1990, Mosby-Wolfe.)

BOX 7-9

Manifestations of Primary Adrenocortical Insufficiency

Cortisol Deficiency

Gastrointestinal
  Anorexia
  Nausea
  Vomiting
  Diarrhea
  Abdominal pain
  Weight loss
Mental
  Confusion
  Psychosis
Metabolic
  Hypoglycemia
  Impaired gluconeogenesis
  Increased insulin sensitivity
Cardiovascular/renal
  Impaired free water clearance
  Impaired pressor response to catecholamines
  Hypotension
Pituitary
  Increased adrenocorticotropic hormone
    secretion
  Hyperpigmentation

Aldosterone Deficiency

Inability to conserve sodium
    Decreased extracellular fluid volume
    Decreased blood volume
    Weight loss
    Decreased cardiac output
    Increased renin production
    Hypotension
    Shock
Impaired renal secretion of potassium and
    hydrogen
    Hyperkalemia
    Metabolic acidosis

Adrenocortical Excess

Cushing's Syndrome Adrenocortical hormone excess is termed **Cushing's syndrome.** Pharmacologic use of exogenous corticosteroids is now the most common cause of Cushing's syndrome. The next most prevalent cause is ACTH-secreting tumors. The form of Cushing's syndrome caused by a functional pituitary adenoma is called **Cushing's disease.** A fourth cause is primary hypercortisolism resulting from a functional adrenal tumor. If the disorder is primary or if it is a result of corticosteroid treatment, ACTH secretion will be suppressed and increased skin pigmentation will not occur. However, if the hypersecretion of the adrenal is a result of an ACTH-secreting nonpituitary tumor, ACTH lev-els sometimes become high enough to increase skin pigmentation. Increased cortisol secretion causes a tendency to gain weight, with a characteristic centripetal fat distribution and a "buffalo hump" (Table 7-4). The face will appear round (fat deposition), and the cheeks may be reddened, in part because of the polycythemia. The limbs will be thin as a result of skeletal muscle wasting (from increased proteolysis), and muscle weakness will be evident (from muscle proteolysis and hypokalemia). Proximal muscle weakness is apparent, so the patient may have difficulty with stair climbing or rising from a sitting position. The abdominal fat accumulation, coupled with atrophy of the abdominal muscles and thinning of the skin, will produce a large, protruding abdomen. Purple abdominal striae are seen as a result of the damage to the skin by the prolonged proteolysis, increased intraabdominal fat, and loss of abdominal muscle tone (Figure 7-12). Capillary fragility is seen as a result of damage to the connective tissue supporting the capillaries. Patients are likely to show signs of osteoporosis and poor wound healing. They have metabolic disturbances that include glucose intolerance, hyperglycemia, and insulin resistance. Prolonged hypercortisolism can lead to manifestations of diabetes mellitus. Because of the suppression of the immune system caused by the glucocorticoids, patients are more susceptible to infection. Mineralocorticoid activities of the glucocorticoids and the possible elevation of aldosterone secretion produce salt retention and subsequent water retention, resulting in hypertension. Excessive androgen secretion in women can produce hirsutism, male pattern baldness, and clitoral enlargement (adrenogenital syndrome).

Conn's Syndrome Primary hyperaldosteronism is called **Conn's syndrome.** It frequently occurs as a result of aldosterone-secreting tumors. Excessive mineralocorticoid secretion results in potassium depletion, sodium retention, muscle weakness, hypertension, hypokalemic alkalosis, and polyuria. Although extracellular fluid volume increases, edema is not common because of hypervolemia-induced ANP release that results in natriuresis.

Congenital Adrenal Hyperplasia Any enzyme blockage that decreases cortisol synthesis will increase ACTH secretion and produce adrenal hyperplasia. The most common form of congenital adrenal hyperplasia occurs as a result of a deficiency of the enzyme **21-hydroxylase** (CYP21). These individuals cannot produce normal quantities of cortisol, **deoxycortisol,** DOC, corticosterone, or aldosterone. Because of impaired cortisol production and resultant elevated ACTH levels,

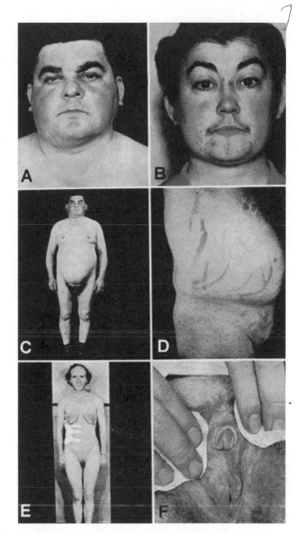

Figure 7-12 ■ A to D, **Cushing's syndrome with typical moon face, reddish cheeks, truncal obesity, and abdominal striae.** E and F, **Woman with adrenogenital syndrome.** (From Wilson JD, Foster DW: *Williams' textbook of endocrinology,* ed 8, Philadelphia, 1992, WB Saunders.)

steroidogenesis is stimulated, increasing the synthesis of those products formed before the blockage. Because this includes the adrenal androgens, a female fetus will be masculinized. Because they are unable to produce the mineralocorticoids, aldosterone, DOC, and corticosterone, patients with this disorder have difficulty retaining salt and maintaining extracellular volume. Consequently, they are likely to be hypotensive. If the blockage is at the next step, **11β-hydroxylase** (CYP11B), DOC will be formed and the levels of DOC will accumulate. Because DOC is a mineralocorticoid and the levels become high, these individuals tend to retain salt and water and become hypertensive. The elevated androgen levels can cause masculinization of a female fetus. If there is a deficiency of 17α-hydroxylase, neither cortisol nor sex hormones are produced. The inability to produce normal androgen levels during fetal development can result in a female phenotype for both males and females. A complete deficiency of **3β-hydroxysteroid dehydrogenase (3β-HSD)** is fatal. An incomplete deficiency results in the inability to produce adequate quantities of mineralocorticoids, glucocorticoids, and strong androgens or estrogens. The adrenal produces large quantities of the weak androgen DHEA. This can result in some masculinization of a female fetus and incomplete masculinization of a male fetus.

Summary

1. The adrenal gland is composed of a cortex, which is of mesodermal origin, and a medulla, which is of neuroectodermal origin. The cortex produces steroid hormones, and the medulla produces catecholamines.

2. Rate-limiting enzymes in medullary catecholamine synthesis are tyrosine hydroxylase and phenylethanolamine *N*-methyltransferase. Cortisol induces the enzyme phenylethanolamine *N*-methyltransferase.

3. Catecholamines increase serum glucose and fatty acid levels. They stimulate gluconeogenesis, glycogenolysis, and lipolysis. The in vivo action of catecholamines on the cardiovascular system depends on the type and dose of the catecholamine.

4. A pheochromocytoma is a tumor of chromaffin tissue that produces excessive quantities of catecholamines. Symptoms of pheochromocytoma are often sporadic and include hypertension, headaches, sweating, anxiety, palpitations, chest pain, and orthostatic hypotension.

5. The zona glomerulosa of the adrenal cortex is the site of aldosterone production. Aldosterone is the strongest naturally occurring mineralocorticoid in humans.

6. Major stimuli for aldosterone production are a rise in angiotensin II and a rise in serum potassium concentration.

7. Major actions of angiotensin II are vasoconstriction, increased growth and vascularity of the zona glomerulosa, increased sidechain cleavage enzyme activity, and increased aldosterone synthesis.

8. Major actions of aldosterone include renal sodium and water retention, increased renal potassium, and hydrogen secretion.

9. Glucocorticoids and sex hormones are produced primarily in the zona fasciculata and zona reticularis of the adrenal cortex. Cortisol is the major glucocorticoid, and dehydroepiandrosterone (DHEA) and androstenedione are the major sex hormones produced in the human adrenal cortex.

10. Major stimuli for cortisol secretion include stress, hypoglycemia, hemorrhage, and adrenocorticotropic hormone (ACTH).

11. Major actions of cortisol include increasing glycogenesis, gluconeogenesis, lipolysis, and proteolysis. Cortisol is hyperglycemic. Cortisol is antiinflammatory, immunosuppressive, and permissive for catecholamine's calorigenic and vasopressive actions.

12. Addison's disease is adrenocortical insufficiency. Common symptoms include hypotension, hyperpigmentation, muscle weakness, anorexia, hypoglycemia, and hyperkalemic acidosis.

13. Cushing's syndrome results from hypercortisolemia. If the basis of the disorder is increased pituitary adrenocorticotropin secretion, the disorder is called *Cushing's disease*. Common symptoms of Cushing's syndrome include centripetal fat distribution, muscle wasting, proximal muscle weakness, thin skin with abdominal striae, capillary fragility, insulin resistance, and polycythemia.

14. Congenital adrenal hyperplasia results from a congenital enzyme deficiency that blocks production of cortisol. The enzyme blockage results in elevated ACTH secretion, which stimulates adrenal cortical growth and secretion of precursors produced before the block. A 21-hydroxylase deficiency is the most common form.

■ KEY WORDS AND CONCEPTS

- Catecholamines
- Epinephrine
- Norepinephrine
- Dopamine
- Mineralocorticoids
- Glucocorticoids
- Chromaffin cells
- Pheochromocytes
- Chromaffin granules
- Chromagranin
- Dihydroxyphenylalanine (DOPA)
- Tyrosine hydroxylase
- Phenylethanolamine *N*-methyltransferase (PNMT)
- Monoamine oxidase (MAO)
- Catechol-*O*-methyltransferase (COMT)
- Vanillylmandelic acid (VMA)
- Metanephrine
- α Receptors
- β Receptors
- Normetanephrine
- Hormone-sensitive lipase (HSL)
- Acetoacetic acid
- β-Hydroxybutyric acid
- Acetone
- Pheochromocytoma
- Fetal zone
- Definitive zone
- Zona glomerulosa
- 17α-Hydroxylase/17,20-lyase (CYP17)
- Zona fasciculata
- Zona reticularis
- Aldosterone
- Deoxycorticosterone (DOC)
- Cortisol
- Dehydroepiandrosterone (DHEA)
- Androstenedione
- Side-chain cleavage (SCC) enzyme (CYP11A1)
- Adrenogenital syndrome
- Hirsutism
- Angiotensin II
- Renin
- Angiotensinogen
- Angiotensin I
- Angiotensin-converting enzyme (ACE)
- Hypokalemic alkalosis
- Aldosterone escape
- Atrial natriuretic peptide (ANP)
- Corticosterone
- Transcortin
- Corticosteroid-binding globulin (CBG)
- Centripetal fat distribution
- Buffalo hump
- Erythropoietin
- Polycythemia
- Addison's disease
- Hyperkalemic acidosis
- Cushing's syndrome
- Cushing's disease
- Conn's syndrome
- Congenital adrenal hyperplasia

- 21-Hydroxylase (CYP21)
- Deoxycortisol
- 11β-Hydroxylase (CYP11B)
- 3β-Hydroxysteroid dehydrogenase (3β-HSD)

■ SELF-STUDY PROBLEMS

1. What is the significance of the anatomic proximity of the adrenal medulla and adrenal cortex?
2. What is the significance of the enzyme tyrosine hydroxylase?
3. Why can the adrenal cortex atrophy when synthetic glucocorticoids are administered?
4. Explain the differences between the cause of orthostatic hypotension in patients with orthostatic hypotension associated with pheochromocytoma and orthostatic hypotension with Addison's disease.

5. Why are the consequences of a secondary pituitary ACTH insufficiency generally less severe than those of a primary adrenal insufficiency?

■ BIBLIOGRAPHY

Bravo EL: Evolving concepts in the pathophysiology, diagnosis, and treatment of pheochromocytoma, *Endocr Rev* 15:356, 1994.

Munck A, Guyre PM: Glucocorticoid hormones in stress:physiological and pharmacological actions, *News Physiol Sci* 1:69, 1987.

Orth DN, Kovacs WJ: The adrenal cortex. In Wilson JD, Foster DW, Kronenberg HM, Larsen PR: *Williams' textbook of endocrinology,* ed 9, Philadelphia, 1998, WB Saunders, pp 517-664.

CHAPTER 8

Male Reproductive System

Objectives

1. Describe the role of hormones in male and female reproductive tract development.
2. Identify the anatomic site of the blood-testis barrier.
3. Describe the relationship between Leydig cells and Sertoli cells.
4. List the functions of the Sertoli cells.
5. List the functions of the Leydig cells.
6. Explain the regulation of Sertoli cell and Leydig cell function.

7. List the major actions of androgens.
8. Describe the role of hormones in the regulation of spermatogenesis.
9. Describe the endocrine changes occurring at puberty and in senescence in the normal male.
10. Describe the physiologic basis for the major symptoms in Klinefelter's syndrome, 5α-reductase deficiency, testicular feminization, and Kallmann's syndrome.

■ DEVELOPMENT OF THE MALE REPRODUCTIVE TRACT

The genetic sex of a fetus depends on the nature of the sex chromosomes contributed by the egg and the sperm. Normally there are 46 chromosomes, consisting of 22 sets of autosomes and a set of sex chromosomes. The **sex chromosomes** are called X and Y chromosomes; XX is the normal pattern for the female, and XY is the normal pattern for the male. The short arm of the Y chromosome contains the gene regulating the differentiation of the primitive gonad into a testis.

Before 6 weeks of gestation, the fetus contains indifferent gonads that have formed from the gonadal ridge. At this stage, the gonads have the potential of becoming either ovaries or testes (Figure 8-1). By 6 weeks of gestation, the gonads contain germ cells, stromal cells that will become **Leydig cells** or thecal cells, and supporting cells that will become either **Sertoli cells** or granulosa cells. Located on the short arm of the Y chromosome is the testis-determining gene referred to as **SRY (sex-determining region Y)**. This gene encodes the putative testicular-determining factor that regulates the development of the testis and is distinct from the gene encoding the H-Y antigen, a male-specific protein once thought to be the protein regulating testicular development. Lack of the H-Y antigen produces problems with

153

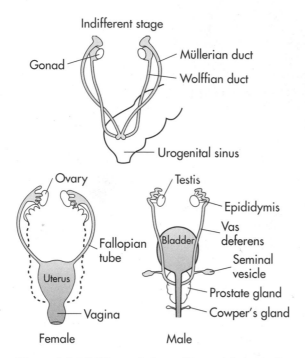

Female   Male

Figure 8-1 ▪ Differentiation of internal genitalia and primordial ducts. (Redrawn from George FW, Wilson JD: Embryology of the genital tract. In Walsh PC, et al, editors: *Campbell's urology,* ed 6, Philadelphia, 1992, WB Saunders.)

spermatogenesis and therefore fertility. If SRY is present, the undifferentiated gonad becomes a testis and the primordial germ cells become the spermatogonia. The testis develops between 6 and 8 weeks of gestation.

Although genes regulate the development of the ovaries and testes, hormones mediate phenotypic gender expression. The fetus originally develops with multipotential internal and external genitalia (Figure 8-2). Internally there are two **wolffian ducts,** which have the potential of becoming male internal genitalia, and two **müllerian ducts,** which have the potential of becoming female internal genitalia. Whether male or female internal genitalia develop depends on the presence or absence of two hormones produced by the fetal testis—**testoster-**

one and **müllerian-inhibiting substance (MIS)** (Box 8-1).

Testosterone is produced by the Leydig cells of the testis, and MIS is produced by the Sertoli cells of the seminiferous tubules. By 8 weeks of gestation, the fetal testis is actively producing testosterone. Because the fetal pituitary is not yet secreting luteinizing hormone (LH), testosterone production is regulated by placental human chorionic gonadotropin (hCG). Testosterone acts in a paracrine manner to unilaterally stimulate growth and development of the wolffian ducts into the epididymis, vas deferens, seminal vesicles, and ejaculatory ducts. The Ser-

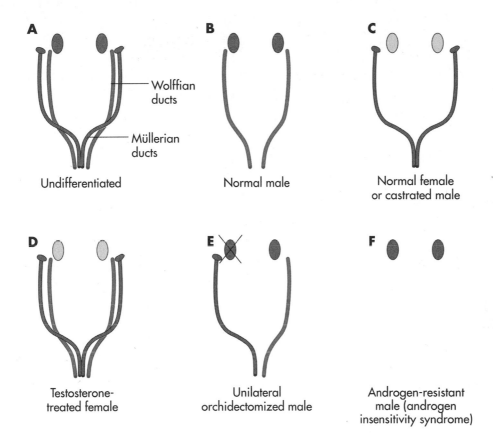

Figure 8-2 ■ **Regulation of development of internal genitalia. Both wolffian and müllerian ducts are originally present in both male and female fetuses (undifferentiated) (A). If functional testes are present, wolffian ducts develop and müllerian ducts regress (B). If no testes are present, müllerian ducts develop and wolffian ducts are lost (C). If a female fetus is exposed to testosterone, both ductile systems can remain (D). If a testis is removed unilaterally (orchidectomized), the müllerian duct will develop and the wolffian duct will regress on one side (E). A male with functional testes but androgen insensitivity will show regression of both ductile systems (F).**

toli cells of the fetal testis produce the peptide hormone MIS, which stimulates regression of the müllerian ducts. In the absence of MIS, the müllerian ducts are retained and become female internal genitalia—fallopian tubes, uterus, cervix, and upper one third of the vagina. In the absence of testosterone, the wolffian ducts regress. This effect is local; if a testis is absent on one side, the müllerian duct will be retained on that side. If high testosterone levels are present in a female fetus because of congenital adrenal disorders, experimentally, or because of maternal endocrine disorders, both sets of ducts can be retained. **Dihydrotestosterone (DHT)** is not involved in the masculinization of these internal genitalia because the enzyme 5α-reductase is not expressed in these tissues at the time of differentiation of the wolffian duct.

Development of the external genitalia is also hormonally regulated, and differentiation occurs between 9 and 12 weeks of gestation (Box 8-2). Androgens, particularly DHT, are respon-

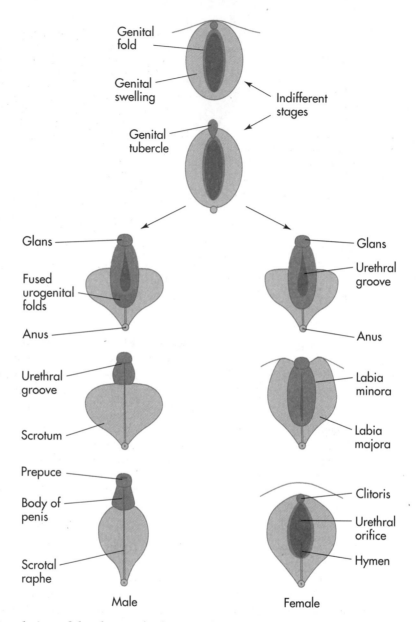

Figure 8-3 ■ **Regulation of development of external genitalia. In the presence of DHT between 9 and 12 weeks' gestation, male external genitalia develop from the genital tubercle, genital fold, genital swelling, and urogenital sinus. In the absence of DHT, female external genitalia develop.**

TABLE 8-1	
Time frame for development of fetal male reproductive system	
6 to 8 weeks' gestation	Differentiation of testes
8 weeks' gestation	Retention of wolffian ducts
	Regression of müllerian ducts
9 to 12 weeks' gestation	Development of male-type external genitalia

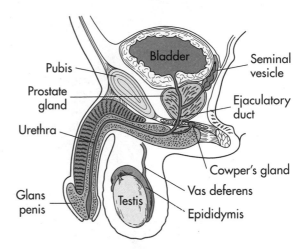

Figure 8-4 ■ Anatomy of male genitalia. (Modified from The Stanford Project [CLASS]: *Clinical anatomy principles,* St Louis, 1996, Mosby.)

sible for transforming the multipotential fetal external genitalia (genital tubercle, genital fold, genital swelling, and urogenital sinus) into the male prostate, penis, penile urethra, and scrotum (Figure 8-3) (Table 8-1). These tissues remain ones in which DHT is produced and where DHT serves as the most potent androgen.

In the absence of androgen exposure, the external genitalia develop into the labia, clitoris, and lower two thirds of the vagina. If **5α-reductase,** the enzyme required to convert testosterone to DHT, is deficient, the external genitalia might be mistaken for female.

The ovary is quiescent during gestation. Ovarian secretions are not involved in fetal differentiation of the female reproductive system. In the absence of either ovary or testis, female internal and external genitalia develop.

■ ANATOMY OF THE TESTIS

During the third trimester, because of the presence of androgens and MIS and possibly increased intraabdominal pressure the testes descend from their retroperitoneal position high in the abdominal cavity through the inguinal canals and into the scrotum (Figure 8-4). The location in the scrotum is essential because it allows for a testicular temperature about 2° C below core temperature. This lower temperature is

necessary for normal spermatogenesis. Failure of the testes to descend results in infertility. Spermatogenesis is so temperature dependent that wearing tight-fitting underwear or frequent bathing in hot water can decrease fertility. The normal adult testis has an average volume slightly more than 18 ml.

The **seminiferous tubules** comprise more than 80% of the mass of the adult testis (Figure 8-5). These tubules are the site of gametogenesis. Between the seminiferous tubules are interstitial cells, or Leydig cells, which are the site of testicular androgen production.

Sperm and tubular fluid are produced in the seminiferous tubules. They enter a series of anastomosing tubules called the **rete testis** and then pass through the **efferent ductules,** which coalesce into a single duct called the **epididymis.** The epididymis, a tightly coiled structure on the surface of the testis, is approximately 5 m long. It is divided into a head (caput), body (corpus), and tail (cauda). The epididymis drains into the **vas deferens.** Sperm entering the head of the epididymis are imma-

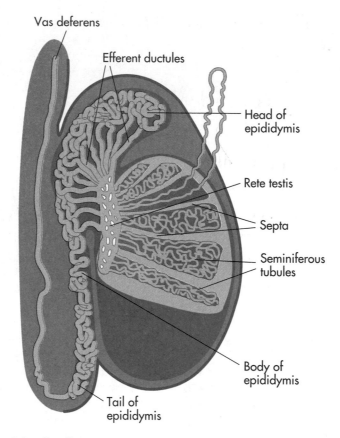

Figure 8-5 ■ **Testis and its ductile system. Septa divide the testis into lobules that are occupied by highly convoluted seminiferous tubules.** (Redrawn from Fawcett DW, editor: *Bloom and Fawcett's textbook of histology,* ed 12, New York, 1994, Chapman & Hall.)

ture and incapable of directional motility or capacitation. While they remain in the epididymis, they mature and acquire these capabilities. However, the chemical composition of seminal fluid inhibits both motility and capacitation. The epididymis and the ampulla of the vas deferens serve as sperm storage sites.

During the sperm's transit through these tubules, its environment is determined by the seminal fluids bathing the sperm. These fluids are produced by the seminiferous tubules, the cells comprising the ductile system, and the ac-

cessory glands of the male reproductive system: **seminal vesicles, prostate,** and **Cowper's (bulbourethral) glands.** The content of these fluids is influenced by the availability of testicular androgens.

Seminiferous Tubules

The testis contains hundreds of tightly packed seminiferous tubules that consist of peritubular cells, a basement membrane, the germinal epithelium, developing germ cells, and Sertoli cells (Figure 8-6).

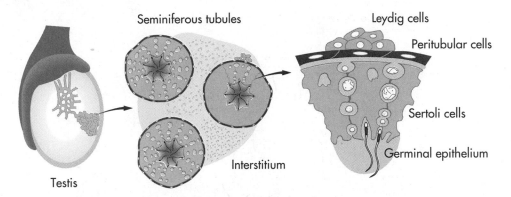

Figure 8-6 ■ **Cell biology of testis.** (Redrawn from Skinner MK: *Endocr Rev* 12:45, 1991.)

BOX 8-3

Functions of Sertoli Cells

- Produce müllerian-inhibiting substance
- Aromatize androgens to estrogen
- Act in supportive role for germ cells
- Form blood-testis barrier
- Produce androgen-binding protein
- Produce inhibin
- Produce seminiferous tubule fluid

Sertoli cells line the basement membrane of the seminiferous tubules and extend the thickness of the tubule wall; they surround and invest the developing germ cells (Box 8-3). Tight junctions between these cells form the anatomic basis for the blood-testis barrier (Figure 8-7).

Testosterone is necessary for the maintenance of the integrity of this tight junction. Sertoli cells restrict transport between the blood and the developing germ cells and in this manner control germ cell nutrient availability. The tight junction separates the seminiferous tubule into two compartments—a **basal compartment,** which is in close contact with extracellular fluids, and an **adluminal compartment,** which is separated from extracellular fluids and contains the more advanced stages of differentiating germ cells. The adluminal compartment is contiguous with the lumen of the seminiferous tubules. Sertoli cells are sometimes referred to as **nurse cells** because they control the germ cell environment. In many respects they are the male counterpart of the ovarian granulosa cells. Sertoli cells have multiple additional functions. Although they lack most of the enzymes necessary for steroidogenesis, they do have P_{450} aromatase (aromatase), the enzyme necessary to convert Leydig cell–derived androgens to estrogens. In addition, on stimulation with follicle-stimulating hormone (FSH) and androgens, they produce **androgen-binding protein.** This binding protein is similar to the plasma protein **sex hormone–binding globulin (SHBG)** except that it is located intratesticularly and serves to maintain high androgen levels within the testis and seminal fluids. This protein is also referred to as **testosterone-estrogen binding globulin (TeBG).** It binds testosterone, estradiol, and DHT with high affinity. FSH stimulates Sertoli cell production of the protein **plasminogen activator,** which activates **plasmin,** a

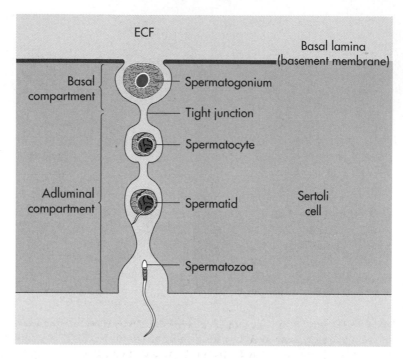

ECF

Basal lamina
(basement membrane)

Basal
compartment

Spermatogonium

Tight junction

Spermatocyte

Adluminal
compartment

Spermatid

Sertoli
cell

Spermatozoa

Figure 8-7 ■ **Sertoli cells form the blood-testis barrier.** *ECF,* **Extracellular fluid.**

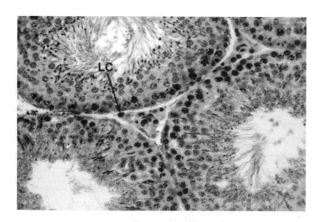

LC

Figure 8-8 ■ **Section of testis showing portions of three seminiferous tubules. Leydig cell** *(LC)* **is indicated in interstitium between tubules.**

protein aiding in **spermiation,** or the final detachment of sperm (Figure 8-8).

Sertoli cells produce seminiferous tubule fluid. This fluid provides an appropriate bathing medium for the sperm; it contains nutrients and inhibits capacitation and motility, thereby prolonging viability. It assists in washing sperm from the tubule lumen into the epididymis. In addition, Sertoli cells produce numerous peptides that act in endocrine, paracrine, or autocrine manners to regulate testicular function. These compounds include inhibin, activin, follistatin, insulin-like growth factor-I, transforming growth factors, transferrin, and numerous cytokines. Many of these compounds are also produced by Leydig cells. Although Sertoli cells have FSH and androgen receptors, they lack LH receptors (Figure 8-9).

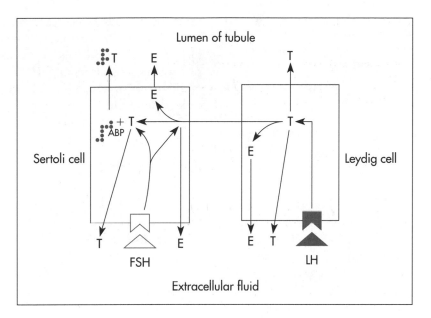

Figure 8-9 ■ **Summary of cooperation of Leydig and Sertoli cells in hormone production. Luteinizing hormone *(LH)* acts on Leydig cells to stimulate androgen production *(T)*. These androgens can serve as substrates for estrogen *(E)* production in either Leydig or Sertoli cells. Follicle-stimulating hormone *(FSH)* acts on Sertoli cells to stimulate estrogen production from testosterone. FSH synergizes with testosterone to stimulate androgen-binding protein *(ABP)* production in Sertoli cells. ABP binds androgens and is important in maintenance of high intratesticular androgen levels.**

Leydig Cells

The primary site of testicular androgen synthesis is the Leydig cells. These **interstitial cells** are interspersed between the seminiferous tubules and have LH receptors but probably not FSH receptors. LH stimulates steroidogenesis by cyclic adenosine monophosphate–mediated processes. Steroidogenesis increases in fetal Leydig cells between 8 and 18 weeks of gestation. By 18 weeks of gestation, Leydig cells represent 50% of testicular volume. The androgens produced at this time are crucial for the development of the male reproductive tract. In the neonate, testicular steroidogenesis again surges, reaching relatively highlevels at 2 to 3 months postpartum. The significance of this brief postnatal rise in androgen production is

not known. Testicular steroidogenesis then remains at low levels until puberty, when an increase in LH secretion activates the testes and androgen production rises sharply. Although there is no true male menopause, testicular androgen production gradually decreases with senescence.

■ TESTICULAR STEROIDOGENESIS

The predominant androgen produced by the testis is testosterone, and the testes produce 95% of the testosterone found in serum of adult men (Table 8-2). The bulk of the remaining testosterone is produced by the adrenal. Although the testis secretes limited quantities of estrogens and DHT, the primary source of these hormones in adult men is peripheral formation from tes-

---

TABLE 8-2

Approximate hormone production rates in adult man

Testosterone	5 mg/day
Estradiol	10-15 μg/day
Dihydrotestosterone	50-100 μg/day
17α-Hydroxyprogesterone	1-2 mg/day

---

ticular androgens. In many tissues, testosterone is converted by the action of the enzyme 5α-reductase to the more potent androgen DHT. Although both hormones interact with the same receptor, DHT has about 2.5 times the potency of testosterone. Testosterone can also be aromatized to estrogens in many tissues; the predominant source of circulating estrogens in the male is adipose tissue aromatization of testicular and adrenal androgens. Sertoli and Leydig cells produce 10% to 15% of serum estrogens in normal adult men. Two other less potent androgens produced in the testis are **dehydroepiandrosterone (DHEA)** and **androstenedione.** Leydig cells also produce progesterone and 17α-hydroxyprogesterone. Figure 8-10 shows the pathways involved in the biosynthesis of androgen and estrogen.

■ CONTROL OF TESTICULAR STEROIDOGENESIS

LH acts on Leydig cells to stimulate steroidogenesis, and FSH synergizes with androgens to stimulate androgen-binding protein production by Sertoli cells. This protein plays an important role in maintaining high intratesticular androgen levels in the vicinity of the developing germ cells. Testosterone acts on the pituitary and hypothalamus to inhibit gonadotropin-releasing hormone (GnRH) production in the hypothalamus and GnRH action on the gonadotrope, which inhibits LH production and secretion. Af-

ter castration, LH levels rise. Androgens, on the other hand, will not return FSH secretion to normal after castration, leading to the search for physiologic regulators of FSH. The protein hormone **inhibin,** which is produced in the Sertoli cells, can inhibit FSH secretion.

Figure 8-11 shows the steps in the regulation of testicular function.

■ ANDROGENS
Transport

Steroid hormones are sparingly soluble in blood, and therefore approximately 87% of the circulating androgens are bound to proteins. Approximately 40% is bound to SHBG, and the other 47% is bound to albumin and other proteins.

Metabolism

Testosterone and its metabolites are primarily excreted in the urine (Figure 8-12). Approximately 50% of excreted androgens are found as urinary **17-ketosteroids,** with most of the remainder being conjugated androgens or diol or triol derivatives.

Only about 30% of the 17-ketosteroids in urine are from the testis; the rest are produced from adrenal androgens. In fact, urinary 17-ketosteroid levels approach normal levels in castrated men. The level of these urinary compounds more appropriately reflects adrenal androgen activity. Androgens are conjugated with glucuronate or sulfate in the liver, and these **conjugated steroids** are excreted in the urine.

Testosterone can be metabolized to two potent hormones. 5α-Reductase converts testosterone to DHT, and aromatase converts it to estradiol. 5α-Reductase occurs primarily in the target organs. Tissues with high levels of this enzyme include the prostate, scrotum, penis, liver, hair follicles, and skin. Unlike testosterone, DHT cannot be aromatized to estrogens.

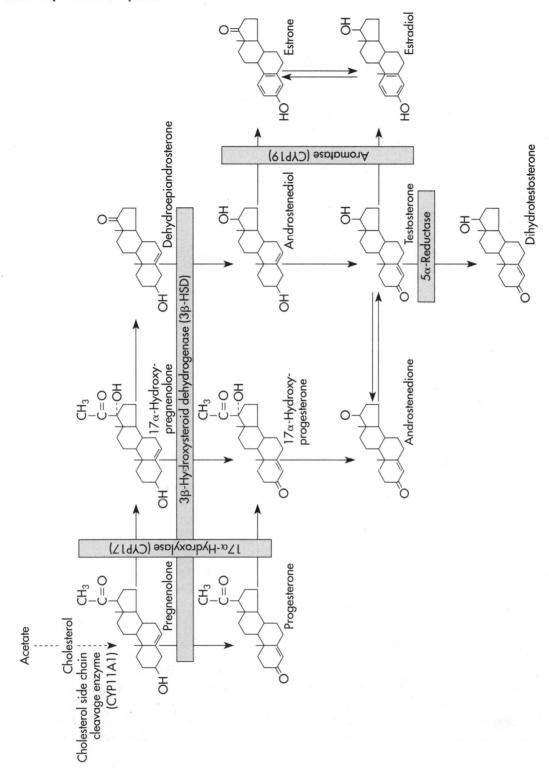

Figure 8-10 ■ **Pathways of testicular androgen and estrogen synthesis.**

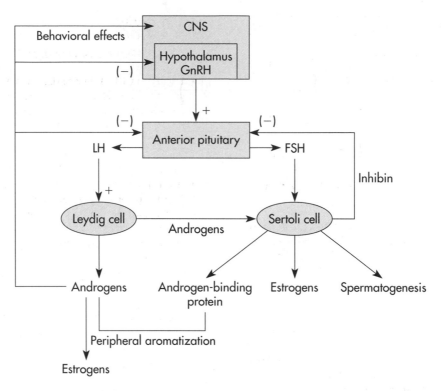

Figure 8-11 ■ **Summary of regulation of testicular function. Gonadotropin-releasing hormone *(GnRH)* stimulates secretion of anterior pituitary hormones—luteinizing hormone *(LH)* and follicle-stimulating hormone *(FSH)*. These hormones act on Leydig and Sertoli cells to stimulate production of hormones, androgen-binding protein, and sperm. Testicular androgens and inhibin can control production of LH and FSH. *CNS,* Central nervous system.**

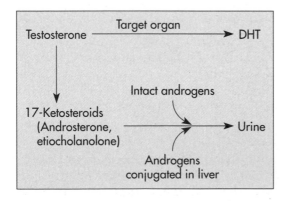

Figure 8-12 ■ **Metabolism of androgens. *DHT,* Dihydrotestosterone.**

Theoretically androgens can be administered orally. However, because the absorption of many naturally occurring androgens is minimal and their half-lives ($t_{1/2}$s) are relatively short, synthetic analogs that are more readily absorbed in the gastrointestinal tract and that have longer $t_{1/2}$s are generally used for oral treatment.

Mechanism of Action

Testosterone freely enters cells and acts either as testosterone, DHT, or estradiol (Figure 8-13). As is typical of steroid hormones, when the hormone binds to the receptor, it produces a con-

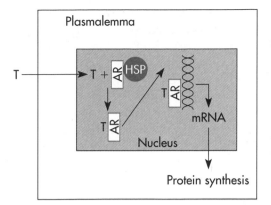

Plasmalemma

T

T + AR HSP

T AR

T AR

mRNA

Nucleus

Protein synthesis

Figure 8-13 ■ **Mechanism of action of testosterone** *(T)*. **Testosterone enters the cell, where it binds to the androgen receptor** *(AR),* **thereby releasing heat shock protein** *(HSP).* **Release of HSP produces conformational change in receptor that increases DNA-binding site availability, thereby permitting binding of ligand-bound receptor to hormone response element of DNA. Ligand-bound receptor acts as transcription factor regulating expression of androgen-sensitive genes.** (NOTE: **Following release of HSP, androgen receptors dimerize** *[not shown].*)

formational change that results in the release of **heat shock protein (HSP)** from the receptor. This increases availability of the DNA-binding sites, thereby permitting binding of the ligand-bound receptor to the **hormone response element (HRE)** of the DNA. From this location, the ligand-bound receptor acts as a transcription factor to regulate gene expression. The androgen receptor is a member of the steroid-thyroid-retinoic acid superfamily of receptors and as such is characterized as having a **DNA-binding domain,** a **ligand-binding domain,** and an **N-terminal region.**

Actions

Because androgens are soluble in lipids, they can diffuse into cells and interact with nuclear receptors. The predominant actions of andro-

---

BOX 8-4

Actions of Androgens

- Regulation of differentiation of male internal and external genitalia in fetus
- Stimulation of growth, development, and function of male internal and external genitalia
- Stimulation of sexual hair development
- Stimulation of sebaceous gland secretion
- Stimulation of erythropoietin synthesis
- Control of protein anabolic effects
- Stimulation of bone growth and closure of epiphyses
- Initiation and maintenance of spermatogenesis
- Stimulation of androgen-binding protein synthesis (synergizes with follicle-stimulating hormone [FSH])
- Maintenance of secretions of sex glands
- Regulation of behavioral effects, including libido

---

gens in males include regulation or reproduction and stimulation of reproductive system growth and maturation (Box 8-4).

In the fetus, testosterone is responsible for the development of the wolffian ducts into epididymis, vas deferens, seminal vesicles, and ejaculatory ducts; DHT is responsible for the development of male external genitalia (penis, scrotum) and the prostate. Exposure of the neonatal rat to aromatizable androgens permanently blocks the ability of the hypothalamus to regulate gonadotropin secretion in a cyclic manner and hence supports an estrous cycle. Gonadotropin secretion in these rats is characterized as tonic.

At puberty, androgens stimulate bone growth but also terminate growth by promoting epiphyseal closure. They stimulate growth and maturation of the external and internal genitalia. In addition, androgens stimulate secretion from the secondary sex glands. They are responsible for the development of the male-type hair pattern that includes pubic hair formation in a diamond-shaped escutcheon, beard growth, and a male scalp hair pattern that includes regression of the hair in the temples and the expression of male-pattern baldness.

Androgens stimulate sebaceous gland secretion and increase the tendency for acne formation at puberty. They stimulate the growth of the larynx, which leads to deepening of the voice. Because androgens are protein anabolic, their use has been abused. Unfortunately, all anabolic steroids presently available retain some androgen activity that cannot be completely isolated from their protein anabolic effects. Both in conjunction with their anabolic effect and through direct renal actions, androgens stimulate retention of nitrogen, sodium, phosphate, potassium, calcium, and sulfate. Because androgens stimulate erythropoietin synthesis, the hematocrit value is greater in men than in women.

Androgens are responsible for male sexual behavior in nonprimate species. Although human sexual behavior is complex and involves many components, androgens, perhaps after aromatization to estrogens within the central nervous system, can influence sexual behavior and libido.

Androgen-binding protein synthesis in the Sertoli cells is stimulated by androgens synergizing with FSH. This protein serves to maintain high androgen levels within the testis, which is important for normal testicular function and spermatogenesis. Intratesticular androgen levels are more than 200 times greater than blood levels, and spermatogenesis ceases if androgen levels are deficient. High levels of exogenously administered androgens can produce infertility because they block LH and FSH production. When LH levels drop, testicular androgen production drops, which can produce an intratesticular androgen deficiency although serum an-

drogen levels are high. In addition, high levels of androgens inhibit secretion of FSH, which is important for Sertoli cell function.

■ SPERMATOGENESIS

Spermatogenesis begins at puberty and continues through the remainder of a normal man's life. The stem cells, or **spermatogonia,** are diploid cells located along the basement membrane (basal lamina) of the seminiferous tubules (Figure 8-14). In this location, they are on the basilar side of the tight junction of the Sertoli cells and therefore are not within the blood-testis barrier. During successive cellular divisions, the developing germ cells remain attached to one another by cytoplasmic bridges that are removed as mature sperm are produced. The three steps in spermatogenesis are (1) mitotic divisions, which provide the cells that will become sperm, (2) meiotic divisions, which produce the haploid spermatids, and (3) spermiogenesis, in which spermatids are differentiated into sperm.

Spermiogenesis

The period of germ cell differentiation from secondary spermatocytes to spermatozoa is termed **spermiogenesis** (Figure 8-15). As the spermatid matures into a sperm, the size of the nucleus decreases and a prominent tail is formed. The tail contains microtubular structures similar to a flagellum; it serves to propel sperm. The chromatin material in the sperm nucleus condenses, and most of the cytoplasm is lost. The **acrosome** (Figure 8-16) is a membrane-enclosed structure on the head of the sperm that acts as a lysosome and contains proteolytic enzymes, including hyaluronic acid, that are important for penetration of the ovum. These enzymes remain inactive until the acrosomal reaction occurs.

Spermatozoa are found at the luminal surface of the seminiferous tubule. Release of sperm, or **spermiation,** requires the action of Sertoli cells. The time from spermatogonia to spermatozoa is approximately 70 days, and although spermatogenesis is continuous within the entire testis, within local regions of the testis all cells are at the same developmental stage. These waves occur in approximately 16-day cycles. There are multiple stages of spermatogenesis and numerous types of germ cells. However, the types can be simplified to include the spermatogonium (stem cell, diploid), spermatocytes (diploid), spermatid (haploid), and spermatozoa.

Sperm in the head of the epididymis are immature and incapable of directional motility or capacitation. Within the epididymis they undergo a 10- to 14-day maturation period. This maturation requires the presence of adequate testosterone levels. During this time, they are nourished by epididymal secretions. Changes occur in the head of the sperm that include condensation of the head and the appearance of *proacrosin* and *hyaluronidase.* By the time the sperm reach the tail of the epididymis, they are capable of directional motility and capacitation if placed in an appropriate environment. Sperm can be stored in the epididymal tail for several days. Sperm are moved through this ductile system by a combination of fluid pressure, ciliary motion, and peristaltic contraction.

Spermatogenesis is hormonally dependent. LH is required to stimulate androgen secretion, and androgens are absolutely essential for spermatogenesis. Without testosterone, spermatogenesis is arrested at the primary spermatocyte stage. FSH is necessary to initiate spermatogenesis and for long-term maintenance of normal levels of spermatogenesis. It facilitates sperm maturation through its action on Sertoli cells. There are no LH or FSH receptors on the germ cells; LH and FSH exert their effects on spermatogenesis through their actions on Leydig and Sertoli cells. In addition to the actions of hormones on spermatogenesis, vitamins A, C, and E are permissive agents in the early stages of spermatogenesis. Vitamins A and E are impor-

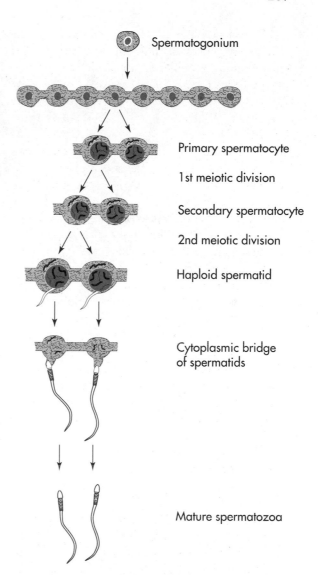

Figure 8-14 ■ Major stages of spermatogenesis. Spermatogonium undergoes mitosis to produce multiple primary spermatocytes. These spermatocytes remain joined by cytoplasmic bridges. Primary spermatocytes undergo the first meiotic division to become secondary spermatocytes and the second meiotic division (reduction-division) to become haploid spermatids. Spermatids mature, are released from cytoplasmic bridge, and differentiate into spermatozoa.

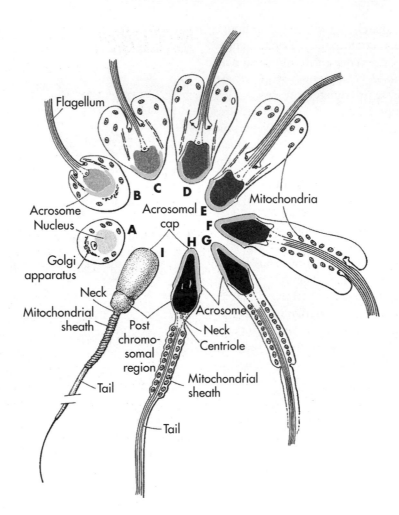

Figure 8-15 ■ **Spermatocyte** (A), **spermatid** (B-F), **and spermatozoon** (G-I). (From Carlson B: *Human embryology and developmental biology,* St Louis, 1994, Mosby.)

tant for the maintenance of the germinal epithelium. Numerous cytokines and growth factors are produced in the testis and appear to play an important role in intratesticular regulation.

■ SEMEN

Semen typically has a volume of 3 to 5 ml per ejaculation. It is primarily a secretion of the seminiferous tubules, prostate (30%), seminal

vesicles, and Cowper's (bulbourethral) glands. It contains nutrients, including fructose, hormones, and decapacitation factors. The seminal vesicles secrete approximately 60% of the volume. These glands are the primary source for semen prostaglandin and fructose. The alkaline secretions of the prostate are high in citrate, zinc, spermine, and acid phosphatase. The predominant buffers in semen are phosphate

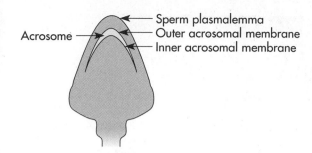

Figure 8-16 ■ **Acrosomal cap of head of sperm. Acrosome consists of two membranes: inner acrosomal membrane and outer acrosomal membrane that is in apposition to plasmalemma.**

BOX 8-5
Functions of Semen
• Provides bulk to sperm
• Maintains alkaline environment
• Buffers vaginal acidity
• Contains prostaglandins
• Prevents capacitation of sperm
• Provides nutrients to sperm
• Inhibits sperm motility in male tract

and bicarbonate. Hormones found in semen include androgens, estrogens, progestogens, and prostaglandins. These compounds are produced in the Leydig cells, Sertoli cells, prostate, and seminal vesicles. Other compounds in semen are **acrosin inhibitor,** which prevents conversion of proacrosin to acrosin in the sperm head, and the protein **spermine,** which is released from deteriorating sperm and is used as a marker for semen. The secretions of the Cowper's glands are high in mucus, and their primary function may be to lubricate the urethra.

Average sperm counts are reported to be from 60 to 100 million/ml semen. Men with sperm counts below 20 million/ml, less than 50% motile sperm, or less than 60% normally conformed sperm are often infertile.

Semen provides fluid bulk to the sperm and serves as a sperm nutrient source (Box 8-5). It contains chemicals that prevent sperm capacitation, thereby prolonging the viability of the sperm. In addition, the high potassium levels inhibit sperm motility, thereby prolonging viability. Semen contains buffers for the acidity of vaginal secretions, and the slightly alkaline pH of semen promotes sperm viability. Prostaglandins in semen may be important stimulators of

female reproductive tract motility, thereby aiding sperm movement in the female reproductive tract.

■ SPERM CAPACITATION

Sperm in semen are incapable of fertilizing an ovum. They acquire this capability after either spending time in the female reproductive tract or being washed free of the contents of semen. These changes in the sperm are referred to as **capacitation.** The ability of semen to inhibit capacitation prolongs sperm viability. There are multiple factors in semen inhibiting capacitation, and various names, such as **decapacitation factor,** have been applied to these compounds. Although visible anatomic changes in sperm do not accompany capacitation, biochemical and physiologic changes do. Sperm metabolic rate, membrane fluidity, intracellular calcium, and motility all increase after capacitation. Capacitation is necessary before the acrosomal reaction can occur.

The **acrosomal reaction** typically occurs when a capacitated sperm reaches the ovum; this reaction is essential for ovum penetration. The zona pellucida glycoprotein **ZP3** might induce the acrosomal reaction. During the acrosomal reaction, the outer acrosomal membrane (see Figure 8-16) fuses with the overlying plasmalemma of the sperm, resulting in progressive vesiculation of the membranes

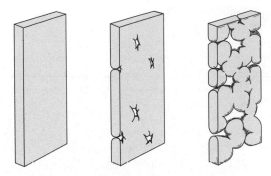

Figure 8-17 ■ Inferred stages in process of vesiculation between two opposed cellular membranes. (Redrawn from Barros C, Bedford JM, Franklin LE, Austin CR: *J Cell Biol* 34:C1, 1967.)

BOX 8-6

Pubertal Changes in Male

- Hypothalamic sensitivity to gonadal steroids decreases, leading to increased GnRH secretion
- Pituitary sensitivity to GnRH increases, leading to increased LH and FSH secretion (reset gonadostat)
- Increased serum LH and FSH levels, leading to increased Leydig cell number and activity, which lead to androgen secretion
- Increased androgen secretion, resulting in anatomic and physiologic changes typical of puberty

GnRH, Gonadotropin-releasing hormone; *LH,* luteinizing hormone; *FSH,* follicle-stimulating hormone.

(Figure 8-17) and exposure of the acrosomal matrix and inner membrane. This change increases extracellular accessibility of acrosomal proteolytic enzymes such as acrosin and hyaluronidase. **Acrosin** is a protease that hydrolyzes the glycoprotein of the zona pellucida surrounding the ovum. It is present in the acrosome as the zymogen proacrosin and is hydrolyzed during the acrosomal reaction. **Hyaluronidase** is a proteolytic enzyme that hydrolyzes the hyaluronic acid binding the cells of the cumulus oophorus.

■ ROLE OF PROLACTIN

The exact role of prolactin in normal reproductive function in the male is not known. However, hyperprolactinemia inhibits male reproductive function. It decreases gonadotropin secretion and gonadotropin action on the testis. Excessive secretion of prolactin can lead to infertility. Hyperprolactinemia can decrease testicular androgen production, decrease spermatogenesis, and produce impotence.

■ PUBERTY

Several years before puberty begins, adrenal androgen levels, under the influence of adrenocor-

ticotropic hormone, begin to rise, resulting in **adrenarche.** The early development of pubic and axillary hair and the early stages of the "growth spurt" are mediated by these androgens in both males and females.

At puberty, the frequency and amplitude of the GnRH pulses increase. This change increases LH and FSH secretion and ultimately testicular androgen production (Box 8-6 and Figure 8-18). Serum FSH and LH levels are relatively low before puberty, and the feedback regulation of androgens on LH is particularly sensitive. Immediately before puberty, intermittent sleep-associated surges in GnRH begin to occur. Gonadotrope sensitivity to GnRH increases, resulting in an increase in GnRH secretion. The sensitivity to negative feedback inhibition of testosterone on GnRH and LH secretion decreases. This change in sensitivity of the system is referred to as **resetting the gonadostat.** The resultant rise in serum LH and FSH levels stimulates growth of the testis, increased Leydig cell testosterone production, and spermatogenesis. The testes and penis enlarge in response to the in-

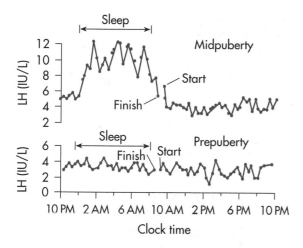

Figure 8-18 ■ Sleep-associated rises in luteinizing hormone *(LH)* secretion in the pubertal male. (Redrawn from Wilson GD, Foster DW, editors: *Williams' textbook of endocrinology,* ed 8, Philadelphia, 1992, WB Saunders.)

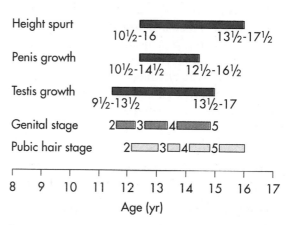

Figure 8-19 ■ Normal sequence of changes of male puberty. Numbers 2 to 5 refer to Tanner stages. (Data from Marshall WA, Tanner JM: *Arch Dis Child* 45:13, 1970.)

TABLE 8-2

Tanner pubertal stages in male

Stage	Genitals	Pubic hair
1	Preadolescent	Preadolescent, no pubic hair
2	Scrotum and testes enlarge, change in scrotal skin texture	Sparse, long, downy pubic hair, chiefly at base of penis
3	Growth of penis in length and further growth of testes and scrotum	Hair darker and coarser
4	Growth of penis in length and breadth, darkening of scrotal skin	Hair adult type but area covered is less than that of an adult
5	Adult-sized genitalia	Adult hair texture and quantity; hair is distributed in diamond-shaped escutcheon with hair extending up linea alba

Data from Marshall WA, Tanner JM: *Arch Dis Child* 45:13, 1970.

---

crease in serum androgen levels, and the physical changes characteristic of male puberty occur (Table 8-2 and Figure 8-19).

Neuronal control of the onset of puberty is a function of control of the pulse generator for GnRH, which resides in the medial basal hypothalamus. This pulse generator is actively functioning in the fetus and neonate but becomes relatively inactive until puberty. These neurons exhibit spontaneous rhythmicity.

■ SENESCENCE

There is no true menopause in men. However, as men age, gonadal sensitivity to LH decreases and androgen production drops. As this occurs, serum LH and FSH levels rise. Although sperm production typically begins to decline after age 50 years, many men can maintain reproductive function and spermatogenesis throughout life. Figure 8-20 shows how plasma testosterone levels change throughout the life span.

■ DISORDERS INVOLVING THE MALE REPRODUCTIVE TRACT

Klinefelter's Syndrome (Seminiferous Tubular Dysgenesis)

Men with an extra X chromosome have the genetic disorder called Klinefelter's syndrome. Although there are multiple permutations of the disorder, the most common form results in a 47,XXY karyotype. Individuals with this syndrome are phenotypically male because of the presence of the Y chromosome, but they typically have small testes and decreased germ cells (Figure 8-21). The testosterone levels are low to normal, and estradiol and gonadotropin levels are high. The high estradiol/testosterone ratio can lead to feminization, including the potential for gynecomastia. Patients with this disorder do not have normal spermatogenesis, and FSH levels are high because of abnormal Sertoli cell function.

5α-Reductase Deficiency

A deficiency of 5α-reductase results in decreased DHT formation. These individuals will typically have normal internal genitalia but incompletely masculinized external genitalia; they are often mistaken for females at birth, thereby potentially producing incomplete male hermaphroditism. The testosterone production is normal, and at puberty, when testosterone production occurs, some masculinization of the ex-

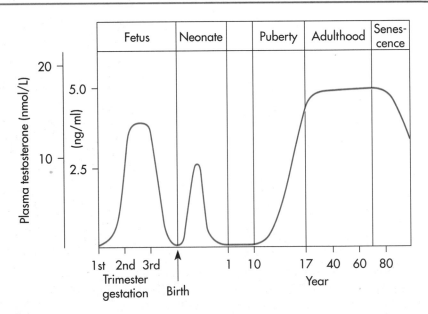

Figure 8-20 ■ Plasma testosterone levels during life span of normal male. (Redrawn from Wilson GD, Foster DW, editors: *Williams' textbook of endocrinology,* ed 8, Philadelphia, 1992, WB Saunders.)

ternal genitalia may occur. Normal development of male-type internal genitalia occurs because of the action of testosterone on wolffian duct development.

Androgen Insensitivity Syndrome

Androgen insensitivity syndrome (AIS; testicular feminization) results from a hereditary defect of the X chromosome gene controlling androgen receptor expression. Because the defect can range from partial to complete inability of the androgen receptor to respond to androgens, the magnitude of symptoms in individuals with the genetic defect is variable. **Male pseudohermaphroditism** can result because,

although the karyotype is 46,XY, the wolffian duct does not develop because androgen action is deficient and the müllerian duct regresses because testes and therefore MIS are present. Consequently, there are no functional internal genitalia.

The external genitalia typically develop as female, thereby giving the individuals a female phenotype (Figure 8-22). People with severe AIS have labia, a clitoris, and a short vagina because these structures do not develop from the müllerian ducts. Pubic and axillary hair is absent or sparse because the development of sexual hair is androgen dependent. Menstruation does not occur, and serum androgen levels are high or

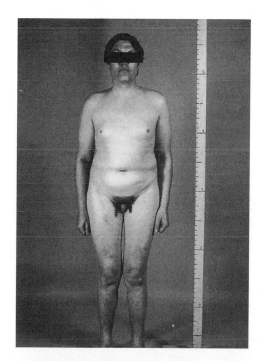

Figure 8-21 ■ **Klinefelter's syndrome in young man. Gynecomastia is present, and body shape is somewhat feminine.** (From Besser GM, Thorner MO: *Clinical endocrinology,* ed 2, London, 1994, Mosby-Wolfe.)

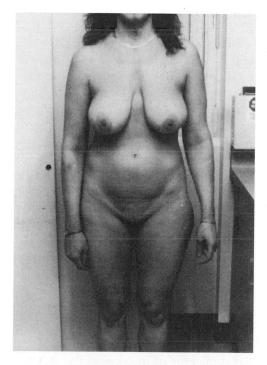

Figure 8-22 ■ **A 46,XY phenotypic woman with complete androgen insensitivity.** (From Quigley CA, et al: *Endocr Rev* 16:271, 1995.)

normal. When androgen production rises at puberty, estradiol production increases, both from the testes and from peripheral aromatization of androgens. Plasma androgen and LH levels are high because the receptor deficiency impairs feedback inhibition of LH secretion. The testes typically remain in the abdomen because androgens stimulate testicular descent.

Kallmann's Syndrome

Kallmann's syndrome is primary isolated gonadotropin deficiency. This genetic disorder is often associated with **anosmia,** or the loss of smell. People affected with this disorder have undescended testes (cryptorchism). Although there is normal embryonic development of the wolffian duct–derived structures, penis development is deficient and microphallus results. These effects probably result from the fact that early fetal development of the internal genitalia is controlled by testicular androgens that are regulated by placental hCG rather than fetal LH. The inability of the fetus to secrete normal quantities of LH has an impact on testicular function later in development, when androgens regulate growth of the external genitalia. The severity of the impairment of LH secretion is variable, as is the severity of the reproductive problems associated with the disorder.

Summary

1. Development of the fetal reproductive system is hormonally regulated. The original fetal reproductive system is multipotential and contains both müllerian and wolffian ducts. If testes are present and produce müllerian-inhibiting substance (MIS) at approximately 8 weeks of gestation, the müllerian ducts regress. If testosterone is produced, the wolffian ducts develop into the epididymis, vas deferens, seminal vesicles, and ejaculatory ducts. If neither MIS nor testosterone is present, the wolffian ducts regress and the müllerian ducts develop into the fallopian tubes, uterus, cervix, and upper one third of the vagina.
2. At approximately 9 to 12 weeks of gestation, the external genitalia develop. If dihydrotestosterone (DHT) is present, a penis and scrotum develop. DHT also regulates the development of the prostate. If DHT is absent, labia, clitoris, and lower two thirds of the vagina develop.
3. Sertoli cells line the basement membrane of the seminiferous tubules. They constitute the blood-testis barrier. Sertoli cells produce MIS, inhibin, seminiferous tubule fluid, and androgen-binding protein. They can aromatize androgens to estrogens and play a supportive role for the germ cells. Sertoli cells have FSH and testosterone receptors.
4. Leydig cells are the primary site of testicular androgen synthesis. They are interspersed among the seminiferous tubules. They have LH receptors.
5. Androgen production in Leydig cells is stimulated by LH.
6. Androgens stimulate growth and development of male secondary sex characteristics. They control sexual hair development, stimulate sebaceous gland secretion, are protein anabolic, and stimulate sex gland secretion.
7. Spermatogenesis is hormonally dependent. LH is required to stimulate androgen secretion, and androgens are essential for spermatogenesis. FSH is necessary to initiate spermatogenesis and for long-term maintenance of normal levels of spermatogenesis.

8. Semen serves to provide bulk to sperm, maintain an alkaline environment for sperm, provide nutrients to sperm, prevent sperm capacitation, and inhibit sperm motility in the male reproductive tract. It contains prostaglandins.

9. At puberty, the gonadostat is "reset" so that the sensitivity to negative feedback inhibition of testosterone on GnRH and LH secretion decreases. LH and FSH secretion rises, which stimulates testicular growth, hormone production, and spermatogenesis.

10. Klinefelter's syndrome results when men have an extra X chromosome.

11. Deficiency of 5α-reductase can result in incomplete male hermaphroditism at birth.

12. Androgen insensitivity syndrome results from a hereditary defect in the gene controlling androgen receptor expression. Male pseudohermaphroditism can result.

13. Kallmann's syndrome is primary isolated gonadotropin deficiency. This genetic disorder is associated with loss of smell and cryptorchism.

■ KEY WORDS AND CONCEPTS

- Sex chromosomes
- Leydig cells
- Sertoli cells
- SYR (sex-determining region Y)
- Wolffian ducts
- Müllerian ducts
- Müllerian-inhibiting substance (MIS)
- Dihydrotestosterone (DHT)
- 5α-Reductase
- Seminiferous tubules
- Rete testis
- Efferent ductules
- Epididymis
- Vas deferens
- Seminal vesicles
- Prostate
- Cowper's (bulbourethral) glands
- Androgen-binding protein
- Sex hormone–binding globulin (SHBG)
- Testosterone-estrogen binding globulin (TeBG)
- Plasminogen activator
- Plasmin
- Spermiation
- Interstitial cells
- Dihydroepiandrosterone (DHEA)
- Androstenedione
- Inhibin
- Conjugated steroids
- Heat shock protein (HSP)
- Hormone response element (HRE)
- DNA-binding domain
- Ligand-binding domain
- N-terminal region
- Spermatogenesis
- Spermatogonia
- Primary spermatocytes
- Secondary spermatocytes
- Spermatids
- Spermatozoa
- Spermiogenesis
- Acrosome
- Acrosin inhibitor
- Spermine
- Capacitation
- Decapacitation factor
- Acrosomal reaction
- ZP3
- Acrosin
- Hyaluronidase
- Adrenarche
- Klinefelter's syndrome
- 5α-Reductase deficiency
- Androgen insensitivity syndrome (AIS)
- Male pseudohermaphroditism
- Kallmann's syndrome
- Anosmia
- Cryptorchism

■ SELF-STUDY PROBLEMS

1. How does FSH regulate spermatogenesis even though germ cells lack FSH receptors?

2. Describe the interactions between Sertoli cells and Leydig cells in estrogen production.

3. Why does a congenital 5α-reductase deficiency have the potential of resulting in a pseudohermaphroditic condition when internal genitalia are male and external genitalia appear female?

4. Why is pubic hair often absent in adult individuals with androgen insensitivity syndrome even though serum estrogen levels are relatively high?

■ BIBLIOGRAPHY

Greenspan FS, Strewler GJ: *Basic and clinical endocrinology,* Norwalk, Conn, 1997, Appleton & Lange.

Griffin JE, Wilson JD: Disorders of the testes and the male reproductive tract. In Wilson JD, Foster DW, Kronenberg HM, Larsen PR, editors: *Williams' textbook of endocrinology,* Philadelphia, 1998, WB Saunders, pp 819-876.

Huhtaniemi I, Pelliniemi LJ: Fetal Leydig cells: cellular origin, morphology, life span, and special functional features, *Proc Soc Exp Biol Med* 201:125, 1990.

Marshall WA, Tanner JM: Variations in the pattern of pubertal changes in boys, *Arch Dis Child* 45:13, 1970.

Quigley CA, DeBellis A, Marschke KB, El-Awady MK, Wilson EM, French FS: Androgen receptor defects: historical, clinical and molecular perspectives, *Endocr Rev* 16:271, 1995.

Saez JM: Leydig cells: endocrine, paracrine, and autocrine regulation, *Endocr Rev* 15:574, 1994.

Skinner MK: Cell-cell interactions in the testis, *Endocr Rev* 12:45, 1991.

Wilson JD, Griffin JE, Russell DW: Steroid 5α-reductase 2 deficiency, *Endocr Rev* 14:577, 1993.

CHAPTER 9

Female Reproductive System

Objectives

1. Describe the role of hormones in female reproductive tract development.

2. Explain the development of the ovarian follicle.

3. Describe the relationship between granulosa and thecal cells.

4. List the functions of granulosa cells.

5. List the major ovarian hormones.

6. Explain the regulation of ovarian steroidogenesis, including the mechanisms underlying the gonadotropin surge.

7. List the major actions of estrogens, progestins, and androgens in the female.

8. Describe the events in the menstrual cycle and explain their physiologic basis.

9. Describe the endocrine changes occurring at puberty and at menopause in the normal female.

■ DEVELOPMENT OF THE FEMALE REPRODUCTIVE TRACT (Box 9-1)

If the testis-determining gene SRY is absent, ovaries develop from the genital ridge. Although the fetal testis begins to develop at 6 weeks of gestation, the fetal ovary remains undifferentiated until after 9 weeks of gestation (Figure 9-1). By this time, the fetal testis is already producing testosterone. In contrast, the fetal ovary remains quiescent during fetal development and, in the absence of testicular müllerian-inhibiting substance (MIS) and testosterone, the müllerian ducts become the fallopian tubes, uterus, and upper vagina, and the genital folds, genital swelling, and genital tubercle become the labia, clitoris, and lower two thirds of the vagina. *Ovaries are not necessary for the fetal development of female internal and external genitalia.*

The female fetus, like the male, shows a peak in luteinizing hormone (LH) and follicle-stimulating hormone (FSH) secretion in utero followed by a second peak 2 to 3 months postpartum. Subsequently, LH and FSH secretion remain relatively low until adolescence.

■ ANATOMY OF THE OVARY

The outer zone, or cortex, of the ovary contains the germ cells (Figure 9-2). These germ cells are

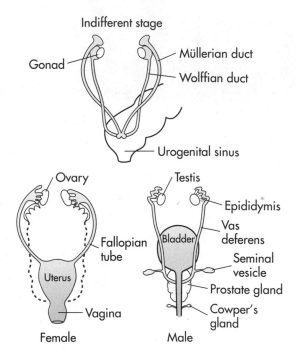

Figure 9-1 ■ Differentiation of internal genitalia and primordial ducts. (Redrawn from George FW, Wilson JD: Embryology of the genital tract. In Walsh PC et al, editors: *Campbell's urology,* ed 6, Philadelphia, 1992, WB Saunders.)

found in numerous **ovarian follicles.** Interspersed among the follicles is the ovarian stroma, which contains connective tissue, blood vessels, and interstitial cells. The inner zone, or medulla, consists primarily of connective tissue and the blood vessels serving the cortex. The mature ovary has follicles of varying sizes and developmental states. Most of these follicles are primordial follicles (see Figure 9-2) that consist of an ovum enveloped by a single layer of granulosa cells. Some of these follicles will develop into primary follicles, and even fewer will develop into mature graafian follicles.

The ovum is released from the ovary into the peritoneum. Fimbriae of the oviduct envelop the ovary, and motility of the fimbriae and ciliary movement in the oviduct pull the ovum into the oviduct.

Folliculogenesis

Ovarian follicular development and steroidogenesis are controlled by gonadotropins, ovarian steroids to some extent, and follicular autocrine and paracrine secretions. Mitosis of primordial oogonia occurs until midgestation, when a peak of approximately 7 million oocytes is present.

After that point, mitosis of oocytes ceases, and there is a progressive loss of oocytes so that at birth there are approximately 2 million and by puberty there are approximately 400,000. Only 400 follicles actually ovulate in the average woman. The remaining 99.9% of the follicles will degenerate and are called atretic follicles.

The oocyte begins the first meiotic division in utero; this first division is arrested in prophase until the time of ovulation. Maturation is thought to be arrested by proposed substances in follicular fluid referred to generically as **maturation-inhibiting factors.** Some MIS is found in follicular fluid and could serve this function. Thus this long, suspended meiosis can last up to 50 years.

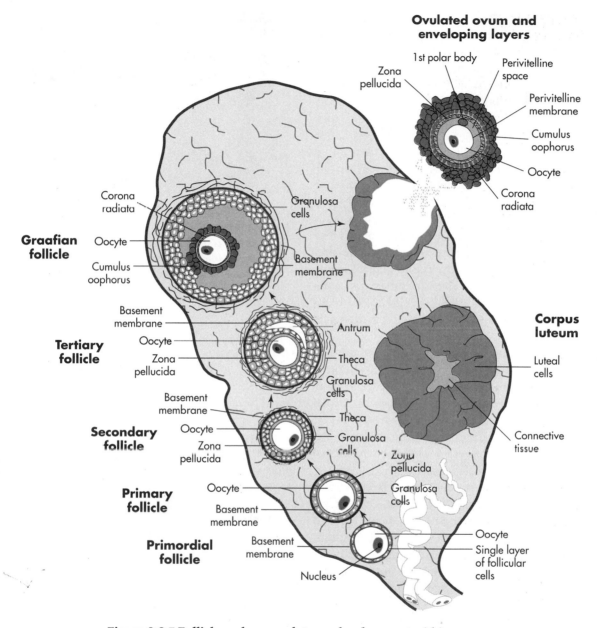

Figure 9-2 ■ Follicle and corpus luteum development within ovary.

Follicular Growth

A resting or inactive oocyte is called a **primordial follicle** (see Figure 9-2). This follicle consists of an oocyte, a one-layer ring of squamous **follicular cells** (which are the precursors to **granulosa cells**), and a basement membrane. As primordial follicles grow and develop, they will either become atretic or ovulate. As the quiescent primordial follicle is transformed into a **primary follicle,** the oocyte grows. The oocyte produces a mucopolysaccharide coating called the **zona pellucida,** and cytoplasmic processes extend from the granulosa cells through the zona pellucida to the oocyte. The zona pellucida was once thought to be produced by granulosa cells. The follicular (granulosa) cells proliferate and become more cuboidal, and multiple layers of granulosa cells develop. Growth to this point is not hormonally dependent.

On stimulation with FSH, a cohort of primary follicles begins to grow and develop. Granulosa cells proliferate, and the follicle grows to its final size of 120 to 200 mm in diameter. Stromal tissue differentiates to form a **thecal layer,** which is located outside the basement membrane. This follicle is now called a **secondary follicle.**

Fluid produced by the granulosa cells accumulates within a cavity, or **antrum.** Once an antrum begins to form, the follicle is considered a **tertiary follicle. Follicular fluid** contains large quantities of ovarian steroids, growth factors, electrolytes, and cytokines. Levels of follicular fluid estrogens and progestins can be 100- to 200-fold greater than levels in serum. This fluid creates the immediate environment for the oocyte.

This follicle matures into a **graafian follicle** (Figure 9-3). By this time, the antrum is large and the follicle is bulging from the surface of the ovary. A projection of granulosa cells extends into the antrum and supports the ovum. These

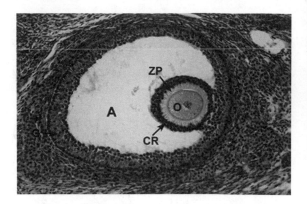

Figure 9-3 ■ **Histologic features of ovarian graafian follicle. Ovum** *(O)* **is surrounded by zona pellucida** *(ZP).* **Shrinkage artifacts result in zona pellucida appearing larger than normal. Corona radiata** *(CR)* **is indicated, as is large antrum** *(A). G,* **Glomerulosa cell;** *T,* **thecal cells.**

cells are referred to as the **cumulus oophorus.** A thin layer of granulosa cells immediately envelops the ovum; this single dense layer of cells is called the **corona radiata.** There are now two thecal layers—an inner **theca interna** and an outer **theca externa.** The thecal layers are vascularized, but because blood vessels do not penetrate the basement membrane, nutrients, hormones, and electrolytes reach the granulosa cells and the oocyte by diffusion.

Ovulation

Ovulation is stimulated by a surge in LH secretion. This surge in LH stimulates completion of the first meiotic division immediately before ovulation. The meiotic division does not form cells of equal size. One cell becomes the large oocyte, and the second cell has minimal cytoplasm and becomes the **first polar body.** It remains in the perivitelline space in close proximity to the oocyte. The second meiotic division occurs on sperm entry into the ovum. The fully mature graafian follicle is located on the surface of the ovary and forms as much as a 1 cm bulge

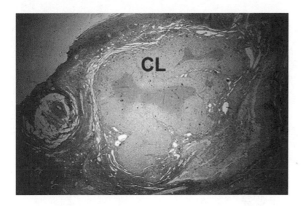

Figure 9-4 ■ Histologic section of ovary shows corpus luteum *(CL).*

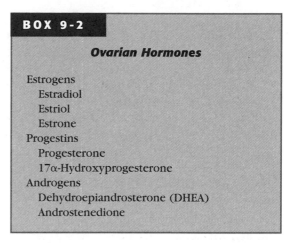

BOX 9-2

Ovarian Hormones

Estrogens
    Estradiol
    Estriol
    Estrone
Progestins
    Progesterone
    17α-Hydroxyprogesterone
Androgens
    Dehydroepiandrosterone (DHEA)
    Androstenedione

on the ovarian surface. The follicular wall thins, and LH and prostaglandins decrease follicular blood flow and stimulate the release of granulosa cell **plasminogen activator,** an enzyme that converts follicular fluid plasminogen to plasmin. LH and progesterone stimulate collagenase production. **Collagenase** and **plasmin** are proteolytic enzymes that break down the remaining follicular wall, thereby allowing release of the ovum. The released ovum is enveloped by the zona pellucida, corona radiata, and loose cumulus oophorus cells, along with follicular fluid.

Corpus Luteum

After ovulation, the collapsed walls of the follicle are transformed into a **corpus luteum** (yellow body) (Figure 9-4). The basement membrane separating granulosa and thecal cells is disrupted, and blood vessels extend to the former granulosa cells. Both the granulosa and theca interna cells become luteal (lutein) cells. The mature corpus luteum can be as large as 3 cm in diameter. If conception does not occur, the corpus luteum remains functional for approximately 14 days and then begins to degenerate **(luteolysis).** The luteal cells become necrotic, and steroid synthesis declines. The corpus luteum fills with connective tissue and becomes a **corpus albi-**

cans (white body). These structures are light and resemble scar tissue.

■ OVARIAN HORMONES

The predominant ovarian steroids are estrogens, progestins, and androgens (Box 9-2). Figure 9-5 shows the steps in the biosynthesis of ovarian steroids. **Estradiol-17β** (estradiol) is both the most potent and most plentiful ovarian estrogen. It is produced primarily in granulosa and luteal cells, but smaller quantities are also produced in theca interna and stromal cells. **Estriol** is a less potent estrogen that is not produced by the ovaries in appreciable quantities except during pregnancy. The major source of estriol in nonpregnant women is the liver, where it is produced from estrone or estradiol. **Estrone** is the least potent of the three estrogens, and although the ovary produces estrone, most estrone in blood is formed from peripheral conversion from estradiol or androstenedione. It is the predominant estrogen in the postmenopausal woman.

The major progestin is **progesterone.** Progesterone is a precursor for androgens and estrogens, and it is produced in all ovarian endocrine cells. The predominant progestins secreted by the ovaries are progesterone and **17α-**

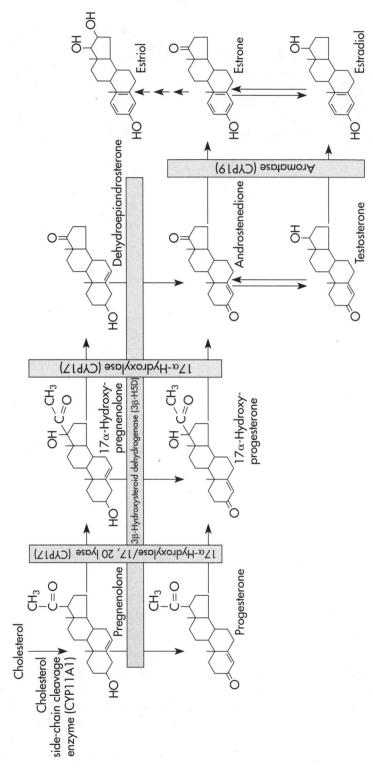

Figure 9-5 ■ Ovarian steroidogenesis.

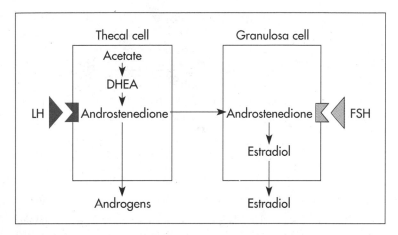

Figure 9-6 ■ **Two-cell theory of early follicular steroidogenesis. Ovarian steroid production in early follicular phase involves synergistic action of thecal and granulosa cells. Luteinizing hormone (LH) stimulates thecal steroidogenesis; primary product is androgen. Follicle-stimulating hormone (FSH) stimulates granulosa cell aromatization of thecal androgens to produce estrogen. DHEA, Dehydroepiandrosterone.**

hydroxyprogesterone. The major ovarian androgens are the weak androgens **dehydroepiandrosterone (DHEA)** and **androstenedione.** Small quantities of testosterone and even dihydrotestosterone are produced in the ovaries. Other hormones produced in the ovary include the peptides inhibins, activins, and relaxin. The ovarian follicle is a site of production of numerous growth factors including insulin-like growth factor-I and transforming growth factors α and β; numerous other paracrine factors such as cytokines are produced in the ovary, and these substances appear to be important in local regulation of ovarian function.

■ OVARIAN STEROIDOGENESIS: THE TWO-CELL HYPOTHESIS

The theca interna is the predominant site of androgen synthesis in the preovulatory follicle. These cells are analogous to the Leydig cells of the testis. They have LH receptors, and LH acts to stimulate steroidogenesis. Although the thecal cells can produce small quantities of estrogens, the predominant hormones are the androgens DHEA and androstenedione.

Granulosa cells are analogous to testicular Sertoli cells. They surround the ovum and regulate the availability of nutrients to these germ cells. Like the Sertoli cells, they have FSH receptors, and FSH stimulates both **inhibin** production and androgen aromatization to estrogen. Granulosa cells are the predominant site of estradiol production in the preovulatory follicle. Preovulatory granulosa cells lack the enzyme 17α-hydroxylase that is necessary for androgen production. Because theca interna cells produce the precursors for granulosa cell estrogen production, both cell types are necessary for optimal estrogen production. Figure 9-6 illustrates the two-cell theory for early follicular steroidogenesis.

Early in the follicular phase, the granulosa cells contain only FSH receptors. As the follicle grows in response to the action of FSH and estrogen production increases as a result of the action of LH on thecal cells and FSH on granulosa cells, serum estrogen levels rise. This estrogen synergizes with FSH to stimulate development of granulosa cell LH receptors. Once LH receptors develop, granulosa cell progesterone secretion increases. After ovulation, granulosa cells and thecal cells become luteal cells. These cells have LH receptors and secrete estrogens and progestins in response to LH stimulation.

Control of Ovarian Steroidogenesis

Both LH and FSH exert their actions by cyclic adenosine monophosphate–mediated mechanisms. LH acts on theca interna cells and luteal cells, and late in the follicular phase it acts on granulosa cells to stimulate cellular growth and steroidogenesis. FSH stimulates granulosa cell aromatization of androgens to estrogens. Estradiol feeds back to inhibit LH and FSH synthesis and secretion at both the hypothalamic and pituitary levels **(negative feedback of estrogen)**

(Figure 9-7). If the woman is ovarectomized, both LH and FSH levels rise, with FSH levels rising more than LH levels. If estrogen is then administered, LH and FSH levels drop and, although LH levels rapidly return to normal, the response of FSH is slower. Inhibin suppresses FSH secretion by acting directly at the gonadotrope.

■ TRANSPORT OF ESTROGENS AND PROGESTINS

Steroids are sparingly soluble in blood and are carried primarily associated with plasma proteins. Approximately 60% of the estrogen is transported bound to **sex hormone–binding globulin (SHBG),** 20% is bound to albumin, and 20% is in the free form.

Progesterone binds primarily to transcortin and albumin. Because it has a relatively low

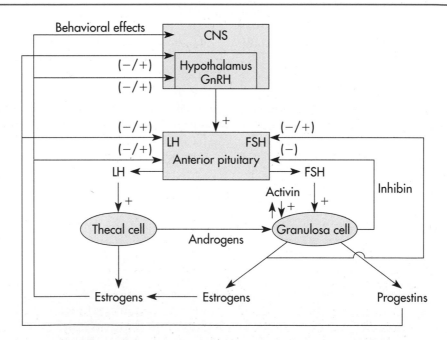

Figure 9-7 ■ Regulation of ovarian function. *CNS,* Central nervous system; *GnRH,* gonadotropin-releasing hormone; *LH,* luteinizing hormone; *FSH,* follicle-stimulating hormone.

binding affinity for these proteins, its circulating half-life (t½) is about 5 minutes.

■ METABOLISM OF ESTROGENS AND PROGESTINS

Estrogens and progestins are degraded in the liver to inactive metabolites, conjugated with sulfate or glucuronide, and excreted in the urine. Major metabolites of estradiol include es-

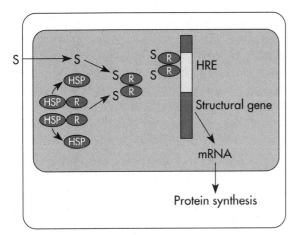

Figure 9-8 ■ Proposed model for action of steroid hormones. Steroids *(S)* diffuse into cell, where they bind to receptors *(R)*, which release heat shock protein *(HSP)*, dimerize, and bind to hormone response element *(HRE)* of DNA.

trone, estriol, and catecholestrogens. The major metabolite of progesterone is pregnanediol, which is conjugated with glucuronide and excreted in the urine.

■ MECHANISM OF ACTION OF ESTROGENS AND PROGESTINS

Estrogens and progestins enter cells by diffusion and bind to nuclear receptors. Although the hormones bind to different receptors, the mechanisms of action of the hormones are similar (Figure 9-8). Binding of the steroid to the receptor leads to dimerization of the receptor. As is typical of steroid hormone action, binding of ligand to the receptor releases heat shock proteins (HSPs), which produces a conformational change in the receptor so that its DNA affinity increases. The ligand-bound receptor associates with the hormone response element (HRE) of the DNA and acts as a transcription factor to regulate gene expression.

■ ACTIONS OF ESTROGENS

At puberty, estradiol stimulates the growth and development of the uterus, fallopian tubes, cervix, vagina, labia, and breasts (Box 9-3). It is an anabolic hormone in these tissues. It stimulates uterine endometrial proliferation and increases spontaneous myometrial electrical activity,

---

BOX 9-3

Actions of Estrogens

Stimulation of growth of uterus, fallopian tubes, vagina
Growth of mammary gland ductile system
Secretion of plentiful, thin cervical mucus
Stimulation of follicular growth
Stimulation of granulosa cell–LH receptor formation
Delay of bone loss at menopause
Stimulation of thin sebaceous gland secretions
Stimulation of bone growth and closure of the epiphyses
Stimulation of endometrial proliferation

↓ Serum cholesterol
↑ Serum high-density lipoprotein
↓ Glucose tolerance
↑ Production of clotting factors
↑ Thyroxine-binding globulin, sex hormone–binding globulin, transcortin synthesis
↑ Progesterone receptors

thereby increasing uterine motility. It also increases uterine sensitivity to oxytocin. Estrogens decrease the viscosity of sebaceous gland secretion and therefore decrease the tendency for acne formation. The increase in progesterone and androgen secretion at puberty is responsible for acne development in women. Both estrogens and androgens stimulate bone growth and closure of the epiphyses at puberty. These actions of androgens might follow local aromatization to estrogens. The shorter stature in women is in part a result of the earlier puberty in females than in males. After menopause, the precipitous decline in estrogen secretion accelerates osteoporosis. Estrogen receptors have been found on osteoblasts, and estrogen treatment after menopause delays age-related bone loss. Estrogens stimulate renal sodium and water retention.

Estrogens have metabolic effects. They antagonize the actions of insulin on peripheral tissues, and estrogen administration decreases glucose tolerance. Estrogens decrease serum cholesterol levels and increase serum high-density lipoprotein (HDL) levels. Estrogens stimulate liver production of many of the hormone-binding proteins in serum such as thyroxine-binding globulin (TBG), transcortin, and SHBG. Consequently, radioimmunoassays of serum thyroid hormones, cortisol, or sex hormones are misleading in pregnancy or after estrogen administration because of this nonspecific action on binding protein levels. The estrogen-induced increase in liver-produced clotting factors can increase the risk of thromboembolic disorders in estrogen-treated women.

Estrogen administration can induce estrous behavior in animals and may increase libido in women. In fact, the action of androgens on libido might occur after androgens' aromatization to estrogens.

■ ACTIONS OF PROGESTINS

Progestins are compounds that have progestational-like effects on the uterus (Box 9-4). The major progestin is progesterone. The sources of these compounds are the ovary, testis, and adrenal. Progesterone stimulates conversion of a proliferative-type endometrium into the secretory-type endometrium, which is optimal for the implantation of the developing embryo. It increases the myometrial transmembrane potential, thereby stabilizing the membrane and decreasing uterine motility. It decreases uterine response to oxytocin. Progesterone stimulates the production of a scanty, viscous, acidic cervical mucus that is hostile to sperm. Because it increases the set-point for thermoregulation, it increases body temperature approximately 0.5° F. This is the basis for using body temperature measurements to determine whether ovulation has occurred. Progesterone secretion from the corpus luteum increases after ovulation. Progesterone synergizes with estrogen in stimulating mammary gland growth and development. However, although estrogens stimulate mammary gland lobular development, progesterone stimulates alveolar development.

BOX 9-4

Actions of Progesterone

Production of secretory endometrium
Stimulation of secretion of scant, viscous cervical mucus
Stimulation of mammary lobular-alveolar growth
Antagonism of aldosterone action; suppression of milk synthesis

↑ Body temperature
↓ Uterine motility
↑ Ventilation
↓ Sodium retention

Progesterone increases the ventilatory response to P_{CO_2} so that ventilation increases and P_{CO_2} decreases. Although estrogen is a central nervous system stimulant, progesterone is a depressant. Because progesterone is a competitive inhibitor of aldosterone at the kidney, it has a natriuretic action.

■ ACTIONS OF ANDROGENS

Adrenal androgens are responsible for pubic and axillary hair development in the female. Androgen secretion increases at puberty, in concert with the increase in estrogen and progesterone secretion. Serum levels of androgens also change in a cyclic manner during the menstrual cycle, with maximal levels occurring at midcycle.

■ ACTIONS OF RELAXIN

Relaxin is a peptide hormone produced in the ovary and placenta. Like insulin, it has an α and β chain connected by two disulfide bridges. Relaxin induces relaxation of the pelvic ligaments and softens the cervix to facilitate childbirth. It inhibits uterine motility.

■ MENSTRUAL CYCLE

The menstrual cycle is a complex of cyclic changes that include changes in the ovaries, uterine endometrium, cervix, vagina, and mammary glands.

Ovarian Cycle

The three phases of the ovarian cycle are the follicular phase, ovulatory phase, and luteal phase (Figure 9-9).

Follicular Phase The follicular phase begins with the growth and development of 6 to 12 primary follicles. Their development depends on FSH levels. Early in the menstrual cycle, FSH levels are rising. LH increases theca interna androgen synthesis. FSH acts on the granulosa cells to stimulate estrogen production from thecal androgens (Box 9-5), and estrogen and FSH synergize to stimulate follicular growth. By about the sixth day of the cycle, one follicle becomes dominant and the others become atretic. It is thought that the follicle that develops fastest begins secreting estrogen, which inhibits FSH production, thereby inhibiting further development of the less mature follicles. Multiple mechanisms have been proposed whereby the dominant follicle might directly inhibit development of the other follicles. These nondominant follicles become atretic.

Estrogen and FSH stimulate granulosa cell–LH receptor production late in the follicular phase. LH then stimulates granulosa cell progesterone production. Because the granulosa cell layers are avascular, intraovarian levels of progesterone increase 100- to 200-fold although circulating levels remain relatively low. By this time, approximately 10 to 13 days into a 28-day cycle, serum estrogen levels reach their highest level.

Ovulation Nine to 24 hours after the estrogen peak, there is a surge in LH secretion, which typically stimulates ovulation of a mature follicle within 24 hours (Box 9-6). The highest levels of LH during the entire cycle occur at this time. The timing of the LH surge is important because it should be coordinated with events in the ovary so that the development of the follicle is

---

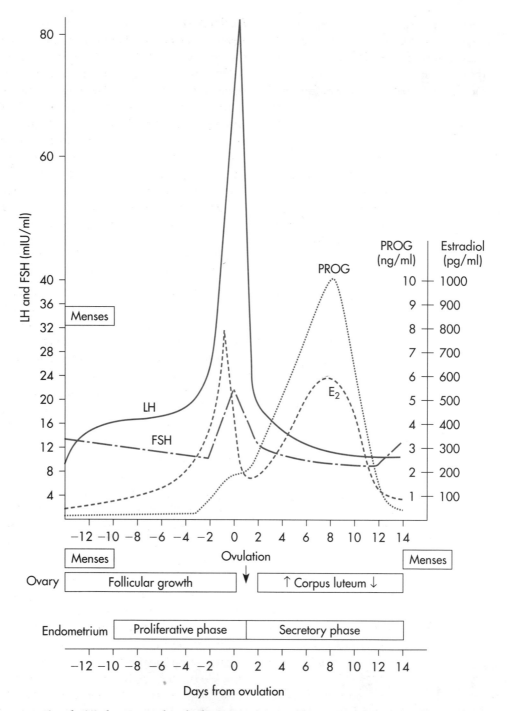

Figure 9-9 ■ Circulating hormone levels during ovarian and endometrial events in human menstrual cycle. *LH,* **Luteinizing hormone;** *FSH,* **follicle-stimulating hormone;** *PROG,* **progesterone;** *E₂,* **estradiol.** (Redrawn from Speroff L, Van de Wiele RL: *Am J Obstet Gynecol* 109:237, 1971.)

BOX 9-7

Luteal Phase

The corpus luteum produces large quantities of progesterone and estrogens.

appropriate at the time of the LH surge. A smaller FSH surge accompanies the LH surge.

Luteal Phase Under the influence of LH, thecal and granulosa cells become the **luteal cells** of the corpus luteum. As the corpus luteum develops, estrogen and progesterone secretion increases in response to LH stimulation (Box 9-7). The high levels of estrogens and progestins produced during this phase inhibit LH and FSH secretion. This phase lasts 10 to 16 days, with an average of 14 days. The duration of the luteal phase is more constant than the duration of the follicular phase as menstrual cycle length changes.

The function and life span of the corpus luteum is determined by hormonal factors. In humans, the corpus luteum lasts only a few days in the absence of LH. Therefore LH is **luteotrophic** for humans because it maintains the life of the corpus luteum. If pregnancy does not occur, the corpus luteum reaches peak steroid production approximately 7 days after ovulation and then begins to undergo **luteolysis.** The uterus produces luteolytic factors in some species, such as swine. A similar situation does not appear to exist in humans because hysterectomy does not lengthen the human ovarian cycle. As corpus luteum production of progesterone, estrogen, and inhibin drops, the hormonal support of the uterine endometrium decreases and menstruation occurs. The decreased inhibin and steroid production by the corpus luteum leads to increased FSH secretion, which stimulates development of the new cohort of follicles destined to regulate the subsequent cycle.

Androgen Secretion

Serum testosterone levels in adult women are typically 0.2 to 0.7 ng/ml. Approximately one half of this testosterone is secreted from the adrenal cortex and ovary. The remainder is formed peripherally from androstenedione and DHEA. Androgen secretion increases at puberty, in concert with the increase in estrogen and progesterone secretion. It also changes in a cyclic manner during the menstrual cycle, with maximal levels occurring at midcycle coincident with the preovulatory estrogen peak. The ovarian androgens serve as precursors for estrogen synthesis.

Neuroendocrine Basis of the Control of LH and FSH Secretion

LH and FSH are secreted in a pulsatile, cyclic manner in the mature, premenopausal woman. These gonadotropins are secreted by the pituitary in response to stimulation by the hypothalamic-releasing hormone gonadotropin-releasing hormone (GnRH). There are numerous regulators of GnRH secretion. These include classic aminergic neurotransmitters such as norepinephrine, amino acids such as glutamate, and neuropeptides such as neuropeptide Y, galanin, neurotensin, angiotensin II, and endogenous opioids. These compounds are produced and localized in regions of the basal hypothalamus involved in the regulation of GnRH secretion. Ovarian steroids are capable of altering levels of these GnRH regulators. It is generally thought that central regulation of gonadotropin secretion by estradiol and progesterone can be mediated by neuroactive amines that are capable of inhibiting or stimulating GnRH release.

The pulsatile pattern of LH and FSH secretion is a result of pulsatile GnRH secretion. The pulse generator resides in the medial-basal hypothalamus in rats. Although the site of this generator is hypothalamic, there are numerous regulators of its activity. Many of these signals originate in other brain regions.

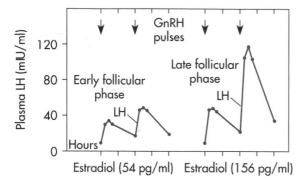

Figure 9-10 ▪ Luteinizing hormone *(LH)* response to gonadotropin-releasing hormone *(GnRH)* administered either early in follicular phase when estrogen levels are relatively low or late in follicular phase when levels are high. (Redrawn from Wang CF, et al: *J Clin Endocrinol Metab* 42:718, 1976.)

Both LH and FSH secretion are regulated by GnRH, and the relative effect on the two gonadotropins depends on the frequency and amplitude of the GnRH pulses. The GnRH pulse has a frequency of one per 70 to 100 minutes. Pulse frequency is greater during the follicular phase than the luteal phase, which is thought to reflect the inhibitory action of progesterone on the pulse generator during the luteal phase.

Positive and Negative Feedback of Estrogens Both estradiol and progesterone regulate gonadotropin secretion in a complex manner. Estradiol produced in the follicular phase alters the pituitary response to GnRH. The slowly rising estradiol levels prime the hypothalamic-pituitary system so that LH levels rise slightly rather than decline (Figure 9-10). Therefore a bolus of GnRH administered early in the follicular phase will produce a smaller rise in LH secretion than would a bolus of GnRH administered later in the follicular phase. In addition, the quantity of GnRH released in the pulses is greater than normal late in the follicular phase. Estradiol administered late in the follicular

phase, if accompanied by progesterone, can stimulate GnRH release, an LH surge, and an accompanying FSH surge. This **positive feedback** of estrogen is mediated at both the hypothalamic and pituitary levels. Serum estradiol levels of at least 200 pg/ml for 2 days are necessary to produce this effect, and a rise in progesterone levels is important for the effect.

An LH surge, resembling that seen in a normal ovulating woman, can be artificially induced in postmenopausal women by administering the estradiol agonist ethinyl estradiol and the progesterone agonist medroxyprogesterone in the appropriate manner, as shown in Figure 9-11.

Although estradiol is generally considered to be the primary trigger for the gonadotropin surge, progesterone increases the magnitude of the surge, accelerates the onset of the surge, and decreases the duration of the surge. Progesterone alone can induce a gonadotropin surge in an estrogen-primed animal. Although progesterone can facilitate the gonadotropin surge, its administration at other periods in the normal cycle can also inhibit gonadotropin secretion.

The increased progesterone, estradiol, and inhibin production resulting from development of the corpus luteum exerts a **negative feedback** on GnRH, LH, and FSH secretion.

The system provides a sensitive servomechanism whereby products produced by the ovary influence the timing of the LH surge. This is important if the surge is to be timed appropriately with the development of the ovarian follicle.

▪ UTERINE CYCLE
Phases of the Uterine Cycle

The phases of the uterine cycle are the **menstrual phase, proliferative phase,** and **secretory phase** (Figure 9-12). The uterus is composed of an outer muscular layer, the **myometrium,** and an inner glandular layer, the **endometrium.** The endometrium is supplied by two types of arteries—straight arteries sup-

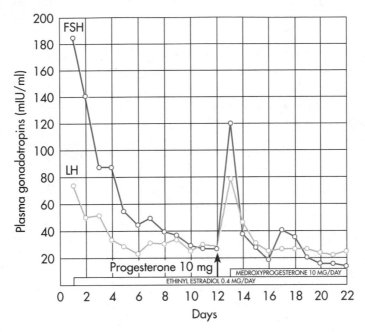

Figure 9-11 ■ Effects of estrogen and progesterone administration on serum luteinizing hormone *(LH)* and follicle-stimulating hormone *(FSH)* levels in postmenopausal woman. (Redrawn from Odell WD: The reproductive system in women. In DeGroot LJ, et al, editors: *Endocrinology,* vol 3, New York, 1979, Grune & Stratton.)

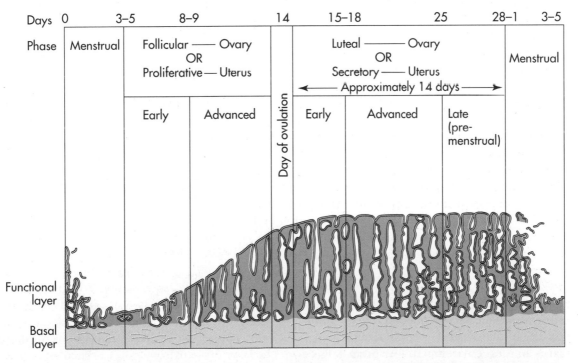

Figure 9-12 ■ Changes in endometrial thickness, glands, and arteries relative to phases of ovarian cycle. (Redrawn from Cunningham FG, et al, editors: *Williams' obstetrics,* Norwalk, Conn, 1993, Appleton & Lange.)

ply the innermost (basal) one third of the endometrium and coiled spiral arteries supply the outermost two thirds. Endometrium proliferates rapidly during the menstrual cycle, and then the outermost two thirds degenerates and is shed each month with menstruation.

During the follicular phase of the ovarian cycle, estrogen stimulates endometrial proliferation. The layer thickens, and the glands and blood vessels of the tissue grow. This endometrium is called a **proliferative endometrium.** After ovulation, progesterone stimulates conversion of the estrogen-primed proliferative endometrium into a **secretory endometrium.** Glandular secretion increases, as does glycogen storage in the endometrial cells. The spiral arteries of the endometrium branch, grow, and become more tortuous. This endometrial stage is referred to as the secretory phase. Maximal development of the secretory endometrium occurs approximately 5 to 7 days after ovulation. This is the time the developing blastocyst would be available for uterine implantation if conception has occurred. If conception does not occur and the corpus luteum regresses, the decline in estrogen and progesterone secretion results in withdrawal of the hormonal support of the secretory endometrium. With inadequate hormonal support, prostaglandins are released, the spiral arteries constrict, uterine ischemia develops, and endometrial necrosis results. **Menstruation** represents the period in which the necrotic outer two thirds of the endometrium is shed. The region of the endometrium that proliferates and is shed during the menstrual cycle is the **functional layer,** whereas the remaining one third is the **basal layer.**

Cervical Mucus Changes

Cervical secretions are hormonally regulated. Estrogen stimulates production of a copious quantity of thin, watery, slightly alkaline mucus that is an ideal environment for sperm. It is de-

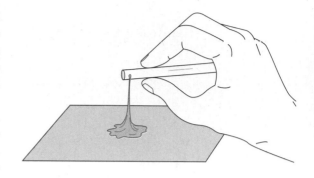

Spinnbarkeit

Figure 9-13 ▪ Spinnbarkeit. Cervical mucus of periovulatory woman is stringy.

scribed as stringy because when the mucus is dropped on a slide and a stick is touched to it and then elevated, a long "string" of mucus can be formed. This characteristic is termed **spinnbarkeit** (Figure 9-13). This occurs because macromolecules in the mucus align themselves in parallel chains when the mucus is "pulled." These macromolecules are thought to facilitate sperm movement through the mucus. When the mucus is allowed to dry on a slide, a fernlike pattern (**ferning**) is formed as a result of the high electrolyte content of the mucus (Figure 9-14). Progesterone stimulates production of a scant, viscous, slightly acidic mucus that is hostile to sperm and does not "fern." During the normal menstrual cycle, the conditions of the cervical mucus are ideal for sperm penetration and viability at the time of ovulation.

▪ VAGINAL CYCLE

The superficial cells of the vaginal epithelium are continually desquamating. For this reason, cells recovered from the vaginal fluids fairly accurately reflect the nature of the intact vaginal cells. The nature of these cells is influenced by the hormonal environment. Estrogens stimulate

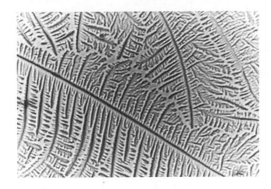

Figure 9-14 ■ **Ferning of cervical mucus on slide.**

BOX 9-8

Puberty Involves

- Thelarche—breast development
- Adrenarche—increase in adrenal androgen secretion
- Menarche—beginning of menstrual cycles
- Decreased gonadostat sensitivity

proliferation of these cells. The estrogen-stimulated vaginal cells are typically large, flat, irregularly shaped, squamous-type cornified cells with relatively small or absent nuclei. This change in the nature of these cells is referred to as **keratinization** or **cornification.** Few leukocytes are present in a vaginal smear. Progesterone, however, tends to have the opposite effect on the epithelium. Progesterone stimulates production of an epithelium that contains smaller basophilic cells with few cornified cells and many leukocytes.

■ PUBERTY

Pubertal changes in the female in many ways resemble those in the male. As in the male, there is a fetal peak for FSH and LH production in midgestation. FSH levels rise more than LH levels, and serum levels for both gonadotropins approach those of a castrated adult (Figure 9-15). These high levels are probably a reflection of immature development of the negative feedback system for gonadotropin regulation. Despite these high gonadotropin levels, the ovaries remain quiescent. There is also a second peak of FSH and to a lesser extent of LH about 2 to 3 months postpartum. LH and FSH levels then drop to relatively low levels until puberty. The prepubertal hypothalamus is extremely sensitive to steroidal inhibition of GnRH. The functionality of this control system is demonstrated by the rise in serum LH and FSH levels that follows the loss of the ovaries or testes. As the female matures, the sensitivity of the **gonadostat** (hypothalamic-pituitary setpoint for gonadal regulation) decreases and GnRH levels rise (Figure 9-16). The exact cause of this change is not understood, but it appears to be independent of steroid action because the same effect is seen in children with gonadal dysgenesis and therefore a deficiency of ovarian steroid production. As with the male, pulsatility increases. Initially there are only bursts of GnRH secretion with sleep. As GnRH secretion increases, LH and FSH secretion increases and the gonadotropins stimulate ovarian follicular growth and steroid secretion. Before puberty, FSH levels exceed LH levels, and at puberty, LH levels exceed FSH levels. This increase in gonadotropin secretion stimulates estrogen and progesterone production. These steroids are responsible for the development of most of the female secondary sex characteristics.

The timing of puberty in females is influenced by the level of body fat. Lean girls tend to enter puberty later. Female athletes with low body fat levels often have **amenorrhea** (absence of menstruation). This is probably because adipose tissue is a site of aromatization of androgens to estrogens. Several years before **menarche** (onset of menstrual cycles), **adrenarche** occurs. This is apparent by the development of pubic and axillary hair (Box 9-8).

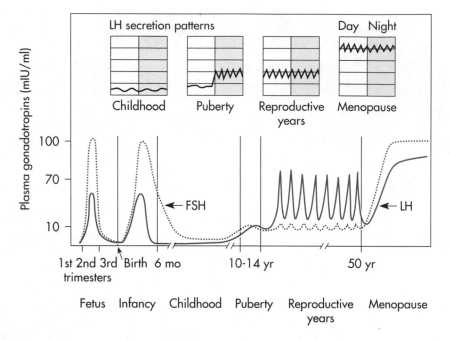

Figure 9-15 ■ Relative serum luteinizing hormone *(LH)* and follicle-stimulating hormone *(FSH)* levels during life in women. (Redrawn from Braunwald E, et al: *Harrison's principles of internal medicine,* ed 4, New York, 1987, McGraw-Hill.)

Breast Development at Puberty (Thelarche)

The increase in estrogen and progesterone secretion at puberty stimulates growth and maturation of the mammary glands. The onset of these mammary gland changes is referred to as **thelarche.** Both hormones stimulate mammary gland growth, but the primary action of estrogen is on the development of the ductile system and the primary action of progesterone is on the lobular-alveolar system. Table 9-1 shows the Tanner stages of pubertal development for women, and Figure 9-17 shows the ages at which these changes occur.

■ MENOPAUSE

Menopause is generally thought to result from primary ovarian deficiency because of depletion of functional follicles. However, the observation that some morphologically normal oocytes can be present in the postmenopausal ovary suggests that oocyte depletion is not the sole cause of menopause. It has been hypothesized that these remaining follicles are less sensitive to gonadotropins. It has been proposed recently that age-related changes in the central nervous system, including critical patterns of GnRH secretion, proceed follicular depletion and could play an important role in menopause. Because follicles do not develop in response to LH and FSH secretion, estrogen and progesterone levels drop. Loss of the negative feedback inhibition of estrogen on GnRH and LH/FSH results in a marked rise in serum LH and FSH. FSH levels rise more than LH levels. This could result from ovarian inhibin loss.

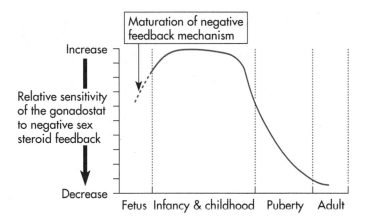

Figure 9-16 ■ **Changes in relative sensitivity of gonadostat during life of man or woman.** (Redrawn from Yen SSC, Jaffe RB, editors: *Reproductive endocrinology,* ed 2, Philadelphia, 1986, WB Saunders.)

TABLE 9-1

Tanner pubertal stages in female

Stage	Breast	Pubic hair
1	Prepubertal	Prepubertal, no pubic hair
2	Breast bud and papilla elevated, small mound present	Slight growth of fine downy hair
3	Enlargement of breast mound, palpable glandular tissue	Hair darker, coiled, denser
4	Areola and nipple elevated	Adult-type hair but area covered is less than adult area
5	Adult breast	Adult-type hair with triangular-shaped distribution

Data from Marshall WA, Tanner JM: *Arch Dis Child* 44:291, 1969.

Menopause typically occurs between 45 and 55 years of age. It extends over several years. Initially the cycles become irregular and are periodically anovulatory. The cycles tend to shorten, primarily in the follicular phase. Eventually, the woman ceases to cycle altogether. The serum estradiol levels drop to about one sixth the mean levels for younger cycling women, and progesterone levels drop to about one third those in the follicular phase of younger women. Production of these hormones does not cease entirely, but the primary source of these hormones in the postmenopausal woman becomes the adrenal, although interstitial cells of the ovarian stroma continue to produce some steroids. Most circulating estrogens are now produced peripherally from androgens. Because estrone is the primary estrogen produced in adipose tissue, it becomes the predominant estrogen in postmenopausal women.

Most of the symptoms associated with menopause result from estrogen deficiency. The vagi-

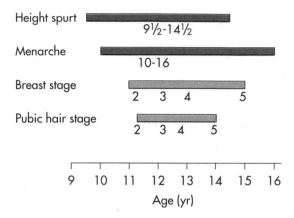

Figure 9-17 ■ **Sequence of events during female puberty indicating ranges of ages at which each event normally occurs. Numbers 2 to 5 refer to Tanner stages.** (Data from Marshall WA, Tanner JM: *Arch Dis Child* 45:13, 1970.)

nal epithelium atrophies and becomes dry, and bone loss is accelerated. The incidence of cardiovascular disease increases markedly after menopause. Hot flashes result from periodic increases in core temperature, which produce peripheral vasodilation and sweating. Hot flashes are now thought to be linked to increases in LH release and are probably associated not with the pulsatile rise in LH secretion but rather with central mechanisms controlling GnRH release. Hot flashes typically subside within 1 to 5 years of the onset of menopausal symptoms. Estrogen therapy generally provides relief from hot flashes, decreases the rate of bone loss, and decreases vaginal atrophy and dryness. Postmenopausal estrogen therapy can decrease the incidence of cardiovascular disease.

■ DISORDERS INVOLVING THE FEMALE REPRODUCTIVE TRACT
Menstrual Problems

Premenstrual Syndrome Although not truly a pathologic disorder in most women, premenstrual syndrome (PMS) produces minor dis-

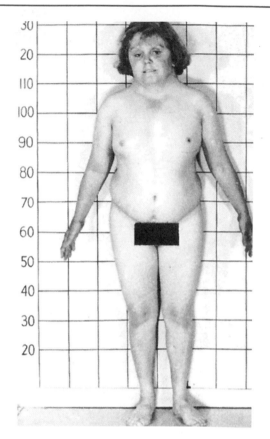

Figure 9-18 ■ **Female with Turner's syndrome. Note characteristically broad "webbed" neck. Stature is reduced, and sexual secondary characteristics are poorly developed.** (From Goodman RM, Gorlin RJ: *Atlas of the face in genetic disorders,* ed 2, St Louis, 1977, Mosby.)

comfort in many women and major discomfort in some women. A multitude of symptoms is associated with PMS, characterized as being manifested cyclically during the luteal phase of the cycle. The symptoms subside at or during menstruation. These symptoms can include irritability, depression, bloating, weight gain, breast tenderness, and headaches. The physiologic basis for the production of these symptoms is

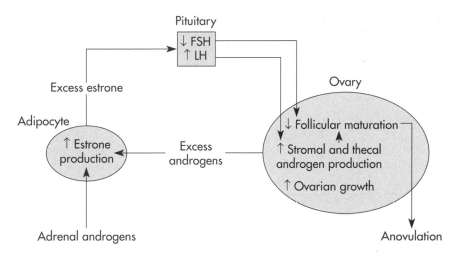

Figure 9-19 ■ **Pathogenesis of polycystic ovarian syndrome.** *FSH,* **Follicle-stimulating hormone;** *LH,* **luteinizing hormone.**

---

probably complex, and the nature of the symptoms is variable among women.

Dysmenorrhea Dysmenorrhea is painful menstruation. Primary dysmenorrhea is a common problem in ovulatory women; it is thought to result from ischemia caused by periodic uterine contractions. The uterine contractions result from uterine prostaglandin production. Pain can be projected to the back and legs and can be accompanied by nausea and diarrhea. Prostaglandin synthetase inhibitors provide relief for some women. Because primary dysmenorrhea is associated with ovulatory cycles, birth control pills administered to prevent ovulation can reduce the discomfort. Secondary dysmenorrhea results from uterine problems such as endometriosis or congenital anomalies.

Turner's Syndrome (Gonadal Dysgenesis)

Turner's syndrome is the most common cause of congenital hypogonadism. In about 50% of cases, it results from the complete absence of the second X chromosome so that the karyotype of the individual is 45,XO. The germ cells do not

develop, and the gonads consist of a connective tissue–filled streak. The major characteristics these individuals express include short stature, a characteristic webbed neck, low-set ears, a shield-shaped chest, short fourth metacarpals, and sexual infantilism resulting from gonadal dysgenesis (Figure 9-18). Internal and external genitalia are typically female.

Polycystic Ovarian Syndrome

Chronically anovulatory women with high circulating androgen, estrogen, and LH levels often have the disorder called **polycystic ovarian syndrome** (Figure 9-19). The continuous gonadotropin secretion leads to ovarian enlargement, and the ovaries typically show a thickened capsule and numerous follicles, many of which are undergoing atresia. FSH levels are low, which inhibits granulosa cell function, and the high intrafollicular androgen level inhibits follicular maturation. A significant portion of the high circulating estrogen levels is estrone formed from peripheral aromatization of androstenedione. These high androgen levels can produce hirsutism and acne. Hirsutism is the abnormal formation of coarse sexual hair in regions atypical for a woman, such as the face, back, and chest. The exact cause of polycystic ovarian syndrome is not well understood, but the primary defect appears to be inappropriate signals between the hypothalamic-pituitary axis and the ovary.

Summary

1. The ovaries are both the site of gametogenesis and a site of steroidogenesis. The granulosa, theca interna, and luteal cells are the sites of the bulk of ovarian steroidogenesis. Steroid synthesis is stimulated by LH and FSH.
2. Ovarian secretions are not necessary for normal fetal development of the female reproductive tract.
3. Early in follicular development, the theca interna cells produce androgens and limited amounts of estrogens in response to LH stimulation. Granulosa cells are capable of aromatizing androgens produced in thecal cells to form estrogens.
4. In the luteal phase of the ovarian cycle, luteal cells produce estrogens and progestins in response to LH stimulation.
5. Estrogens, under the appropriate circumstances, can either inhibit or facilitate LH secretion.
6. Major actions of estrogens include stimulation of uterine, fallopian tube, and vaginal growth and development. Estrogens stimulate granulosa cell–LH receptor formation, long-bone growth, and epiphyseal closure. Estrogens stimulate production of many liver proteins such as thyroxine-binding globulin (TBG) and sex hormone–binding globulin (SHBG).
7. Progestins stimulate formation of a secretory uterus. They antagonize aldosterone's actions on the kidney, increase body temperature, decrease uterine motility, and increase pulmonary ventilation.
8. Ovulation is stimulated by a surge in LH secretion.
9. The uterine cycle consists of the menstrual phase, proliferative phase, and secretory phase.
10. Puberty in females consists of thelarche, adrenarche, and menarche. The sensitivity of the gonadostat decreases in puberty.
11. Menopause results from depletion of functional follicles.
12. Turner's syndrome (gonadal dysgenesis) is the most common cause of congenital hypogonadism. It typically results from the absence of the second X chromosome, so that the karyotype of the individual is 45,XO.
13. Polycystic ovarian syndrome produces chronic anovulation. Circulating androgen, estrogen, and LH levels are typically high.

■ KEY WORDS AND CONCEPTS

- Ovarian follicles
- Maturation-inhibiting factors
- Primordial follicle
- Follicular cells
- Granulosa cells
- Primary follicle
- Zona pellucida
- Thecal layer
- Secondary follicle
- Antrum
- Tertiary follicle
- Follicular fluid
- Graafian follicle

- Cumulus oophorus
- Corona radiata
- Theca interna
- Theca externa
- First polar body
- Plasminogen activator
- Plasmin
- Corpus luteum
- Estradiol-17β
- Estriol
- Estrone
- Progesterone
- 17α-Hydroxyprogesterone
- Dehydroepiandrosterone (DHEA)
- Androstenedione
- Inhibin
- Progestins
- Negative feedback of estrogen
- Sex hormone–binding globulin (SHBG)
- Relaxin
- Follicular phase
- Luteal phase
- Luteal cells
- Positive feedback
- Negative feedback
- Proliferative phase
- Secretory phase
- Myometrium
- Endometrium
- Spiral arteries
- Secretory endometrium
- Menstruation
- Functional layer
- Basal layer
- Spinnbarkeit
- Ferning
- Keratinization (cornification)
- Menarche
- Adrenarche
- Thelarche
- Menopause
- Premenstrual syndrome (PMS)
- Dysmenorrhea

- Turner's syndrome (gonadal dysgenesis)
- Polycystic ovarian syndrome

■ SELF-STUDY PROBLEMS

1. Describe the ovarian control of development of the internal genitalia in the female.
2. What is the relationship between a primordial follicle, primary follicle, graafian follicle, corpus luteum, and corpus albicans?
3. How do granulosa cells and thecal cells work together to produce estrogens?
4. What is thought to be the physiologic basis for the midcycle gonadotropin surge?
5. What is meant by the expression "resetting the gonadostat" when applied to puberty?

■ BIBLIOGRAPHY

Brann DW, Mahesh VB: Excitatory amino acids: function and significance in reproduction and neuroendocrine regulation, *Frontiers Neuroendocrinol* 15:3, 1994.

Carr BR: Disorders of the ovary and female reproductive tract. In Wilson JD, Foster DW, editors: *Williams' textbook of endocrinology,* Philadelphia, 1992, WB Saunders.

Fauser BCJM, Van Heusden AM: Manipulation of human ovarian function: physiological concepts and clinical consequences, *Endocr Rev* 18(1):71-106, 1997.

Fawcett DW: *Bloom and Fawcett, a textbook of histology,* ed 12, New York, 1994, Chapman & Hall.

Goldfien A, Monroe SE: Ovaries. In Greenspan FS, Baxter JD, editors: *Basic and clinical endocrinology,* Norwalk, Conn, 1994, Appleton & Lange.

Graham JD, Clark CL: Physiological action of progesterone in target tissues, *Endocr Rev* 18(4):502-519, 1997.

Hoek A. Schoemaker J, Drexhage HA: Premature ovarian failure and ovarian autoimmunity, *Endocr Rev* 18(1):107-134, 1997.

Kalra SP: Mandatory neuropeptide-steroid signaling for the preovulatory luteinizing hormone-releasing hormone discharge, *Endocr Rev* 14:507, 1993.

Korach KS, Couse JF, Curtis SW, Washburn TF, Lindzey J, Kimbro KS, Eddy EM, Migliaccio S, Snedeker SM, Lubahn DB, Schomberg DW, Smith EP: Estrogen receptor gene disruption: molecular characterization and experimental and clinical phenotypes, *Rec Prog Horm Res* 51:159-188, 1996.

Wise PH: Menopause: aging of pacemakers, *News Physiol Sci* 12:143, 1997.

10

Endocrinology of Pregnancy

Objectives

1. Describe the physiologic basis for conception.

2. List the major factors controlling implantation.

3. Explain the role of the syncytiotrophoblast and cytotrophoblast in placental development and function.

4. List the major functions of amnionic fluid and explain how it is formed.

5. Explain why the fetus is essential for placental estrogen synthesis.

6. List the major placental hormones and explain their primary roles in pregnancy.

7. Explain, when possible, the physiologic basis for the cardiovascular, renal respiratory, and endocrine changes that occur in pregnancy.

8. Explain the physiologic basis of gestational diabetes.

9. Describe the major theories of parturition in humans.

10. Describe the physiologic basis of contraception with oral contraceptives.

■ CONCEPTION (Box 10-1)

Sperm transport in the female reproductive tract is governed by numerous factors. In humans, sperm can traverse the distance from the cervix to the site of fertilization, typically the ampulla of the fallopian duct, in as little as 5 minutes. Although tail-wagging is probably important for sperm penetration of the cervical mucus and ovum, animal experiments suggest that movement through the female reproductive tract is faster than can be accounted for by flagellar movement alone. Prostaglandins and oxytocin released in the woman at sexual inter-course and prostaglandins in semen stimulate female reproductive tract motility. This increase in motility assists sperm movement.

Fertilization depends on the activities of multiple sperm. Approximately 200 of the 2 to 6 million sperm ejaculated reach the vicinity of the ovum in humans. Multiple sperm are necessary for disruption of the cumulus oophorus and corona radiata, thereby divesting the ovum of some of its envelopments. Acrosomal **hyaluronidase** is important at this step. The sperm binds to human-specific glycoprotein sperm receptors on the zona pellucida and then proteolytically

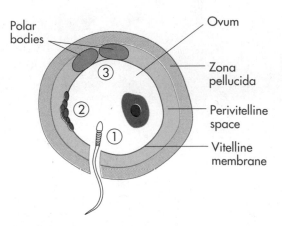

Figure 10-1 ■ Fertilization of ovum. Sperm enters zona pellucida and vitelline membrane (*1*). After fertilization, cortical granules are extruded into perivitelline space (*2*). Entry of sperm triggers completion of second meiotic division with release of second polar body into perivitelline space (*3*).

cleaves a narrow path through the zona pellucida (Figure 10-1). The acrosomal enzyme **acrosin** is important for zona pellucida penetration. When a sperm penetrates the zona pellucida and enters the vitelline membrane, ovum calcium uptake increases and enzyme-containing **cortical granules** are extruded from the ovum. These lysosome-like granules are ejected into the perivitelline space, where the proteolytic enzymes alter the zona pellucida so that further sperm penetration cannot occur. These changes in the zona pellucida are called the **zonal reaction.** The zona pellucida is necessary to prevent **polyspermia** (penetration of the ovum by multiple sperm).

Ovum penetration is the stimulus for completion of the second meiotic division. Consequently, the appearance of the second polar body in the perivitelline space is an index of fertilization. The actual period when fertility is possible is limited because the ovum remains viable for only about 24 hours, and sperm in the female reproductive tract have a maximum survival of 2 to 3 days. The fertilized ovum is called a **zygote.**

The zygote rapidly begins mitotic divisions and forms a ball of cells called a **morula,** within the zona pellucida (Figure 10-2, *A*). The morula remains in the fallopian tubes for approximately 3 to 4 days, and most of this time it is in the ampulla. During this time it is nourished by fallopian tube secretions.

Movement of the morula in the fallopian tube is hormonally regulated. The morula is retained in the ampulla for several days because of circular muscle contraction in the isthmus of the ampulla. This delay allows ample time for progesterone-stimulated development of the secretory endometrium. Estrogen stimulates circular muscle contraction in the isthmus, leading to retention of the morula in the ampulla. As progesterone levels rise, the circular muscle relaxes, permitting advancement of the morula through the fallopian tubes. Zygote motility within the fallopian duct is also regulated by ciliary activity within the fallopian tube. Estrogens accelerate development of these cilia and increase their beating. Ciliary action is the primary mechanism drawing the ovulated ovum into the fallopian tube. If fallopian tube motility is abnormal, either the morula can arrive at the uterus at an inappropriate time for implantation or implantation can occur in the fallopian tube, producing a tubal pregnancy. Occasionally implan-

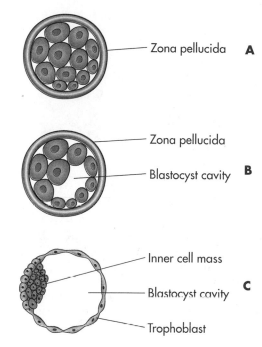

Figure 10-2 ■ Early cleavage stages in embryos. A, **Morula**. B, **Early blastocyst with zona pellucida intact.** C, **Late blastocyst shows inner cell mass and blastocyst cavity.**

tation occurs in the peritoneal cavity rather than the fallopian tube. It is possible for a blastocyst to implant in an area other than the uterus and for the fetus to grow and develop. However, the uterus is effectively designed for vascular constriction after delivery and separation of the placenta from the decidua; excessive bleeding is thus avoided. A major complication of ectopic pregnancy (implantation at a location other than the uterus) is hemorrhage.

Shortly after the morula enters the uterus, the cells secrete fluid into a cavity called the **blastocyst cavity** (Figure 10-2, B and C). On formation of this cavity, the morula becomes a **blastocyst.** The blastocyst contains two types of cells; there is an asymmetrically located **inner cell mass** that will become the embryo and an outer con-

centric layer of **trophoblast** cells. The trophoblast will form the chorion. The portion of the trophoblast adjacent to the inner cell mass becomes the **chorion frondosum,** and the remainder of the trophoblast forms the **chorion laeve** (smooth chorion).

The free-floating blastocyst is nourished by uterine secretions for 2 to 3 days, and then the zona pellucida is shed (constituents of uterine fluid may lyse the zona pellucida). Figure 10-3 shows the cleavage stages up to about 5 days after fertilization. Implantation occurs 6 to 7 days after conception (Figure 10-4). By 7 days, the blastocyst is producing human chorionic gonadotropin (hCG) in sufficient quantities to be measurable in maternal serum.

If the embryo arrives at the uterus before or after optimal secretory endometrial development, implantation might not occur and the embryo would be sloughed from the body. The mother would probably never realize conception had occurred.

■ IMPLANTATION

Implantation occurs in a properly prepared endometrium by a complex series of steps controlled by secretions of the ovary and the blastocyst that include steroids, growth factors, and prostaglandins. Although the hormonally primed endometrium is the ideal implantation site, it is not essential for implantation. The most common implantation site is the upper posterior surface of the uterine wall.

Implantation depends on normal uterine motility, which is a function of estrogen and progestin levels. High progestin levels at this time produce a relatively quiescent uterus. At the implantation site, characteristic endometrial changes, referred to as the **decidual reaction,** occur. These changes can be artificially produced in a rat by irritating the hormonally prepared endometrium with a metal or glass object. The endometrial stromal cells enlarge, and the

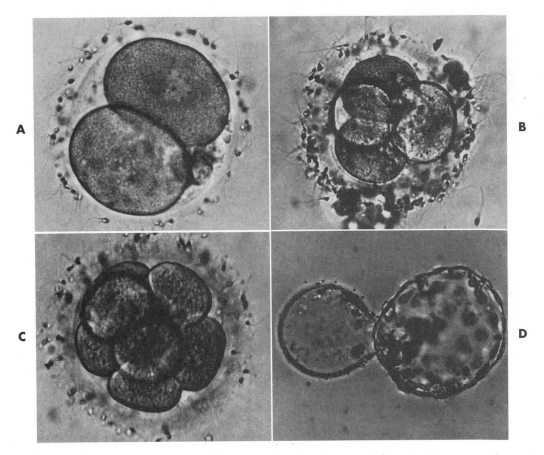

Figure 10-3 ■ **Cleavage stages of human eggs fertilized in vitro. A, Two cells 39 hours after fertilization. Polar body is at right of boundary between the two cells. B, Four cells 42 hours after fertilization. C, Eight cells 49 hours after fertilization. D, Hatching blastocyst 123 hours after fertilization. In A to C, numerous spermatozoa can be seen clinging to zona pellucida.** (From Veeck LL: *Atlas of the human oocyte and early conceptus,* vol 2, Baltimore, 1991, Williams & Wilkins.)

endometrium thickens. The term **decidua** is applied to the endometrium of pregnancy. The area of the decidua immediately associated with the trophoblast is the **decidua basalis,** which forms the **basal plate** (maternal portion) of the placenta. As the blastocyst becomes embedded in the endometrium, the portion of endometrium covering the blastocyst is called the **decidua capsularis.** The remaining layer of the endometrium is called the **decidua parietalis.**

■ DEVELOPMENT OF THE PLACENTA

The placenta is derived from maternal decidua basalis (endometrium) and chorion frondosum.

At implantation, the embryonic blastocyst invades the endometrium by phagocytosis (Figure 10-5, *A*). Nourishment is obtained from uterine secretions and endometrial phagocytosis. Initially, the trophoblast consists of **cytotrophoblastic cells** (Figure 10-5, *B*). After implantation, the **syncytiotrophoblast** differentiates

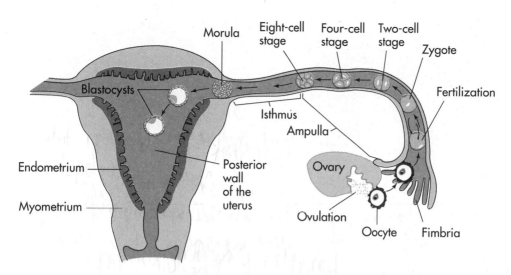

Figure 10-4 ■ Fertilization and human development during first week.

from the **cytotrophoblast.** The syncytiotrophoblast, or outer layer of the trophoblast, is a multinucleate syncytium of cells without defined cell borders. It is this layer that is in direct contact with the decidua. The trophoblast surrounds the developing embryo and contains the blastocyst cavity with it (Figure 10-5, *C*).

By about 9 days of gestation, cavities, called **lacunae,** form within the projections of the syncytiotrophoblast that penetrate the decidua (Figure 10-5, *D*). These fingerlike projections of the syncytiotrophoblast represent the earliest forms of the placental villi.

Penetration of the endometrial veins establishes the initial circulation to the placenta by about day 15 of gestation. Shortly thereafter, the endometrial spiral arteries are invaded, thereby establishing maternal blood flow to the intervillous spaces. Maternal blood is now in direct contact with the villous syncytiotrophoblast.

Invasion of the endometrium ceases once uterine arterioles have been invaded and development of maternal circulation to the placenta has been completed. The increased Po_2 at the syncytiotrophoblast might inhibit further invasion. Fetal blood vessels form within the mesenchyme of the villi, and by day 17, fetal circulation to the villi is established, thereby providing both maternal and fetal circulations to the placenta. The villi are now called **chorionic villi** (Figure 10-6). The human placenta is **hemochorial** because the villous syncytiotrophoblast is directly bathed in extravasated maternal blood in these large sinuses. The lacunae coalesce to form the intervillous spaces. As the chorionic villi mature, the cytotrophoblast becomes discontinuous, leaving a diffusion barrier consisting of the syncytiotrophoblast, mesenchyme, and capillary endothelium. In some regions the mesenchyme is lost, leaving two layers.

Eventually, extraembryonic mesoderm differentiates from the cytotrophoblast and invades and lines the blastocyst cavity (Figure 10-7). Thus the **chorion,** composed of three layers—mesoderm, cytotrophoblast, and syncytiotrophoblast—is formed. The blastocyst cavity is now called the **extracoelomic cavity.** The ex-

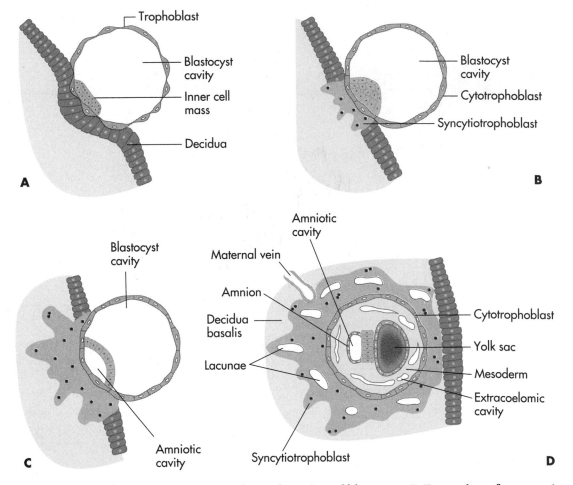

Figure 10-5 ■ Steps in implantation. A, Early implantation of blastocyst. B, Formation of cytotrophoblast and syncytiotrophoblast. C, Formation of amniotic cavity. D, Formation of lacunae with maternal venous penetration.

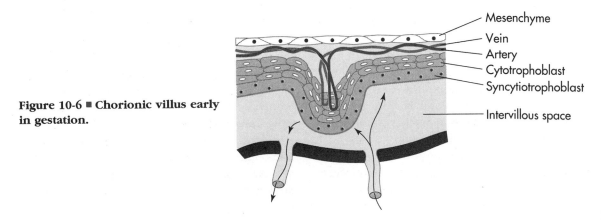

Figure 10-6 ■ Chorionic villus early in gestation.

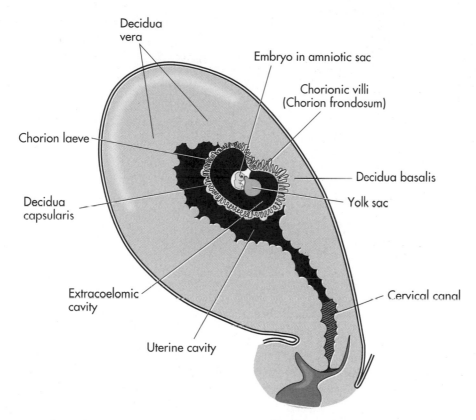

Figure 10-7 ■ Early embryonic development showing embryo relative to decidua, amnion, and chorion. (Redrawn from Cunningham FG, et al, editors: *Williams' obstetrics,* ed 19, Norwalk, Conn, 1993, Appleton & Lange.)

tracoelomic cavity is eventually obliterated as the embryo and the amnion grow. Initially the villi entirely surround the embryo. The villi in contact with the decidua basalis are called the **chorion frondosum,** and the villi associated with the decidua capsularis are called the **chorion laeve.** Eventually villi are lost from the chorion laeve. The chorion frondosum forms the fetal component of the placenta (Figure 10-8).

A space develops between the trophoblast and the inner cell mass. This space becomes lined with cells produced from the trophoblast that form the **amnion.** As the amniotic cavity

grows, this layer eventually lines the trophoblast and extends over the surface of the placenta, umbilical cord, and embryo. It is contiguous with the chorion. A part of the amniotic cavity is lined by the ectoderm of the embryo.

A clear fluid called **amniotic fluid** accumulates within the cavity formed within the amnion. It eventually envelops the fetus. This fluid serves many important roles during fetal development. It cushions and therefore protects the fetus from physical blows to the mother's abdomen. This fluid compartment is often considered an extension of the fetal fluid compartment

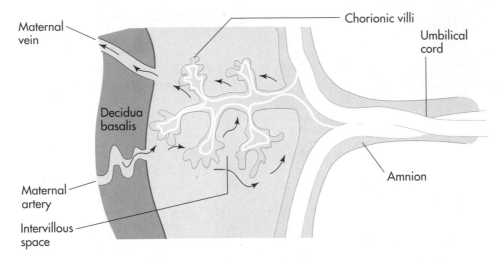

Figure 10-8 ■ **Placenta. Although intervillous space is indicated for illustrative purposes, chorionic villi are actually so numerous that they almost completely fill the space, leaving a space not much wider than the diameter of a capillary.**

because it more closely resembles fetal than maternal fluids. The fluid is formed from maternal fluids of the uterus and fetal fluids diffusing through the thin fetal skin and lungs and from fetal urine and gastrointestinal secretions. It contains fetal and uterine endocrine and paracrine secretions and desquamated fetal tissue. Fetal "breathing" movements are important for normal fetal lung development, and amniotic fluid is inspired and expired by the immature lungs.

■ PLACENTAL ENDOCRINE FUNCTION
Fetoplacental Unit (Box 10-2)

Maternal serum progesterone levels increase as the pregnancy progresses. Serum levels of estradiol, estriol, and estrone all rise (Figure 10-9). Although there is minimal estriol production in nonpregnant women, estriol becomes a major estrogen during pregnancy. Most estrogens are produced by the corpus luteum early in the first trimester. At this time, hCG is the major regulator of corpus luteum steroid production. How-

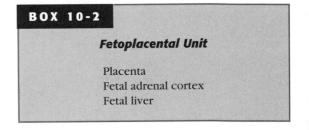

BOX 10-2

Fetoplacental Unit

Placenta
Fetal adrenal cortex
Fetal liver

ever, as the placenta develops, placental steroid production from the syncytiotrophoblast increases so that by 8 weeks of gestation placental steroidogenesis is sufficient to support the pregnancy without steroidogenesis by the ovaries. Although ovarian steroidogenesis continues throughout pregnancy in the normal woman, during the latter two thirds of the pregnancy, placental steroidogenesis far exceeds ovarian steroidogenesis.

Placental steroidogenesis requires the concerted action of the fetal adrenal, fetal liver, and the placenta. Therefore steroidogenesis in pregnancy is a function of the **fetoplacental**

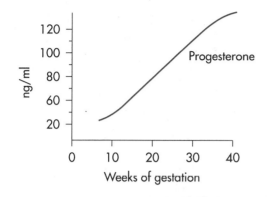

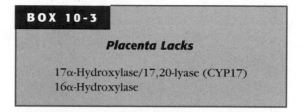

BOX 10-3

Placenta Lacks

17α-Hydroxylase/17,20-lyase (CYP17)
16α-Hydroxylase

BOX 10-4

Fetus Lacks

3β-Hydroxysteroid dehydrogenase (3β-HSD)
Aromatase (CYP19)

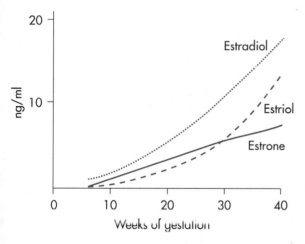

Figure 10-9 ■ Maternal serum progesterone and estrogen levels during pregnancy.

unit (Figure 10-10). Although the placenta can synthesize cholesterol from acetate, most placental cholesterol comes from the mother. The placenta can produce pregnenolone and progesterone. However, because it lacks the enzyme **17α-hydroxylase/17,20-lyase (CYP17),** which is needed to convert pregnenolone to **dehydroepiandrosterone (DHEA),** it cannot produce androgens and estrogens without involving the fetus (Box 10-3). The androgen precursors for placental estrogen production are derived from both fetal and ma-

ternal circulations. The fetal adrenal cortex has 17α-hydroxylase/17,20-lyase and therefore can convert pregnenolone produced in the placenta to DHEA or progesterone to androstenedione. The fetal adrenal lacks **3β-hydroxysteroid dehydrogenase (3β-HSD),** and therefore the fetus cannot convert DHEA to androstenedione. It also lacks the aromatase enzyme necessary for estrogen production (Box 10-4). DHEA and androstenedione produced in the fetus from placental pregnenolone and progesterone can be converted in the placenta to estradiol and estrone. The placenta has the enzyme **aromatase (CYP19),** which is necessary for estrogen production.

The fetal liver is essential for **estriol** production because it has the enzyme **16α-hydroxylase,** which converts DHEA to **16α-OH DHEA.** Placenta then converts 16α-OH DHEA to estriol. Consequently, maternal serum estriol levels reflect the functions of the fetal liver, fetal adrenal cortex, and the placenta, whereas progesterone levels can reflect only a functional placenta.

Fetal steroids are commonly sulfated, and sulfation serves to protect the fetus from the high steroid levels in pregnancy because sulfation

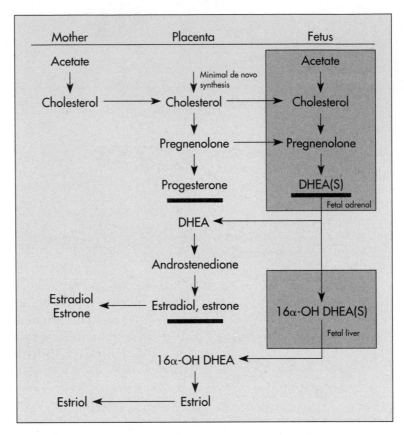

Figure 10-10 ■ **Fetoplacental unit.** *Solid bar,* **Enzyme block;** *DHEA,* **dehydroepiandrosterone;** *16α-OH DHEA,* **16α-hydroxydehydroepiandrosterone.**

decreases the biologic activity of the steroid. The placenta is able to use these sulfated precursors because it has high concentrations of the enzyme **sulfatase,** which removes the sulfate moiety.

Alpha-Fetoprotein

Alpha-fetoprotein (AFP) is a glycoprotein synthesized in the fetal yolk sac and liver and excreted into amnionic fluid via the urine. It probably serves many roles in the fetus. This compound binds estrogens and thereby decreases the availability of free estrogens in the

fetus. Like sulfation, AFP decreases fetal steroid exposure. High levels of AFP in amnionic fluid can indicate the presence of a fetal neural tube defect, whereas low levels can indicate genetic aberrations such as Down syndrome.

Fetal Adrenal Cortex

The fetal adrenal cortex contains an outer **definitive zone,** which will become the zona glomerulosa, zona fasciculata, and zona reticularis, and an inner **fetal zone.** The fetal zone is the predominant portion of the adrenal cortex in the fetus, constituting as much as 80% of the bulk of the large fetal adrenal. It is the site of most fetal adrenal steroidogenesis, and its major product is the weak androgen DHEA, which is secreted as DHEA sulfate. DHEA sulfate is desulfated in the placenta, where it is a crucial precursor for placental estrogen production. Involution of the fetal zone occurs subsequent to delivery, and the bulk of this region is lost within the first 2 neonatal months. Both the fetal adrenal and the placenta work together to produce cortisol. Cortisol production occurs in the definitive zone rather than the fetal zone of the adrenal cortex.

■ NONSTEROIDAL PLACENTAL HORMONES

Human Chorionic Gonadotropin

(Box 10-5)

Human chorionic gonadotropin (hCG) is a glycoprotein that is structurally and functionally similar to luteinizing hormone (LH). Like LH, it stimulates ovarian steroid hormone synthesis. hCG is the major hormone preventing luteolysis and is therefore essential for the initial maintenance of pregnancy. It is often used clinically in place of LH because its 24- to 30-hour half-life ($t_½$) is much longer than that of LH. It is produced by the cells of the syncytiotrophoblast. The hormone can be detected in maternal serum within 1 week of conception, and levels increase rapidly after implantation, typically reaching peak serum levels by 9 to 12 weeks of gestation (Figure 10-11, *A*). During this period, hCG is important to maintain the corpus luteum. By 8 weeks, the ovaries are no longer essential for pregnancy,

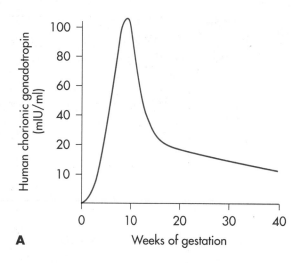

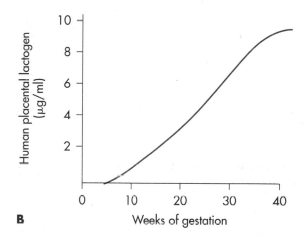

Figure 10-11 ■ Maternal serum human chorionic gonadotropin levels (A) **and human placental lactogen levels** (B) **during pregnancy.**

and hCG levels fall during the second and third trimesters. Fetal testis steroid production is regulated by hCG (see Chapter 8).

Human Placental Lactogen (Box 10-6)

Human placental lactogen (hPL), also called **human chorionic somatomammotropin**, is a 191–amino acid protein hormone produced in the syncytiotrophoblast that is structurally simi-

BOX 10-6

Major Functions of Human Placental Lactogen

- Mobilizes maternal nutrients for fetus
- Is lipolytic, insulin antagonistic
- Stimulates mammary gland growth and development

lar to growth hormone (GH) and prolactin (PRL). Its function overlaps those of both GH and PRL. It can be detected within the syncytiotrophoblast by 10 days after conception and in maternal serum by 3 weeks of gestation (Figure 10-11, *B*). Maternal serum levels rise progressively throughout the remainder of the pregnancy. The quantity of hormone produced is directly related to the size of the placenta, so that as the placenta grows during gestation, hPL secretion increases. As much as 1 g/day of hPL can be secreted late in gestation.

Like GH, hPL is protein anabolic and lipolytic. Its antagonistic action to insulin is the major basis for the diabetogenicity of pregnancy. Like PRL, it stimulates mammary gland growth and development. Mammary gland development in pregnancy results from the actions of hPL, PRL, estrogens, and progestins. hPL inhibits maternal glucose uptake and use, thereby increasing serum glucose levels. Glucose is a major energy substrate for the fetus, and hPL increases fetal glucose availability (Figure 10-12).

As with hCG, far less hPL is found in fetal circulation than in maternal circulation. This suggests that the hormones may play a more important role in the mother than in the fetus. hPL is not essential for the pregnancy.

Both hPL and PRL act as fetal growth hormones and stimulate production of the fetal growth-promoting hormones: insulin-like growth factors (IGF-I and IGF-II). Ironically, fetal

GH does not appear to regulate growth, and anencephalic infants and GH-deficient children typically have normal birth weights.

Other Placental Hormones

The placenta is a source of many other hormones, including placental adrenocorticotropic hormone (ACTH), placental thyroid-stimulating hormone (TSH), and relaxin. The role of placental ACTH and TSH is not understood. The placenta produces **parathyroid hormone–related protein (PTHrP),** which increases placental calcium transport. Cytotrophoblastic PTHrP production increases in response to decreased extracellular calcium concentration. All the hypothalamic releasing and inhibiting hormones have homologs produced in the placenta, and placental gonadotropin-releasing hormone (GnRH) might regulate hCG secretion. The exact role of these placental releasing and inhibiting hormones remains to be conclusively established.

■ OTHER HORMONAL CHANGES OF PREGNANCY
Thyroidal Changes

Thyroid size increases during pregnancy, and serum total thyroxine (T_4) and triiodothyronine (T_3) levels can double. The primary basis for the increase in serum thyroid hormone levels is an estrogen-induced increase in liver **thyroxine-binding globulin (TBG)** production, which leads to an increase in hormone binding. However, serum *free* T_4 and T_3 levels do not increase markedly during gestation because hormone turnover rate is increased. The increased thyroidal growth and hormone synthesis during pregnancy are not caused predominantly by placental TSH. Instead, thyroidal stimulation is thought to reflect the actions of hCG. The increased thyroid function parallels the first-trimester serum hCG rise. Late in the first trimester, when maternal serum hCG levels peak, maternal thyroid

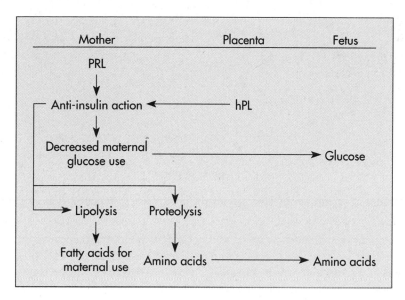

Figure 10-12 ■ Role of human placental lactogen *(hPL)* and prolactin *(PRL)* in altering maternal metabolism to provide amino acids and glucose to fetus.

size and hormone synthesis peak and maternal serum TSH levels are at their lowest. Because the α chains of hCG are identical to those of TSH and the β chains are similar, hCG can cross-react with TSH receptors when hCG levels are high. There is a transient drop in serum TSH levels at this time because of the rise in serum T_4 and T_3 levels. Free thyroid hormone levels do increase slightly at this time.

Adrenal Changes

Estrogens not only stimulate liver TBG production but also nonspecifically stimulate liver production of many other serum proteins, such as **transcortin.** Consequently, serum cortisol levels rise. Although maternal serum ACTH levels increase slightly during pregnancy, they typically remain within the normal nonpregnant range. However, late in pregnancy, serum free cortisol levels rise steadily to a peak at parturition that is about twofold nonpregnancy levels.

This surge in cortisol production is important for the initiation of lactation.

Estrogen stimulates liver angiotensinogen production and renal renin production. Consequently, angiotensin II and aldosterone synthesis increases. Estrogens potentiate the adrenal action of angiotensin II but inhibit the vascular actions. Although aldosterone secretion in pregnancy increases, symptoms of hyperaldosteronism are not typically present in pregnancy because progesterone is antagonistic to the action of aldosterone on the kidney.

Prolactin Levels

PRL levels rise during pregnancy because estrogen stimulates PRL synthesis and secretion (Figure 10-13). Pituitary enlargement in pregnancy reflects growth of PRL-secreting lactotropes. Secretion of other anterior pituitary hormones decreases or remains relatively constant. Pituitary enlargement during pregnancy makes the

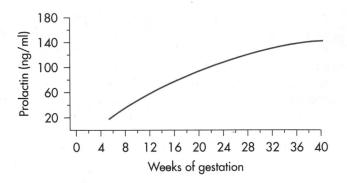

Figure 10-13 ▪ Maternal serum prolactin concentration during gestation. (Redrawn from Rigg LA, Yen SSC: *Am J Obstet Gynecol* 128:215, 1977.)

pituitary susceptible to vascular insult and necrosis at parturition (Sheehan's syndrome, see Chapter 2).

Luteinizing Hormone and Follicle-Stimulating Hormone Levels

Pituitary LH and FSH production decrease during pregnancy because of negative feedback inhibition by the high placentally produced estrogen and progestin levels.

Growth Hormone Levels

Maternal GH levels are comparable to, or slightly lower than, those in nonpregnant women.

▪ FETAL ENDOCRINE SYSTEM
Pituitary Gland

The fetal anterior pituitary develops relatively early in gestation. Typically the pituitary hormones are present and secreted before establishment of the feedback control systems mediated through the hypothalamus. By 12 weeks after conception, all the anterior pituitary hormones can be detected in the gland, and hypothalamic releasing or inhibiting hormones are present in the hypothalamus. The hypophyseal portal system is not functional until approxi-

mately 18 weeks of gestation. Typically, at midgestation, anterior pituitary hormone levels are high because of immature feedback control systems. The fetal pituitary is not necessary for the early development and secretion of the endocrine target organs. Although fetal serum GH levels are high late in gestation, GH is not thought to be an important regulator of fetal growth, and the high serum levels probably reflect the immaturity of the control systems for GH regulation. Fetal PRL is secreted early in development, and by birth, fetal levels exceed maternal levels. In addition, PRL levels are particularly high in amnionic fluid; much of this PRL is produced by the decidua. Both fetal and decidual PRL might be important in osmoregulation of amnionic fluid. PRL and hPL have been proposed as fetal growth regulators.

The fetal posterior pituitary secretes oxytocin and antidiuretic hormone (ADH) by midgestation. Fetal oxytocin has been proposed to play a role in parturition.

Parathyroid Gland

Fetal serum calcium levels are typically higher than maternal levels because placental PTHrP mobilizes maternal calcium and increases placental calcium transport. Although the fetal parathyroid is functional by the end of the first trimester, the high fetal serum calcium levels resulting from the transport of calcium across the placenta suppress fetal parathyroid function. In response to the calcium demands of the growing fetus, maternal parathyroid hormone (PTH) secretion increases. Maternal serum PTH increases are generally sufficient to maintain relatively normal maternal serum calcium levels despite the drain of calcium to the fetus.

Testes and Ovaries

Fetal testicular development and function are regulated primarily by hCG, rather than fetal LH, during midgestation. The presence of a functional feedback system for the control of gonadal steroidogenesis is demonstrated by the rise in LH secretion in the immediate postnatal period, when maternal steroids are no longer present. The role of the ovaries during fetal development is not known; they appear to be relatively quiescent in utero.

Thyroid Gland

The fetal thyroid is capable of producing thyroid hormones between 10 and 12 weeks after conception, and fetal serum levels of T_4 increase rapidly in midgestation. The initial function of the thyroid does not depend on fetal TSH secretion. Although very little T_3 can be detected in fetal serum, the hormone is present in fetal tissues. Fetal and perhaps maternal thyroid hormones are important for normal fetal brain development in utero.

Adrenal Gland

As mentioned earlier, the fetal adrenal is essential for key steps in placental hormone synthesis. The fetal adrenal becomes large during prenatal development, and the greatest portion of the adrenal cortex consists of the fetal zone. Fetal adrenal steroid production is present by 7 weeks after conception. During the first few postnatal months, the fetal zone regresses and the definitive zone eventually becomes the sole steroidogenic region of the adrenal cortex.

Pancreas

The fetal pancreas can secrete insulin and glucagon by 15 weeks after conception. However, in the fetus, blood glucose is determined more by the glucose transported across the placenta than by fetal metabolism or fetal insulin production. The ability of the fetal pancreas to respond to chronically elevated glucose levels in the latter half of gestation is demonstrated by pancreatic hyperplasia and hyperinsulinemia that develop in neonates of poorly regulated hyperglycemic mothers.

■ PLACENTAL TRANSPORT

As placental development continues, the cytotrophoblast becomes discontinuous so that the minimal placental barrier to transport consists of the syncytiotrophoblast, sometimes mesenchyme, and fetal capillary endothelium. The complexity of the mature placental villi markedly increases the surface area for transport between maternal and fetal blood. Depending on the substance involved, transport can occur by simple diffusion, facilitated diffusion, active transport, and endocytosis.

Gases, water, and many electrolytes cross the placenta by simple diffusion. Because the placental membrane is considerably thicker than the diffusional surface of the lungs, placental gas transport efficiency is only about 1/50th that of the lung on a per unit weight basis. A sizable gradient exists for oxygen between maternal and fetal blood. It is debatable whether the steep gradient results from lack of oxygen equilibration or high placental oxygen consumption, or both. The Po_2 of blood in placental venous blood (oxygenated blood) is approximately 30 mm Hg (maternal arterial Po_2 is approximately 105 mm Hg). Fetal compensation

---

BOX 10-7

Placental Transport

Glucose transport—Carrier-mediated facilitated diffusion
Amino acid transport—Carrier-mediated secondary active transport
Low-density lipoprotein (LDL) transport—LDL receptor–mediated endocytosis
Gas transport—Simple diffusion

BOX 10-8

Physiologic Changes in Pregnancy

Cardiovascular Changes

↑Vascular volume
↓Peripheral resistance
↑Stroke volume
↑Heart rate
↑Contractility
↑Cardiac output

Respiratory Changes

↑Minute volume
↑Tidal volume
↓P_{CO_2}
↓Functional residual capacity
↓Inspiratory reserve volume

Renal Changes

↑Antidiuretic hormone, renin, angiotensin II, aldosterone secretion
Respiratory alkalosis

---

for the low P_{O_2} is aided by a high fetal blood flow rate and the high oxygen affinity of fetal hemoglobin.

Carbon dioxide, on the other hand, is more soluble in body tissues, and the diffusion capacity is greater. Placental vein P_{CO_2} is about 43 mm Hg (maternal arterial blood P_{CO_2} is approximately 32 mm Hg).

Amino acids are transported by carrier-mediated secondary active transport (Box 10-7). Glucose is transported by carrier-mediated facilitated diffusion and is a major substrate for energy metabolism in the fetus. Although there is limited fatty acid transport, neutral fats do not cross the placenta, and low-density lipoproteins (LDLs) are transported across the placenta by LDL receptor–mediated endocytosis.

The fat-soluble steroid hormones cross relatively readily, but protein hormone transport is minimal. Limited thyroid hormone transport occurs, and carrier-mediated systems may be involved.

■ PHYSIOLOGIC CHANGES OF PREGNANCY

Physiologic changes occur in the pregnant woman both as a consequence of the size of the developing fetus and as a result of the endocrine and cardiovascular changes associated with the pregnancy (Box 10-8).

Cardiovascular Changes

Both heart rate and stroke volume, and therefore cardiac output, increase in pregnancy to approximately 40% more than preconception levels, with most of this increase occurring by 8 weeks of gestation. Blood volume increases 50% during pregnancy.

As the pregnancy progresses, the placental circulation requires a progressively larger portion of the maternal cardiac output. The additional vasculature of the maternal side of the placenta produces a large increase in the capacity of the vascular system. Uteroplacental blood flow near term is estimated to be as much as 900 ml/min. Much of the increase in blood volume occurs between 6 and 32 weeks of gestation. It is in part a result of the estrogen-stimulated increase in renin-angiotensin-aldosterone secretion. Progesterone, hPL, and PRL stimulate erythropoiesis, but because late in pregnancy blood volume expands faster than increased red blood cell synthesis, the hematocrit value drops slightly.

Because the placenta is essentially an arteriovenous shunt, vascular resistance is low. Therefore total peripheral resistance drops and diastolic pressure tends to drop. Blood pressure typically does not rise until late in pregnancy unless preeclampsia develops. Because the growing uterus exerts pressure on the veins of the legs where these veins enter the abdomen, venous pressure in the lower extremities rises on standing, and edema and venous damage can occur.

In part, these changes can be attributed to the need for increased blood flow to the growing uterus and placenta; however, significant cardiovascular changes occur relatively early in gestation when the uterus and placenta are still small. Although the arteriovenous shunt through the placenta is the basis for some of the cardiovascular changes, the basis for the early development of the cardiovascular changes has not been definitively established.

Respiratory Changes

As pregnancy proceeds, the functional residual capacity (volume of air in the lungs at the end of a quiet expiration) and residual volume (volume remaining at the end of a maximal expiration) decrease and respiratory rate remains unchanged. Minute volume increases and tidal volume increases, so Pco_2 decreases.

There are three major causes of the respiratory changes associated with pregnancy. The bulk of the growing fetus and uterus increases intraabdominal pressure and forces the diaphragm upward. The high metabolic rate of the growing fetus increases maternal oxygen consumption and carbon dioxide production. In addition, progesterone acts directly on the central nervous system (CNS) to lower the set-point for regulation of respiration by carbon dioxide,

thereby increasing ventilation. Consequently, Pco_2 decreases from 40 to approximately 32 mm Hg. The increased need for fetal oxygen and release of carbon dioxide and the direct CNS actions of progesterone all act to alter respiration during pregnancy. The progesterone-induced hyperventilation of pregnancy produces a mild, compensated respiratory alkalosis with a decrease in serum Pco_2 and therefore a drop in serum HCO_3^-.

Renal Changes

Water retention occurs in normal pregnancies. This is caused in part by changes in the set-points for regulation of ADH secretion and thirst so that both increase, with a resultant decrease in serum osmolality. The cause of this change is not known, but it could be related to actions of hCG.

The glomerular filtration rate (GFR) increases approximately 60% over nonpregnant levels. The exact cause of the increased GFR is not known. As GFR increases, the filtered load of filtered substances increases, and the increased filtered loads of glucose and amino acids can lead to glucosuria and aminoaciduria in pregnancy. Glucosuria in pregnancy also results from impaired distal tubule glucose absorption. The mechanisms underlying this change are not known.

Plasma renin, angiotensin II, and aldosterone increase, at least in part because of the decrease in blood pressure resulting from the decreased vascular resistance. Because "effective circulating blood volume" tends to decrease with growth of the placental circulation, mean arterial pressure drops, resulting in increased renin release. The uterus also produces renin in pregnancy. Angiotensin II stimulates aldosterone production, and aldosterone increases renal salt and water retention. In addition, estrogen stimulates liver synthesis of angiotensinogen, the precursor of angiotensin I. Estrogen and progesterone both directly increase the secretion of renin, the enzyme converting angiotensinogen to angiotensin I. Consequently, as placental estrogen and progesterone production increases, angiotensin II formation increases. Although angiotensin II stimulates aldosterone synthesis, the vasculature appears refractory to its vasopressive actions.

Maternal serum levels of the mineralocorticoid **deoxycorticosterone (DOC)** increase during pregnancy. This increase in circulating DOC levels does not result from increased adrenal secretion but from renal conversion of placental progesterone to DOC. DOC stimulates renal salt and water retention. Maternal aldosterone secretion increases to levels about 20-fold those of nonpregnant women. The increased secretion of the mineralocorticoids aldosterone and DOC is important for the volume expansion seen in the mother during pregnancy.

Gastrointestinal Changes

Gastric emptying rate and intestinal transit times are decreased in pregnancy. These changes might be a result of progesterone actions decreasing smooth muscle motility. Heartburn, or reflux of acidic gastric secretions into the esophagus, occurs for multiple reasons. The increased intraabdominal pressure increases intragastric pressure, which increases the likelihood of reflux into the esophagus. Progesterone also decreases lower esophageal sphincter tone, thereby increasing reflux tendency.

■ METABOLIC CHANGES OF PREGNANCY
Diabetogenicity of Pregnancy

During the last half of pregnancy, when hPL levels are highest, maternal energy metabolism shifts from an anabolic state in which nutrients are stored, to a catabolic state, sometimes described as **accelerated starvation,** in which maternal energy metabolism shifts toward fat utilization with glucose sparing. As maternal glucose use for energy decreases, lipolysis increases and fatty acids become major energy

sources. The peripheral response to insulin decreases and pancreatic insulin secretion increases. Beta cell hyperplasia occurs in pregnancy. Pregnancy aggravates existing diabetes mellitus, or diabetes mellitus can develop for the first time in pregnancy. If the diabetes resolves spontaneously with delivery, the condition is referred to as **gestational diabetes.** Other hormones contributing to the diabetogenicity of pregnancy are estrogens and progestins, because both of these hormones decrease insulin sensitivity.

■ PARTURITION

Human pregnancy lasts an average of 40 weeks from the beginning of the last menstrual period (gestational age). This corresponds to an average fetal age of 38 weeks. Parturition is the process whereby uterine contractions lead to childbirth. Parturition control in humans is complex, and the exact mechanisms underlying parturition control are not well understood (Box 10-9). In many species, such as sheep, the timing of parturition is fetally controlled, and fetal regulation is at least a factor in humans.

Fetal Adrenal Changes

Sheep parturition is initiated by maturational changes in the hypothalamic-pituitary axis that increase fetal ACTH secretion. ACTH stimulates fetal adrenal cortisol synthesis. Cortisol stimu-

---

BOX 10-9

Possible Stimuli for Parturition

↑Uterine size
↑Fetal adrenocorticotropic hormone (ACTH) production
↑Oxytocin receptor concentrations
↑Uterine prostaglandin production
↑Estrogen/progesterone ratio (sheep)

lates placental 17α-hydroxylase production (the human placenta lacks 17α-hydroxylase), which increases the conversion of progesterone to androgen. These androgens are estrogen precursors, and therefore, when their production increases, it shifts the balance of estrogen and progesterone production toward estrogen production. The change in the estrogen/progesterone ratio increases uterine motility both directly and indirectly by stimulating prostaglandin production (Figure 10-14). ACTH or glucocorticoid treatment of the pregnant sheep initiates parturition.

In humans, progesterone secretion does not decline immediately before parturition. Progesterone administration cannot delay parturition. The role of fetal ACTH production in the control of human parturition is not clear. ACTH or glucocorticoid treatment of a pregnant woman

does not induce parturition as it does in sheep. However, there is the possibility that a fetal signal involving the hypothalamus-pituitary-adrenal system in humans initiates parturition in humans as is suggested by the observation that anencephalic fetuses or those with adrenal hypoplasia tend to have a prolonged gestation.

Cortisol production from the definitive zone of the fetal adrenal is important for maturation of fetal lungs and fetal enzyme systems.

Estrogen and Progesterone Secretion

Although a rise in maternal serum estrogen and a drop in progesterone levels are seen late in gestation in some species, no change in the ratio of the two hormones is seen in human serum. However, the amnion, chorion, and decidua produce estrogens and progesterone, and estrogen inhibits formation of progesterone from

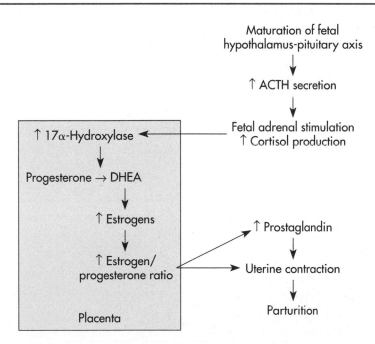

Figure 10-14 ■ Control of parturition in sheep. *DHEA,* Dehydroepiandrosterone; *ACTH,* adrenocorticotropic hormone.

pregnenolone. It is possible that locally produced estrone could alter myometrial estrogen/progesterone ratios and local prostaglandin production and oxytocin receptor levels.

Uterine Size

Uterine size is thought to be a factor regulating parturition because stretch of smooth muscle, including the uterus, increases muscle contraction. In addition, uterine stretch stimulates uterine prostaglandin production. Multiple births generally occur prematurely. The tendency for early delivery can be a result of increased uterine size, increased fetal production of chemicals stimulating delivery, or both.

Oxytocin

Oxytocin, which stimulates powerful uterine contractions, plays a major role in parturition (Figure 10-15). It is released in response to stretch of the cervix, and it stimulates uterine contractions and thereby facilitates delivery. Oxytocin can be used to induce parturition, and uterine sensitivity to oxytocin increases before parturition. Because maternal serum oxytocin levels do not increase until after parturition has begun, oxytocin is not thought to initiate

parturition. However, progesterone inhibits and estrogen stimulates synthesis of oxytocin receptors, and, although maternal serum progesterone levels do not decrease immediately before human parturition, estrogen levels rise and oxytocin receptor synthesis increases.

Prostaglandins

Prostaglandins and other cytokines increase uterine motility, and levels of these compounds increase during parturition, thereby facilitating delivery. Their exact role in the initiation of parturition is not known. Prostaglandin levels in amnionic fluid, fetal membranes, and uterine decidua increase before the onset of labor. Prostaglandins $F_{2\alpha}$ and E_2 increase uterine motility. Large doses of these compounds have been used to induce labor. Because estrogens stimulate prostaglandin synthesis in the uterus, amnion, and chorion, the rising estrogen levels late in gestation can increase uterine prostaglandin formation before parturition.

Fetal Role in Initiation of Labor

Fetal signals are thought to initiate parturition in many species, including man. Although the fetal signal in sheep is well established and, as men-

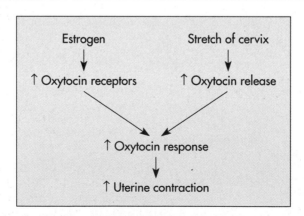

Figure 10-15 ■ Role of oxytocin in parturition.

tioned earlier, involves an increase in fetal pituitary ACTH secretion, the exact signal in humans is not known. It is likely that the fetal signal for parturition acts through alterations in steroid and cytokine production locally in the fetal membranes and decidua, which are not readily apparent in maternal serum.

■ HORMONAL CONTROL OF FETAL SURFACTANT PRODUCTION

The fetal type II pneumocyte begins production of surfactant late in gestation. **Surfactant** contains multiple compounds, but the primary constituent is phospholipids, of which phosphatidylcholine (60%) and phosphatidylglycerol (10%) are the most prevalent. Phosphatidylglycerol production does not occur until about 35 weeks' gestation, and the progressive rise in the surfactant phosphatidylglycerol level is used as an index of lung maturation. Surfactant reduces alveolar surface tension in the postnatal lung. Both corticosteroids and thyroid hormones accelerate fetal lung surfactant production in vivo and in vitro. Consequently, one or both of the groups of compounds have been used to prevent anticipated **respiratory distress syndrome (RDS)** in premature deliveries. Corticosteroids induce lung structural maturation, resulting in increased diffusional surface area, and stimulate synthesis of enzymes regulating surfactant production. Other hormones, such as insulin and transforming growth factor-β, can block lung maturation (Box 10-10).

■ MAMMOGENESIS AND LACTATION

Mammary gland growth and development during pregnancy is stimulated by hPL, PRL, progesterone, and estrogens. The mammary gland is composed of lobules that have numerous milk-producing alveoli. These alveoli represent the functional unit of the mammary gland (Figure 10-16). They are composed of secretory epi-

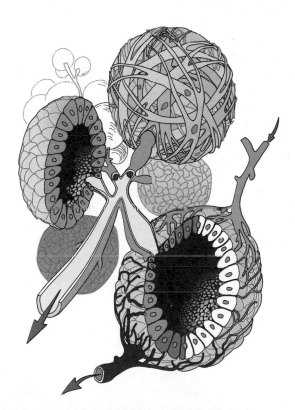

Figure 10-16 ■ Alveolar and ductal system of breast. Myoepithelial cells surround mammary gland alveolus. (Redrawn from Cunningham FG, et al, editors: *Williams' obstetrics,* ed 19, Norwalk, Conn, 1993, Appleton & Lange.)

BOX 10-10

Control of Fetal Surfactant Production

Increase
  Corticosteroids
  Thyrotropin-releasing hormone (TRH),
   thyroid hormones
Decrease
  Insulin
  Transforming growth factor-β (TGF-β)

thelial cells surrounded by specialized contractile epithelial cells called myoepithelial cells. These cells surround the alveolus, and when they contract, milk is expelled from the lumen of the alveolus into the larger ducts of the mammary gland. This process of milk expulsion, called **milk ejection** or **let-down,** is stimulated by oxytocin.

Although the mammary gland develops during pregnancy, copious lactation does not typically occur because the high estrogen and progesterone levels suppress milk synthesis. After parturition, when maternal estrogen and progesterone levels decrease, milk synthesis begins. The rise in cortisol at parturition is important in the initiation of lactation. Cortisol is thought to act by regulating key enzymes in milk synthesis.

■ CONTRACEPTION

There are multiple methods of contraception. These methods include the age-old rhythm method, which relies on abstinence from sexual intercourse during fertile periods around the time of ovulation. (The fertile period is considered the period extending from 3 to 4 days before the time of ovulation until 3 to 4 days afterward.) A second method is withdrawal before ejaculation, **coitus interruptus.** Both of these methods have higher failure rates (20% to 30%) than the **barrier methods** (2% to 12%), **intrauterine devices (IUDs)** (<2%), and **oral contraceptives** (<1%).

Barriers such as condoms or diaphragms are more effective as contraceptives when used with spermicidal jellies.

IUDs are relatively effective. They are thought to prevent implantation by locally producing an inflammatory response in the endometrium. Some forms of IUDs contain copper, zinc, or progestins, which inhibit sperm transport or viability in the female reproductive tract.

Oral contraceptives have been marketed in the United States since the early 1960s. The doses of steroids used are manyfold lower than those used 35 years ago. Properly used, oral contraceptives have a low failure rate.

Many forms of oral contraceptives are marketed today. The trend over the years has been to decrease the dosage of steroids used because the side effects are dose dependent. All oral steroidal contraceptives contain a progestin. Five Food and Drug Administration–approved synthetic progestins are used in oral contraceptives. These are **norgestrel, norethindrone, norethindrone acetate, ethynodiol diacetate,** and **norethynodrel.** These compounds have some androgenic activity. In addition, all oral contraceptives except the **mini-pill** contain an estrogenic compound. The two commercially approved estrogens are **ethinyl estradiol** and **mestranol.** Therefore all oral steroidal contraceptives contain either a combination of an estrogen and a progestin or a progestin alone. The differences between the various pills are a result of varying patterns and doses of hormone administration or variation among the five progestins and two estrogens used. The treatment regimens include **fixed-dose combination pills,** progestin-only mini-pills, and **biphasic** or **triphasic pills,** in which the estrogen level typically remains constant but the progestin levels vary during the cycle. The dose of steroids can be decreased by use of the more complicated biphasic and triphasic regimens.

Oral contraceptives work through multiple mechanisms. Most block the LH surge that triggers ovulation. However, some pills, such as the progestin-only mini-pill, do not prevent LH surges. Fertility is also blocked by changing the nature of cervical mucus, by altering endometrial development, and by regulating fallopian tube motility. Because these contraceptives suppress FSH, they impair early follicular development.

Summary

1. Fertilization normally occurs in the ampulla of the fallopian tube. It requires the activities of multiple sperm. Enzymes in the acrosome of the sperm are important in penetration of the cumulus oophorus, corona radiata, and zona pellucida. Ovum penetration by sperm stimulates the completion of the second meiotic division.

2. Implantation occurs 6 to 7 days after fertilization. It typically occurs in the upper posterior surface of the uterine wall.

3. The fetoplacental unit consists of the placenta, fetal adrenal cortex, and fetal liver. All three tissues are necessary to produce the full complement of placental steroid hormones. The placenta lacks 17α-hydroxylase/17,20-lyase and 16α-hydroxylase. The fetus lacks 3β-hydroxysteriod dehydrogenase and aromatase.

4. hCG is structurally and functionally similar to LH. It stimulates ovarian steroid hormone synthesis and is used as an index of pregnancy.

5. hPL is structurally and functionally similar to both GH and PRL. It stimulates mammary gland development during pregnancy and mobilizes maternal nutrients for the fetus. It is an insulin antagonist and is lipolytic.

6. Glucose crosses the placenta by carrier-mediated facilitated diffusion. Amino acid transport is by carrier-mediated secondary active transport, and low-density lipoprotein transport is by receptor-mediated endocytosis. Gas transport is by simple diffusion.

7. Cardiovascular changes in pregnancy include increased vascular volume; decreased peripheral resistance; and increased heart rate, cardiac contractility, and cardiac output.

8. Respiratory changes in pregnancy include increased minute volume and increased tidal volume. The hyperventilation of pregnancy produces a mild compensated respiratory alkalosis.

9. During pregnancy, ADH, renin, angiotensin II, and aldosterone secretion increases. These changes produce water retention. GFR increases, thereby increasing the filtered load of filtered substances. This increased load can result in a greater tendency for aminoaciduria and glucosuria in pregnancy.

10. The exact mechanism underlying initiation of parturition in humans has not been defined. Possible stimuli include increased uterine size, increased fetal ACTH production, increased oxytocin receptor concentration, and increased uterine prostaglandin production.

11. Corticosteroids and TRH(or thyroid hormones) can accelerate surfactant production in late-gestational fetuses.

12. Mammary gland development in pregnancy is regulated by hPL, PRL, estrogens and progestogens. Copious milk production in pregnancy is blocked by estrogens and progestogens.

■ KEY WORDS AND CONCEPTS

- Hyaluronidase
- Acrosin
- Cortical granules
- Zonal reaction
- Polyspermia
- Zygote
- Morula
- Blastocyst cavity
- Blastocyst
- Inner cell mass
- Trophoblast

- Decidual reaction
- Decidua
- Decidua basalis
- Basal plate
- Decidua capsularis
- Decidua parietalis
- Cytotrophoblastic cells
- Syncytiotrophoblast
- Cytotrophoblast
- Lacunae
- Chorionic villi
- Hemochorial
- Chorion
- Extracoelomic cavity
- Chorion frondosum
- Chorion laeve
- Amnion
- Amniotic fluid
- Fetoplacental unit
- 17α-Hydroxylase/17,20-lyase (CYP17)
- Dehydroepiandrosterone (DHEA)
- 3β-Hydroxysteroid dehydrogenase (3β-HSD)
- Aromatase (CYP19)
- Estriol
- 16α-Hydroxylase
- 16α-OH DHEA
- Sulfatase
- Alpha-fetoprotein (AFP)
- Definitive zone
- Fetal zone
- Human chorionic gonadotropin (hCG)
- Human placental lactogen (hPL)
- Human chorionic somatomammotropin
- Parathyroid hormone–related protein (PTHrP)
- Thyroxine-binding globulin (TBG)
- Transcortin
- Deoxycorticosterone (DOC)
- Accelerated starvation
- Gestational diabetes
- Surfactant
- Respiratory distress syndrome (RDS)
- Milk ejection (let-down)

- Coitus interruptus
- Barrier methods
- Intrauterine devices (IUDs)
- Oral contraceptives
- Norgestrel
- Norethindrone
- Norethindrone acetate
- Ethynodiol diacetate
- Norethynodrel
- Mini-pill
- Ethinyl estradiol
- Mestranol
- Fixed-dose combination pills
- Biphasic pills
- Triphasic pills

■ SELF-STUDY PROBLEMS

1. Why are multiple sperm necessary for fertilization to occur?
2. How does implantation occur?
3. What is the fate of the lacunae that form in the syncytiotrophoblast?
4. What constitutes the minimal diffusion barrier across the mature placenta?
5. Why does placental estriol production cease while progesterone production continues after the in utero death of a fetus?
6. What is the primary basis for maternal pituitary enlargement during pregnancy?
7. What is the endocrine basis for the diabetogenicity of pregnancy?

■ BIBLIOGRAPHY

Ahokas RA, Anderson GD: The placenta as an organ of nutrition. In Lavery JP, editors: *The human placenta: clinical perspectives,* Rockville, Md, 1987, Aspen, pp 207-220.

Albrecht ED, Pepe GJ: Placental steroid hormone biosynthesis in primate pregnancy, *Endocr Rev* 11:124, 1990.

Casey ML, MacDonald PC, Simpson ER: Endocrinological changes of pregnancy. In Wilson JD, Foster DW, editors: *Williams' textbook of endocrinology,* ed 8, Philadelphia, 1992, WB Saunders, pp 977-991.

Creasy RK, Resnik R: *Maternal-fetal medicine: principles and practice,* ed 3, Philadelphia, 1994, WB Saunders.

Cunningham FG, MacDonald PC, Gant NF, Leveno KJ, Gilstrap LC: *Williams' obstetrics,* ed 19, Norwalk, Conn, 1993, Appleton & Lange.

Goodman HM: *Basic medical endocrinology,* ed 2, New York, 1994, Raven Press.

Greenspan FS, Baxter JD: *Basic and clinical endocrinology,* Norwalk, Conn, 1994, Appleton & Lange.

Griffin JE, Ojeda SR: *Textbook of endocrine physiology,* ed 2, 1992, Oxford University Press.

Hacker NF, Moore JG: *Essentials of obstetrics and gynecology,* Philadelphia, 1992, WB Saunders.

Larsen WJ: *Human embryology,* New York, 1993, Churchill Livingstone.

Metcalfe J, Stock MK, Barron DH: Maternal physiology during gestation. In Knobil E, Neill, JD, editors: *The physiology of reproduction,* vol 2, New York, 1988, Raven Press, pp 2145-2177.

Moore KL, Persaud TVN: *The developing human: clinically oriented embryology,* ed 5, Philadelphia, 1993, WB Saunders.

Murro HN: The placenta in nutrition, *Annu Rev Nutr* 3:97, 1983.

Murro HN: Role of the placenta in ensuring fetal nutrition, *Fed Proc* 45:2550, 1985.

Peppler RD, Thompson CC: Anatomy, embryology, and physiology of the fallopian tube. In Stovall TG, Ling FW, editors: *Extrauterine pregnancy: clinical diagnosis and management,* 1993, McGraw-Hill, pp 9-26.

Porterfield SP, Hendrich CH: The role of thyroid hormones in prenatal and neonatal neurological development—current perspectives, *Endocr Rev* 14:94, 1993.

Riggs LA, Yen SSC: Multiphasic prolactin (PRL) secretion during parturition in humans, *Am J Obstet Gynecol* 128:215, 1977.

Schneider H, Proegler M, Sodha R, Dancis J: Asymmetrical transfer of a-aminoisobutyric acid (AIB), leucine and lysine across the in vitro perfused human placenta, *Placenta* 8:141, 1987.

List of Abbreviations and Symbols

ACE	angiotensin-converting enzyme	cAMP	cyclic adenosine monophosphate
ACh	acetylcholine	CBG	corticosteroid-binding globulin
ACTH	adrenocorticotropic hormone		
ADH	antidiuretic hormone (arginine vasopressin)	CCK	cholecystokinin
		cGMP	cyclic guanosine monophosphate
AFP	alpha-fetoprotein		
AIS	androgen insensitivity syndrome	CLIP	corticotropin-like intermediate peptide
Ala	alanine	CO	cardiac output
ANF	atrial natriuretic factor (atrial natriuretic peptide)	COMT	catechol-O-methyltransferase
		CNS	central nervous system
ANP	atrial natriuretic peptide (atrial natriuretic factor)	CREB	cAMP response element-binding protein
Arg	arginine	CRH	corticotropin-releasing hormone
ATP	adenosine triphosphate		
AVP	arginine vasopressin (antidiuretic hormone)	CV	cardiovascular
		D_3	vitamin D (cholecalciferol)
BCAA	branched-chain amino acid	DAG	diacylglycerol
BMR	basal metabolic rate	DHEA	dehydroepiandrosterone
Ca^{2+}	calcium ion	DHT	dihydrotestosterone

DIT	diiodotyrosine	IDDM	insulin-dependent diabetes mellitus
DKA	diabetic ketoacidosis		
DOC	deoxycorticosterone	I/G ratio	insulin/glucagon ratio
DOPA	dihydroxyphenylalanine	IGF-I	insulin-like growth factor-I
dP/dt	rate of tension development	IGF-II	insulin-like growth factor-II
E	estrogen	IGFBP	insulin-like growth factor–binding protein
E_1	estrone		
E_2	estradiol	Ile	isoleucine
E_3	estriol	IP_3	inositol triphosphate
ECF	extracellular fluid	IRS-1	insulin receptor substrate–1
EGF	epidermal growth factor	IUD	intrauterine device
Enk	enkephalin	LDL	low-density lipoprotein
FFA	free fatty acid	Leu	leucine
FGF	fibroblast growth factor	LH	luteinizing hormone
FSH	follicle-stimulating hormone	LHRH	luteinizing hormone–releasing hormone (gonadotropin-releasing hormone)
GAG	glycosaminoglycan		
GH	growth hormone, somatotropin		
GIH	growth hormone–inhibiting hormone; somatostatin	LPH	lipotrophic hormone
		Lys	Lysine
GI	gastrointestinal	MAO	monoamine oxidase
GIP	gastroinhibitory peptide	MIS	müllerian-inhibiting substance
Gln	glutamine	MIT	monoiodotyrosine
GLP-1; GLP-2	glucagon-like peptide-1; glucagon-like peptide-2	mRNA	messenger ribonucleic acid
		MSH	melanocyte-stimulating hormone
Glu	glutamate		
GLUT	glucose transporter	NAD	nicotinamide adenine dinucleotide
GnRH	gonadotropin-releasing hormone (luteinizing hormone–releasing hormone)		
		NGF	nerve growth factor
		NIDDM	non–insulin-dependent diabetes mellitus
GRPP	glucagon-related polypeptide		
GTP	guanosine triphosphate	NSILA	nonsuppressible insulin-like activity
Hb	hemoglobin		
hCG	human chorionic gonadotropin	P	progestin
		PDGF	platelet-derived growth factor
HLA	human leukocyte antigen	PG	prostaglandin
hPL	human placental lactogen	PIH	prolactin-inhibiting hormone (dopamine)
HR	heart rate		
HRE	hormone response element	PIP_2	phosphatidylinositol bisphosphate
3β-HSD	3β-hydroxysteroid dehydrogenase		
		PKA	protein kinase A
HSL	hormone-sensitive lipase	PKC	protein kinase C
HSP	heat shock protein	PLC	phospholipase C
ICF	intracellular fluid	PMS	premenstrual syndrome

PNMT	phenylethanolamine-*N*-methyltransferase	TeBG	testosterone-estrogen binding globulin (sex hormone–binding globulin)
POMC	pro-opiomelanocortin		
PRF	prolactin releasing factor	TG	thyroglobulin
PRL	prolactin	TGF	transforming growth factor
PSNS	parasympathetic nervous system	Tm	tubular maximum
		TNF	tumor necrosis factor
PTH	parathormone, parathyroid hormone	TPO	thyroid peroxidase
		TR	thyroid receptor
PTHrP	parathyroid hormone–related protein (peptide)	TRH	thyrotropin-releasing hormone
PTU	propylthiouracil	TSAb	thyroid-stimulating antibody (thyroid-stimulating immunoglobulin)
RAIU	radioactive iodide uptake		
RBC	red blood cell		
RDS	respiratory distress syndrome	TSH	thyrotropin, thyroid-stimulating hormone
REM	rapid eye movement	TSI	thyroid-stimulating immunoglobulin (thyroid-stimulating antibody)
rT_3	reverse triiodothyronine		
SCC	side-chain cleavage enzyme		
SGLT-1	sodium-dependent glucose transporter-1	$T/S[I^-]$	thyroid to serum ratio of iodide
SHBG	sex hormone–binding globulin (testosterone-estrogen binding globulin)	$t_{1/2}$	half-life
		TTR	transthyretin (thyroxine-binding prealbumin)
SIADH	syndrome of inappropriate antidiuretic hormone secretion	Val	valine
SNS	sympathetic nervous system	VIP	vasoactive intestinal peptide
SRY	sex-determining region Y	VLDL	very-low-density lipoprotein
SS	somatostatin	VLN	ventral lateral nucleus
T_3	triiodothyronine	VMA	vanillylmandelic acid
T_4	thyroxine, tetraiodothyronine	VMN	ventral medial nucleus
TBG	thyroxine-binding globulin	ZP3	zona pellucida glycoprotein

Answers to Self-Study Problems

■ CHAPTER 1

1. A protein hormone cannot be administered orally because it would be digested. It must be administered by injection. Small peptides such as oxytocin may be administered through mucous membranes (e.g., sublingually).

2. They are packaged in membrane-bound secretory vesicles (granules) within the cytoplasm of the cell.

3. Binding to serum-transport proteins increases the quantity of hormone that can be carried in serum for any hormone that is sparingly soluble in blood. It increases the half-life of the hormone by delaying entry into cells and therefore delaying metabolism. It decreases renal clearance of the hormone by decreasing the quantity of hormone filtered in the glomerulus.

4. A compound that binds to the promoter of the gene upstream from the TATA box and regulates gene transcription.

5. The first messenger is the hormone that carries the signal from the endocrine gland to the target organ. The second messenger is a substance produced within the target cell in response to the interaction of the hormone and the receptor. Second messengers include compounds such as cAMP, calcium, IP_3, and DAG.

■ CHAPTER 2

1. GH and PRL have similar structures, and there is some overlap in activity between the two hormones.

2. In most cases, synthesis and secretion of anterior pituitary hormones can be influenced by negative feedback directly at the pituitary level. However, the predominant control of many of the anterior pituitary hormones is mediated by releasing and inhibiting hormones. These releasing and inhibiting hormones are produced in the hypothalamus and are transported in blood through the hy-

pophyseal portal system to the anterior pituitary where they can influence the synthesis and release of the anterior pituitary hormones. This system serves as an important link between the nervous system and the anterior pituitary.

3. Secondary disorder.

4. GH stimulates the production of the IGFs. However, it is only one of a group of regulators of the IGFs. The IGFs are thought to mediate most of the growth-promoting actions of GH.

5. Although GH is a lipolytic hormone, when insulin is present, it can prevent the development of ketoacidosis.

6. TSH is the thyroid growth stimulator, and by definition in panhypopituitarism, there is TSH deficiency.

7. Hyperprolactinemia is often a result of a PRL-secreting pituitary adenoma. As the adenoma grows, it can extend out of the sella turcica and compress adjacent nervous tissue. The optic chiasma is located immediately anterior to the pituitary stalk. Pressure in the region of the optic chiasma would affect those fibers crossing at the chiasma first. These fibers have their origin from the nasal portion of the retina, which corresponds to the temporal visual fields.

8. In a secondary endocrine deficiency, the target endocrine gland (e.g., thyroid) continues to produce some, albeit less, hormone. However, in a primary deficiency, the problem originates with the target endocrine gland.

■ CHAPTER 3

1. ADH is not synthesized in the posterior pituitary; it is synthesized in the hypothalamus. If the hypothalamus remains intact, secretion can be restored from above the site of the damage.

2. ADH is released by parvicellular neurons in the median eminence. It is carried in the hy-

pophyseal portal circulation to the anterior pituitary where it can directly influence the response of the corticotropes.

3. ADH secretion is no longer regulated according to normal servomechanisms. The inappropriately high ADH levels result in water reabsorption in excess of that which would be appropriate to produce a normal serum osmolality.

4. If you withhold water from a person with psychogenic diabetes insipidus, urine volume and osmolality will return to normal and ADH can be measured in serum. However, in a person with neurogenic diabetes insipidus, ADH secretion does not increase when water is withheld, urine volume continues to remain higher than normal, and osmolality is lower than normal.

■ CHAPTER 4

1. In hypothyroidism, cholesterol synthesis decreases. However, the LDL receptor levels also decrease. These receptors play a crucial role in cellular uptake and hence use of the cholesterol-rich LDLs. Consequently, serum cholesterol levels rise, not because more cholesterol is synthesized, but because cholesterol cannot be cleared effectively from the circulation.

2. The metabolism of administered drugs decreases in hypothyroidism. Therefore medication dosages frequently need to be decreased to prevent overmedication.

3. As the binding affinity decreases, serum free T_4 rises, which results in lower levels of TSH released. T_4 secretion drops until total serum T_4 drops to a point at which free T_4 is returned to normal. Total serum T_4 remains low as long as the binding affinity is low.

4. The increased estrogen production resulting from the pregnancy increases liver TBG production. As TBG levels increase, serum hormone binding increases. To maintain normal

serum free T_4 levels, more T_4 is secreted until a new equilibrium is established in which free hormone levels are close to normal and total levels (bound plus free) are high. Normal pregnant women have significant thyroidal changes during pregnancy, but they are not considered to be hyperthyroid.

5. The size of the thyroid decreases because TSH is suppressed, and TSH stimulates growth of the gland. Because TSH secretion decreases, T_4 synthesis and secretion decrease.

■ CHAPTER 5

1. Insulin released in the early phase is preformed insulin, whereas insulin released in the late phase is newly synthesized insulin.

2. A hormone that acts to lower blood glucose concentration.

3. Insulin regulates muscle uptake and use of branched-chain amino acids. When insulin is deficient, levels of branched-chain amino acids tend to rise in serum.

4. Insulin increases clearance of triglycerides in VLDL from serum by increasing the activity of the enzyme lipoprotein lipase. Insulin increases cholesterol clearance by increasing LDL receptors, which are important for removing cholesterol from serum.

5. In the presence of a low I/G ratio, more fatty acids are released from adipose tissue. These fatty acids are transported to the liver where they are metabolized. Beta oxidation increases. The low I/G ratio inhibits glycolysis and hence production of malonyl CoA. Malonyl CoA is a competitive inhibitor of carnitine palmitoyltransferase I, therefore, as malonyl CoA levels drop, carnitine palmitoltransferase I activity increases. This enzyme transesterifies fatty acyl CoA to fatty acylcarnitine, the form in which it traverses the inner mitochondrial membrane. Mitochondria contain the enzymes for beta oxidation and

ketogenesis. The elevated acetyl CoA production from beta oxidation along with the decreased TCA cycle activity caused by NAD depletion results in increased ketone body production.

6. Glucose taken orally is absorbed in the gastrointestinal tract, where it stimulates the release of gastrointestinal hormones such as GIP, secretin, and glucagon, which are potent stimulators of pancreatic insulin secretion.

7. Glucagon secretion is suppressed.

■ CHAPTER 6

1. PTH increases the filtered load because it increases serum calcium levels. Even though PTH increases the distal nephron calcium reabsorption and therefore the fractional reabsorption of calcium, the increase in calcium filtered generally exceeds the increase in the quantity of calcium reabsorbed.

2. Paget's disease is characterized by high bone turnover. Calcitonin decreases bone resorption, which would decrease turnover rate.

3. Excess PTH increases serum calcium levels. The high calcium levels can increase intracellular calcium levels in cardiac cells, which can lead to cardiac arrest in systole.

4. Hyperparathyroidism increases renal excretion of calcium and phosphate, and the presence of the additional osmotically active electrolytes decreases renal water reabsorption.

5. PTH decreases HCO_3^- reabsorption in the kidney, which could produce metabolic acidosis. Because HCO_3^- reabsorption is inversely related to chloride (Cl^-) reabsorption, the decrease in HCO_3^- absorption would increase Cl^- reabsorption and produce hyperchloremia.

6. PTH acts on the distal nephron by increasing cAMP. The elevated urinary cAMP level

reflects this mechanism of action of PTH.

7. The urinary calcium level is low because the low serum calcium levels result in a decreased filtered load for calcium even though fractional reabsorption of calcium is low in the absence of PTH.

8. Alkalosis increases protein binding of calcium, which decreases free calcium levels.

9. Cardiac contractility depends on the availability of intracellular calcium. Because much of the calcium involved in excitation-contraction coupling in cardiac cells comes from ECFs, when extracellular calcium drops, myocardial contractility decreases.

10. Alkaline phosphatase is produced by osteoblasts; elevated serum alkaline phosphatase levels indicate high bone turnover. Elevation of osteocalcin and hydroxyproline levels suggests that bone resorption has increased. Hydroxyproline is an amino acid that is a constituent of collagen.

■ CHAPTER 7

1. Blood flows from the adrenal cortex to the medulla, and cortisol induces the enzyme PNMT. Consequently, the medulla is exposed to high levels of cortisol, which act to increase the proportion of epinephrine to norepinephrine produced.

2. It is a rate-limiting enzyme in the synthesis of catecholamines.

3. Synthetic glucocorticoids inhibit CRF and ACTH secretion, and ACTH is trophic for the zona fasciculata and zona reticularis.

4. Orthostatic hypotension can occur in patients with pheochromocytoma because the high circulating catecholamine levels down regulate the norepinephrine receptors at the sympathetic nervous system nerve terminals in the efferent limb of the baroreceptor reflexes. Orthostatic hypotension occurs in patients with Addison's disease for two reasons. Cortisol is necessary for the manifestation of the action of catecholamines on vasoconstriction and the aldosterone deficiency results in hypovolemia.

5. When ACTH is deficient, the zona glomerulosa continues to produce aldosterone, but if the entire adrenal gland fails, aldosterone secretion is lost. Some limited function of the adrenal zona fasciculata and zona reticularis continues even with a pituitary ACTH deficiency.

■ CHAPTER 8

1. FSH binds to receptors on Sertoli cells. It synergizes with testosterone to stimulate production of androgen-binding protein. This protein, which is released into the tubular lumen, binds Leydig cell–produced androgens and thereby keeps androgen levels high within the testis. FSH also stimulates production of Sertoli cell P_{450} aromatase. This enzyme converts Leydig cell–produced testosterone to estrogens in the Sertoli cell. Sertoli cells regulate the transport of nutrients to the developing germ cells.

2. Sertoli cell estrogen production requires androgens that are produced in Leydig cells. Leydig cells have all the enzymes necessary for the production of estrogens.

3. Pseudohermaphroditic individuals have normally functioning testes that produce the testosterone necessary for wolffian duct development and müllerian inhibiting substance necessary for müllerian regression. This differentiation occurs before the development of 5α-reductase activity in many fetal tissues. However, by the time differentiation of the external genitalia occurs, 5α-reductase is present in the undifferentiated external genitalia. DHT is the major androgen regulating development of these genitalia.

4. Pubic hair development is regulated by androgens, not estrogens.

■ CHAPTER 9

1. The ovary does not regulate development of the internal genitalia. In fact, the müllerian ducts differentiate before the onset of ovarian steroidogenesis.

2. The primordial follicle develops into a primary follicle, which matures to become a graafian follicle. Following ovulation of the graafian follicle, the follicle becomes a corpus luteum. A corpus albicans is the degenerated remains of a corpus luteum.

3. Early in the follicular phase, the granulosa cells lack the enzymes necessary to produce androgens. They do, however, have aromatase and are capable of aromatizing androgens produced in the thecal cells to estrogens. FSH regulates aromatase activity in the granulosa cells. Thecal cells can produce a limited quantity of estrogens, but they produce large quantities of androgens that diffuse to the granulosa cells to serve as a substrate for estrogen production. LH regulates steroidogenesis in the thecal cells.

4. The LH surge is timed appropriately with follicular development because of the intricate interplay between ovarian steroids produced in the developing follicle and the hypothalamic-pituitary mechanisms controlling gonadotropin secretion. At the time of the midcycle surge, estrogen is thought to exert a positive feedback on LH secretion at both the hypothalamic level (where it increases GnRH secretion) and the pituitary level (where it increases pituitary sensitivity to GnRH). Progesterone is thought to also be important in this response. Progesterone increases the magnitude of the response, accelerates the timing of the response, and decreases the duration of the LH surge. There are multiple mechanisms of this action of progesterone. Progesterone alone can produce an LH surge in an estrogen-primed rat.

5. At the time of puberty, the sensitivity of the hypothalamus and pituitary to negative feedback inhibition by estrogens is decreased. This allows serum estrogen levels to rise. The exact mechanism underlying resetting of the gonadostat is not yet firmly established, but multiple models have been proposed.

■ CHAPTER 10

1. The odds of a single sperm reaching the ampulla of the fallopian tube are poor. Many sperm never even penetrate the uterus. It takes numerous sperm in the ampulla to have ample acrosomal enzymes to dissociate the cumulus oophorus and corona radiata. If sperm counts are too low, the odds are against sufficient sperm ever reaching the ampulla and divesting the ovum of its cellular investments.

2. Implantation occurs in a hormonally prepared endometrium by phagocytic invasion of the endometrium by a blastocyst that has been divested of the zona pellucida.

3. The lacunae coalesce and eventually become the intervillous spaces of the mature placenta.

4. The syncytiotrophoblast, mesenchyme, and fetal capillary endothelium.

5. Progesterone can be made entirely within the placenta. However, estriol requires the participation of the placenta, fetal adrenal, and fetal liver.

6. Estrogens stimulate PRL synthesis and secretion. As placenta estrogen production increases, pituitary PRL secretion increases. PRL is the only pituitary hormone with large gestational increases in secretion.

7. Rising serum levels of hPL, estrogens, and progesterone antagonize the actions of insulin.

Comprehensive Multiple-Choice Examination

1. Which hormone has a receptor that is structurally similar to the estrogen receptor?
   a. Insulin
   b. Epinephrine
   c. FSH
   d. Thyroid hormone

2. According to the second-messenger hypothesis, the second messenger is the:
   a. Hormone carrying the signal to the target organ
   b. Receptor located on the cell membrane
   c. Intracellular chemical messenger
   d. Receptor located in the cell nucleus

3. Which hormone would have an N-signal peptide as a portion of the original gene transcript?
   a. GH
   b. Cortisol
   c. Epinephrine (catecholamine)
   d. T_4 (thyroid hormone)

4. G_s proteins serve as transducers in the actions of:
   a. Testosterone
   b. PRL
   c. GH
   d. TSH

5. Which one of the following hormones does not have intracellular receptors?
   a. T_3
   b. Estrogens
   c. Cortisol
   d. Epinephrine

6. Transcription factors include:
   a. Estrogen receptors
   b. The hormone response element
   c. Heat shock proteins
   d. Phosphodiesterase

7. Which hormone is *not* biologically effective if administered orally?
   a. T_4 (thyroid hormone)
   b. Estradiol (an estrogen)

  c. GH
  d. Cortisol

8. You have discovered a "new" hormone that it is a protein with a molecular size of 180 amino acids. Which statement is most likely to be correct about this hypothetical hormone?
   a. It will probably have its action by entering the cell and binding to a nuclear receptor.
   b. It will probably need to be relatively tightly associated with plasma proteins to be carried in any appreciable quantities in blood.
   c. It can be effectively administered orally.
   d. It will be stored in the cell in membrane-bound secretory vesicles.

9. You learn that the new hormone discussed in question 8 activates phospholipase C. Given this information, which one of the following changes is most likely to occur following hormone administration?
   a. Intracellular DAG levels will increase.
   b. Cytosolic calcium concentrations will decrease.
   c. Calcium association with calmodulin will decrease.
   d. Phosphorylation of protein tyrosine residues will increase.

10. Factors known to increase ACTH secretion include all of the following *except:*
    a. Stress
    b. ADH
    c. Hyperglycemia
    d. CRH

11. Ketosis is not likely to occur in acromegaly because:
    a. GH is not a lipolytic hormone.
    b. GH inhibits beta oxidation
    c. GH stimulates lipoprotein lipase.
    d. Most individuals with acromegaly have sufficient insulin production to suppress ketosis.

12. Adults with gigantism characteristically have disproportionately long arms and legs relative to their height. This occurs because:
    a. They frequently have delayed puberty because of decreased gonadotropin secretion.
    b. GH stimulates long bone growth but not membranous or appositional bone growth.
    c. GH acts on bone by stimulating IGF production, and IGFs act only on long bones.
    d. GH acts preferentially on distal appendages, and hence the term *acromegaly* is applied to adults with hypersecretion of GH.

13. A patient had a difficult delivery 6 months ago with excessive blood loss. When she returns to her obstetrician for her 6-month follow-up visit, she mentions that her menstrual cycles have not resumed even though she is not nursing her infant. Her physician suspects postpartum pituitary necrosis. If correct, all of the following would be present *except:*
    a. Thyroid atrophy
    b. Low serum cortisol levels ·
    c. Diabetes insipidus .
    d. Low serum LH levels ·

14. Correct statements about POMC include all of the following *except:*
    a. It is a prohormone for β-LPH.
    b. It contains the amino acid sequences of MSH.
    c. Its synthesis is regulated by CRH in the adult human pituitary.
    d. It is synthesized from ACTH.

15. In a normal individual with a typical sleep/wake cycle, the highest cortisol levels occur at:
    a. 6 AM
    b. 11 AM
    c. 5 PM
    d. 11 PM

16. Which statement best describes the relationship between GH and IGF-I?
    a. There is always a direct relationship between serum concentrations of GH and IGF-I.
    b. IGF-I mediates most, if not all, of the growth-promoting actions of GH.
    c. GH is protein anabolic, whereas IGF-I is not.
    d. GH is produced only in the pituitary, whereas IGF-I is produced only in the liver.

17. A 40-year-old man presents with severe joint pain. His teeth are widely spaced, and his hands, nose, and feet are unusually large. He comments that over the last 10 years, his shoe size has grown from a 10 to a 16. You order a detailed serum profile. Which of the following results would you expect from the blood analyses, and what is the correct reason?
    a. Serum IGF-I levels are high secondary to high GH levels.
    b. Serum TSH levels are high, and excessive thyroid function is responsible for the bone pain.
    c. Serum IGF I levels are low because of an insulin deficiency.
    d. Serum glucose levels are low because of increased insulin sensitivity.

18. Increased insulin sensitivity in panhypopituitarism is caused by:
    a. High serum insulin-induced receptor down regulation
    b. Low serum thyroid hormone levels
    c. High serum cortisol levels
    d. Low serum GH levels

19. IGF-I acts to:
    a. Increase blood glucose
    b. Stimulate lipolysis
    c. Stimulate cellular division (hyperplasia)
    d. Inhibit cartilage growth

20. ADH is:
    a. Produced in the posterior pituitary
    b. A neural hormone
    c. Carried in the blood bound to the protein neurophysin
    d. A large protein that must be administered by injection

21. Actions of ADH include:
    a. Stimulation of ACTH synthesis and secretion
    b. Inhibition of renal cAMP production
    c. Antagonism of the actions of oxytocin
    d. Inhibition of the sensation of thirst

22. Your patient has an ADH-secreting pulmonary carcinoma (syndrome of inappropriate ADH secretion—SIADH). As a result of unregulated ADH secretion, you would expect to find:
    a. Retention of water resulting in volume expansion
    b. A low urinary osmolality
    c. Increased renal sodium reabsorption
    d. A high serum sodium concentration

23. A 25-year-old woman develops a nonfunctional hypothalamic tumor that results in a complete inability to produce oxytocin. The most likely pathological response to this deficiency is:
    a. Inability to ovulate
    b. Amenorrhea
    c. Hypertension
    d. Inability to lactate normally
    e. Inability to deliver a child vaginally

24. T_4 rather than T_3 is generally thought to be the most appropriate treatment for hypothyroidism. T_4 normally is the most appropriate hormone to use because it:
    a. Is the more potent hormone
    b. Has a higher binding affinity for the thyroid hormone receptor
    c. Has a larger extrathyroidal pool with a slower turnover rate

d. Is the only form of thyroid hormones that can be transported into cells

25. Which pathologic condition would most likely cause increased thyroidal radioactive iodide uptake?
    a. Primary hypothyroidism
    b. Secondary hypothyroidism
    c. Graves' disease

26. All but one of the answers below list common symptoms of hyperthyroidism and the correct physiological basis for the symptom. For an answer to be correct, both the symptom and the explanation must be correct. Which answer is *incorrect?*
    a. The resting heart rate increases because circulating levels of catecholamines increase. Excess thyroid hormones stimulate the release of more adrenal catecholamines.
    b. Myocardial contractility increases because thyroid hormones act directly on the heart and act indirectly by potentiating the effect of catecholamines on the myocardium.
    c. Peripheral resistance decreases because of cutaneous vasodilation as a thermoregulatory response.
    d. The circulating half-lives of most exogenously administered drugs decrease because the rate of metabolism increases and drug inactivation is more rapid.

27. Mrs. J is a 58-year-old postmenopausal woman weighing 186 pounds. The serum T_4 is 8 μg/dl (normal is 6 to 12 μg/dl), TSH is 4 μU/ml (normal is 2 to 10 μU/ml), and she complains of depression. Her doctor prescribes a low dosage of T_4 to "pep her up." What changes would you expect to see 4 weeks after the initiation of treatment?
    a. The size of the thyroid will be reduced.
    b. Serum TSH will be greater than 4 μU/ml.

c. Serum T_4 will be less than 8 μg/dl.
    d. The basal metabolic rate will be elevated.

28. If a person with normal thyroid function is treated with T_3, which of the following changes will become apparent within 48 hours?
    a. Serum T_4 will drop.
    b. TG synthesis will increase.
    c. Iodide uptake by the thyroid will increase.
    d. Serum TG levels will rise.

29. Mr. Z is a 27-year-old man with a readily apparent thyroid goiter. He comments that he has gained 3 pounds in the last year, and you notice that his weight is approximately 15 pounds greater than normal for his age and frame. What can you conclude about this patient's thyroid function?
    a. The goiter indicates that he is hyperthyroid.
    b. The combination of the excessive weight and the goiter indicates that he is hypothyroid.
    c. He is probably euthyroid because, although a goiter can occur in both euthyroid and hyperthyroid individuals, the weight gain eliminates the possibility of hyperthyroidism.
    d. It is not possible to draw any conclusions about his thyroid status from the information provided.

30. Which of the following relationships between the disorder indicated below and the probable clinical observations is the most appropriate?
    a. Primary (thyroidal) hypothyroidism: ↓ serum T_4; ↓ serum TSH; ↓ radioactive iodide uptake (RAIU); ↓ response of TSH to TRH following a TRH challenge
    b. Secondary (pituitary) hypothyroidism: ↓ serum T_4; ↓ serum TSH; ↓ RAIU; little

or no change in TSH secretion following a TRH challenge

  c. Primary (thyroidal) hypothyroidism: $\downarrow$ serum T_4; $\uparrow$ serum TSH; $\downarrow$ RAIU; $\downarrow$ TSH secretion following a TRH challenge

  d. Tertiary (hypothalamic) hypothyroidism: $\downarrow$ serum T_4; $\uparrow$ serum TSH; $\downarrow$ RAIU; $\downarrow$ TSH secretion following a TRH challenge

31. Biologic actions of thyroid hormones include all of the following *except:*

  a. Stimulate protein synthesis and proteolysis

  b. Increase Na-KATPase activity

  c. Stimulate glycogenesis

  d. Increase oxidative phosphorylation

  e. Stimulate growth and vascularity of the thyroid gland

32. Which pair of symptoms and causes is most appropriate for hypothyroidism?

  a. The skin is warm and moist because of peripheral vasodilation.

  b. Diarrhea occurs because of increased GI secretion and motility.

  c. Puberty is delayed or absent because TSH crossreacts with LH and FSH receptors.

  d. Myxedema occurs because mucopolysaccharides accumulate in the extracellular spaces.

  e. There is a tendency to gain weight because appetite increases.

33. If you withdraw insulin from an insulin-dependent diabetic patient, you would expect to see all of the following *except:*

  a. A decrease in urinary bicarbonate levels

  b. An increase in renal ammonium production

  c. An increase in the release of alanine and glutamate from skeletal muscle

  d. A decrease in BUN (blood urea nitrogen)

  e. A decrease in Pa_{CO_2}

34. Correct cause-and-effect relationships following insulin withdrawal in a person with diabetes mellitus include:

  a. The ratio of potassium concentration inside the cell to potassium concentration outside the cell decreases in untreated diabetes for multiple reasons, including decreasing secondary to intracellular H^+ buffering, which results in a shift of potassium to the extracellular compartment.

  b. Ketonemia (excess ketone bodies in serum) per se does not increase urine flow because it is entirely reabsorbed in the renal tubule.

  c. Urinary phosphate decreases because renal excretion of H^+ results in increased phosphate reabsorption.

  d. Serum sodium rises because of hemoconcentration that results from a net fluid shift from the extracellular compartment to the intracellular compartment.

  e. Glomerular filtration rate increases as a result of increased serum glucose concentration.

35. The most effective direct stimulus for the release of glucagon is:

  a. A decrease in serum alanine

  b. An increase in serum glucose

  c. Somatostatin

  d. Insulin (direct action on the alpha cell)

36. People with non–insulin-dependent diabetes mellitus are generally not ketosis prone. This is thought to be a result of:

  a. The lack of an increase in glucagon in these individuals

  b. The presence of insulin in these individuals

  c. Their obesity

  d. The fact that, unlike insulin-dependent diabetic patients, their blood glucose levels do not tend to rise significantly

37. Metabolic actions of insulin include all of the following *except:*
    a. Increased glycogenesis
    b. Decreased gluconeogenesis
    c. Increased basal metabolic rate
    d. Increased skeletal muscle amino acid uptake (especially branched-chain amino acids)

38. The hormone *least* likely to be diabetogenic in excess is:
    a. Cortisol
    b. GH
    c. hCG
    d. hPL

39. Which of the following relationships about glucose transport into cells is correct?
    a. Glucose transport into the cells of the renal proximal tubule is via an insulin-sensitive transport system.
    b. Whereas the transport of glucose into skeletal muscle is regulated by insulin, the transport into adipocytes is independent of direct insulin actions.
    c. Exercise can increase the rate of glucose transport into skeletal muscle cells, even in the absence of insulin.
    d. Most areas of the brain have insulin-sensitive glucose transport systems.

40. In the statements below, which is the correct cause-and-effect relationship for diabetes mellitus?
    a. Ketoacidosis occurs when acetyl CoA entry into TCA cycle exceeds acetyl CoA production.
    b. Ketoacidosis occurs when beta oxidation depletes NAD.
    c. Osmotic diuresis occurs as a result of glucosuria, but not ketonuria, because ketone bodies are readily reabsorbed in the kidney.
    d. Hypertension occurs because ketone bodies are vasoconstrictors.

41. A decrease in the I/G ratio in serum will produce:
    a. A fall in blood glucose
    b. A rise in serum branched-chain amino acids
    c. A decrease in hormone-sensitive lipase activity
    d. An increase in lipoprotein lipase activity

42. An 8-year-old child with diabetes mellitus of 1 year's duration has had two severe episodes of diabetic ketoacidosis that have required hospitalization. Which of the following statements is most likely to be correct about his condition?
    a. He has increased frequency of certain HLA types.
    b. He would not be likely to have high titers of anti-islet cell antibodies.
    c. The serum fatty acid levels would have been low at the time of admission to the hospital.
    d. The pancreas would have fewer functioning alpha cells.

43. Secretion of PTH is increased by:
    a. An increase in serum magnesium concentration
    b. An increase in serum phosphate concentration
    c. An increase in dietary calcium
    d. A decrease in urinary calcium levels
    e. Treatment with thiazide diuretics

44. Hyperparathyroidism results in:
    a. Alkalosis
    b. Hyperchloremia
    c. Hyperphosphatemia
    d. Hypophosphaturia
    e. Hypocalcemia

45. Which cause-and-effect relationship is correct for a deficiency of active vitamin D (calcitriol)?
    a. Hypercalcemia occurs because of decreased intestinal calbindin levels.

b. Hypophosphatemia occurs because of decreased intestinal phosphate absorption.

c. Bone formation is increased because vitamin D blocks the action of PTH on bone resorption.

d. Osteoporosis, but not osteomalacia, is associated with a calcitriol deficiency because calcitriol synergizes with PTH in its action on bone.

46. A 50-year-old man has low serum calcium and high serum phosphate levels. His urinary cAMP levels are low. He most likely suffers from:

a. Hypoparathyroidism
b. Hyperparathyroidism
c. Vitamin D deficiency
d. Cushing's syndrome

47. Renal osteodystrophy (bone problems associated with renal failure) is characterized by:

a. A decrease in serum PTH levels
b. An increase in urinary phosphate levels
c. An increase in serum calcium levels
d. A decrease in 1α-hydroxylase activity

48. Which set of serum values would be most typical of a patient with a calcium-mobilizing tumor?

a. High serum phosphate, high serum calcium, and high serum PTH
b. Low serum phosphate, high serum calcium, and high serum PTH
c. Low serum phosphate, high serum calcium, and low serum PTH
d. Low serum phosphate, low serum calcium, and high serum PTH
e. High serum phosphate, low serum calcium, and low serum PTH

49. Which set of serum values would be most typical of a patient with hyperparathyroidism?

a. High serum phosphate, high serum calcium, and high serum PTH

b. Low serum phosphate, high serum calcium, and high serum PTH
c. Low serum phosphate, high serum calcium, and low serum PTH
d. Low serum phosphate, low serum calcium, and high serum PTH
e. High serum phosphate, low serum calcium, and low serum PTH

50. Which set of serum values would be most typical of a patient with a vitamin D deficiency?

a. High serum phosphate, high serum calcium, and high serum PTH
b. Low serum phosphate, high serum calcium, and high serum PTH
c. Low serum phosphate, high serum calcium, and low serum PTH
d. Low serum phosphate, low serum calcium, and high serum PTH
e. High serum phosphate, low serum calcium, and low serum PTH

51. 1,25-dihydroxycholecalciferol:

a. Increases bone mineralization by increasing serum calcium levels
b. Decreases bone resorption by antagonizing the action of PTH on bone
c. Decreases serum phosphate levels by decreasing renal phosphate reabsorption
d. Decreases serum alkaline phosphatase levels by decreasing bone turnover

52. Bone loss associated with renal failure occurs because:

a. The failing kidney is no longer capable of PTH production.
b. Renal phosphate clearance decreases in renal failure.
c. The failing kidney increases activation of vitamin D.
d. Renal calcium clearance increases in renal failure.

53. A patient has hypercortisolism, and the MRI results indicate that there is hyperplasia of

the right adrenal but the left adrenal appears smaller than normal. What does this generally indicate about the origin of the adrenal disorder?

a. The adrenal hyperfunction most likely results from a secondary or tertiary disorder producing pituitary ACTH hypersecretion.

b. The adrenal hyperfunction is most likely a result of an ACTH-secreting nonadrenal tumor.

c. The adrenal hyperfunction is most likely a primary disorder resulting from malfunction of the adrenal gland.

d. The hypercortisolism is probably not a result of an adrenal disorder but rather is the result of exogenous administration of glucocorticoids.

54. Mrs. Q is a 39-year-old woman complaining of polyuria and nocturia, and her fasting blood glucose level is high. Her hematocrit value is exceptionally high even though she is not dehydrated, and she has difficulty with deep knee bends. You notice that her face appears round and puffy, and, although her weight is slightly above normal for her frame, her arms and legs appear thin. Which one of the following conditions would be most likely to be correct about her condition?

a. The liver glycogen levels would probably be low.

b. Hypertension is a common occurrence in this disorder.

c. Her cardiac output is likely to be lower than normal.

d. She will probably have orthostatic hypotension.

55. Which of the following cause-and-effect relationships is correct?

a. Weight gain in Cushing's syndrome is a result of the lipogenic action of cortisol.

b. A person with adrenal insufficiency has difficulty excreting a water load in a normal period of time because of the actions of aldosterone on sodium and hence water reabsorption.

c. Anemia occurs in Addison's disease because of the action of cortisol on GI iron absorption and on erythropoietin release.

d. Skin darkening in Addison's disease indicates that the site of the disorder is in the pituitary rather than the adrenal.

e. Synthetic glucocorticoids are useful in the treatment of arthritis because they stimulate bone growth.

56. Mr. Jones is a 49-year-old brick mason who has come to you complaining of intermittent periods of cardiac palpitations accompanied by excessive sweating and headaches. You suspect he suffers from a pheochromocytoma. If you were to examine him shortly after one of these episodes, you would expect to find:

a. Postural hypotension

b. Hypoglycemia

c. Depressed serum FFAs

d. Low serum cortisol levels

The figure below shows the relationship between serum ACTH levels and serum cortisol levels under different conditions. The normal relationship is shown as a reference. Answer questions 57 to 59 using this figure.

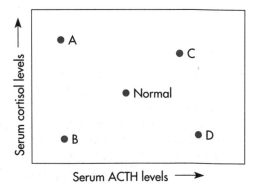

57. A patient with an ACTH-secreting pulmonary tumor would most likely be represented by:
    a. Point A
    b. Point B
    c. Point C
    d. Point D
58. A patient with Cushing's disease and bilateral adrenal hyperplasia would most likely be represented by:
    a. Point A
    b. Point B
    c. Point C
    d. Point D
59. A patient with a functional adrenal cortical tumor would most likely be represented by:
    a. Point A
    b. Point B
    c. Point C
    d. Point D
60. In humans, total adrenalectomy is fatal without replacement therapy whereas hypophysectomy is not. This is because, after hypophysectomy:
    a. The adrenal cortex undergoes compensatory hypertrophy.
    b. The adrenal catecholamines compensate for the metabolic actions of cortisol.
    c. The secretion of aldosterone is not markedly decreased.
    d. Tissue requirements for corticosteroids decrease markedly.
61. Factors that increase serum cortisol concentrations include all of the following *except:*
    a. Stress
    b. Eating a high-carbohydrate meal
    c. Pregnancy
    d. Exercise
62. A 72-year-old man is suffering from nocturia, difficulty with urination, including decreased flow, and inability to completely empty the bladder. The prostate is symmetrically enlarged, nontender, and smooth. The predominant androgen associated with this enlargement is:
    a. DHEA
    b. Androstenedione
    c. DHT
    d. Testosterone
    e. Androsterone
63. People with androgen insensitivity syndrome show developmental abnormalities. Which of the following primary or secondary sexual characteristics is most likely to be seen in these individuals? The presence of:
    a. A prostate
    b. A penis
    c. Breast development at puberty
    d. Descended testes
    e. Pubic and axillary hair
64. Which serum patterns, relative to normal, are most likely to occur in androgen insensitivity syndrome?
    a. ↑ LH, ↑ FSH, ↑ testosterone, ↑ estrogen
    b. ↓ LH, ↓ FSH, ↑ testosterone, ↑ estrogen
    c. ↓ LH, ↓ FSH, ↓ testosterone, ↑ estrogen
    d. ↓ LH, ↓ FSH, ↓ testosterone, ↓ estrogen
    e. ↑ LH, ↑ FSH, ↓ testosterone, ↓ estrogen
65. Characteristics of inhibin include that it:
    a. Is a steroid hormone
    b. Inhibits FSH secretion
    c. Is produced in the testis but not the ovary
    d. Contains two β chains
66. Which of the following is true regarding the determinants of sexual development?
    a. The presence of the gene for HY antigen on the Y chromosome determines whether a testis develops from the gonadal ridge.
    b. The presence of MIS determines whether the wolffian ducts develop.
    c. The presence of estrogen determines whether a vagina develops.
    d. The presence of DHT determines whether a prostate develops.

67. The anatomic site of the blood-testis barrier is the:
    a. Tight junction of the Sertoli cells
    b. Basal lamina (basement membrane) of the seminiferous tubules
    c. Testicular capsule
    d. Testicular interstitium
    e. Testicular capillary endothelium
68. Menopause results from:
    a. Ovarian failure
    b. Pituitary failure
    c. Hypothalamic failure
    d. All of the above
69. Which hormonal relationship most closely resembles that of inhibin and FSH?
    a. Estrogen and progesterone
    b. Estrogen and LH
    c. Somatostatin and estrogen
    d. GnRH and FSH
70. The most significant source of serum testosterone in the normal woman is:
    a. Liver production from ovarian estradiol
    b. Peripheral production from adrenal DHEA
    c. Ovarian granulosa cell production
    d. Luteal cell production
71. Cessation of growth after adolescence is a result primarily of:
    a. A decrease in GH secretion
    b. An increase in androgen and estrogen secretion
    c. An increase in cortisol secretion
    d. A decrease in thyroxine secretion

The figure at the top of the page represents serum levels of a hormone during the menstrual cycle. This is a typical 28-day cycle, and the graph begins on day 1 of the cycle. Answer questions 72 to 74 using this graph.

72. Ovulation will most likely occur 12 to 36 hours after this time:
    a. Point A

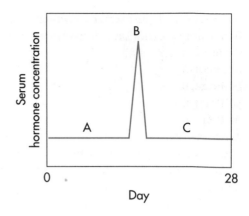

    b. Point B
    c. Point C
73. There should be an optimally developed secretory endometrium at this time:
    a. Point A
    b. Point B
    c. Point C
74. Both estrogen and progesterone levels in serum are high at this time:
    a. Point A
    b. Point B
    c. Point C
75. Progesterone acts to stimulate:
    a. Uterine contraction
    b. Endometrial proliferation
    c. Mammary gland lobular-alveolar development
    d. Production of a thin, watery, slightly alkaline cervical mucus
    e. Keratinization (cornification) of the vaginal epithelium
76. Which of the following observations would be the most effective indicator that ovulation has occurred?
    a. A drop in body temperature
    b. A rise in serum progesterone levels
    c. A rise in serum estrogen levels
    d. A surge in serum LH levels
    e. A surge in serum FSH levels

77. The most effective early test for pregnancy involves measuring serum or urinary levels of which hormone?
    a. Estradiol
    b. Progesterone
    c. hPL
    d. hCG
    e. Estriol

78. Which maternal serum hormonal changes would most effectively indicate death or impairment of the fetus?
    a. Decreased estradiol levels
    b. Decreased estriol levels
    c. Decreased progesterone levels
    d. Decreased hCG levels
    e. Decreased hPL levels

79. What is the predominant cause of the diabetogenicity of pregnancy?
    a. Increased pancreatic insulin secretion
    b. Increased placental hPL secretion
    c. Increased pancreatic glucagon secretion
    d. Increased maternal GH secretion
    e. Increased placental ACTH secretion

80. Amnionic fluid is best described as:
    a. More closely approximating the constituency of maternal extracellular fluids than that of fetal extracellular fluids
    b. Being formed primarily as an excretory product of the amnionic membrane
    c. Containing fetal urine
    d. Having production regulated by hCG levels

Answers to Multiple-Choice Examination

1. d	22. a	43. b	64. a
2. c	23. d	44. b	65. b
3. a	24. c	45. b	66. d
4. d	25. c	46. a	67. a
5. d	26. a	47. d	68. a
6. a	27. a	48. c	69. b
7. c	28. a	49. b	70. b
8. d	29. d	50. d	71. b
9. a	30. b	51. a	72. b
10. c	31. e	52. b	73. c
11. d	32. d	53. c	74. c
12. a	33. d	54. b	75. c
13. c	34. a	55. c	76. b
14. d	35. a	56. a	77. d
15. a	36. b	57. c	78. b
16. b	37. c	58. c	79. b
17. a	38. c	59. a	80. c
18. d	39. c	60. c	
19. c	40. b	61. b	
20. b	41. b	62. c	
21. a	42. a	63. c	

Index

A

Acetoacetic acid, conversion of acetyl CoA into, 136

Acetone, conversion of acetyl CoA into, 136

Acidosis
  hyperchloremic, in hyperthyroidism, 121
  hyperkalemic, 147

Acromegaly, 37
  progression of, *39*

Acrosin
  in sperm capacitation, 170
  in zona pellucida penetration, 201

Acrosin inhibitor in semen, 169

Acrosomal reaction, 169-170

Activins, 46-47

Addison's disease, 147

Adenohypophysis, 21-47
  control of, 23-24, *25*
  growth and, 43-44

Itals = figures and boxes
t = tables

Adenohypophysis—cont'd
  hormones of, 21-22, 27-42
    adrenocorticotropic hormone as, 29
    follicle-stimulating hormone as, 27
    growth hormone as, 29, 31-38
    luteinizing hormone as, 27
    pro-opiomelanocortin as, 28-29
    structures of, 22-23
    thyroid-stimulating hormone as, 27-28

Adenylyl cyclase system, *8, 9*

Adipose tissue
  fat metabolism in, glucagon and, 96
  insulin actions on, 91-93

Adrenal cortex, 137-150
  aldosterone produced by, 139, 141-142
  anatomy of, 137-139
  androgens produced by, 146
  corticosteroids produced by, synthesis of, 139, *140*
  cortisol and, 142-146
  definitive zone of, 137
  fetal, 210-211

251